Handbook of
Hepato-Pancreato-Biliary Surgery

T0323295

Handbook of
Hepato-Pancreato-Biliary Surgery

Editor

Nicholas J. Zyromski, MD

Associate Professor
Department of Surgery
Indiana University School of Medicine
Indianapolis, Indiana

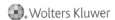

. Wolters Kluwer

Philadelphia • Baltimore • New York • London
Buenos Aires • Hong Kong • Sydney • Tokyo

Acquisitions Editor: Keith Donnellan
Product Development Editor: Brendan Huffman
Production Project Manager: Joan Sinclair
Design Coordinator: Teresa Mallon
Senior Manufacturing Manager: Beth Welsh
Marketing Manager: Daniel Dressler
Prepress Vendor: SPi Global

Copyright © 2015 Wolters Kluwer

All rights reserved. This book is protected by copyright. No part of this book may be reproduced or transmitted in any form or by any means, including as photocopies or scanned-in or other electronic copies, or utilized by any information storage and retrieval system without written permission from the copyright owner, except for brief quotations embodied in critical articles and reviews. Materials appearing in this book prepared by individuals as part of their official duties as U.S. government employees are not covered by the above-mentioned copyright. To request permission, please contact Wolters Kluwer Health at Two Commerce Square, 2001 Market Street, Philadelphia, PA 19103, via email at permissions@lww.com, or via our website at lww.com (products and services).

9 8 7 6 5 4 3 2 1

Printed in China

Library of Congress Cataloging-in-Publication Data
Handbook of hepato-pancreato-biliary surgery / edited by Nicholas J. Zyromski.
   p. ; cm.
  Includes bibliographical references and index.
  ISBN 978-1-4511-8501-0
 I. Zyromski, Nicholas J., editor.
  [DNLM: 1. Pancreatic Diseases–surgery–Handbooks. 2. Biliary Tract Diseases–surgery–Handbooks. 3. Digestive System Surgical Procedures–Handbooks. 4. Liver Diseases–surgery–Handbooks. WI 39]
  RD546
  617.5′562–dc23

             2014005744

This work is provided "as is," and the publisher disclaims any and all warranties, express or implied, including any warranties as to accuracy, comprehensiveness, or currency of the content of this work.

   This work is no substitute for individual patient assessment based upon healthcare professionals' examination of each patient and consideration of, among other things, age, weight, gender, current or prior medical conditions, medication history, laboratory data and other factors unique to the patient. The publisher does not provide medical advice or guidance and this work is merely a reference tool. Healthcare professionals, and not the publisher, are solely responsible for the use of this work including all medical judgments and for any resulting diagnosis and treatments.

   Given continuous, rapid advances in medical science and health information, independent professional verification of medical diagnoses, indications, appropriate pharmaceutical selections and dosages, and treatment options should be made and healthcare professionals should consult a variety of sources. When prescribing medication, healthcare professionals are advised to consult the product information sheet (the manufacturer's package insert) accompanying each drug to verify, among other things, conditions of use, warnings and side effects and identify any changes in dosage schedule or contradictions, particularly if the medication to be administered is new, infrequently used or has a narrow therapeutic range. To the maximum extent permitted under applicable law, no responsibility is assumed by the publisher for any injury and/or damage to persons or property, as a matter of products liability, negligence law or otherwise, or from any reference to or use by any person of this work.

LWW.com

To my family: Jennifer, Anna, Jake, Maddy, J.R., and Sarah.
Thank you for defining my life so completely.

CONTRIBUTORS

Thomas A. Aloia, MD
Assistant Professor
Department of Surgical Oncology
The University of Texas MD Anderson Cancer Center
Houston, Texas

Massimo Arcerito, MD
Fellow
Division of HPB and Advanced GI Surgery
Department of Surgery
University of Michigan
Ann Arbor, Michigan

Chandrakanth Are, MD
Associate Professor
Fellow Division of Surgical Oncology
Department of Surgery/Genetics, Cell Biology and Anatomy
University of Nebraska Medical Center
Program Director
General Surgery Residency
University of Nebraska Medical Center
Omaha, Nebraska

Marshall S. Baker, MD, MBA
Assistant Clinical Professor of Surgery
Division of Surgical Oncology
University of Chicago Pritzker School of Medicine
NorthShore University Health System
Chicago, Illinois

Chad G. Ball, MD, MSC, FRCSC, FACS
Assistant Professor
Department of Surgery
University of Calgary
Foothills Medical Center
Calgary, Alberta, Canada

Danielle A. Bischof, MD
Clinical Fellow
Department of Surgery
Johns Hopkins Hospital
Baltimore, Maryland

Jordan P. Bloom, MD
Resident
Department of Surgery
Massachusetts General Hospital
Boston, Massachusetts

Rebecca A. Busch, MD
Resident
Department of Surgery
University of Wisconsin School of Medicine and Public Health
Madison, Wisconsin

Eugene P. Ceppa, MD
Assistant Professor
Department of Surgery
Division of Hepatopancreatobiliary Surgery
Indiana University School of Medicine
Indianapolis, Indiana

Clifford S. Cho, MD
Assistant Professor
Section of Surgical Oncology
Division of General Surgery
Department of Surgery
University of Wisconsin School of Medicine and Public Health
Madison, Wisconsin

Kathleen K. Christians, MD
Professor of Surgery
Division of Surgical Oncology
Department of Surgery
Medical College of Wisconsin
Milwaukee, Wisconsin

Gregory A. Coté, MD, MS
Assistant Professor of Medicine
Division of Gastroenterology and Hepatology
Indiana University School of Medicine
Indianapolis, Indiana

Rachelle N. Damle, MD
Resident in General Surgery
Department of Surgery
University of Massachusetts Medical School
Worcester, Massachusetts

Jashodeep Datta, MD
Resident in General Surgery
Department of Surgery
University of Pennsylvania Perelman School of Medicine
Philadelphia, Pennsylvania

Mashaal Dhir, MBBS
Resident in General Surgery
Department of Surgery
Nebraska Medical Center
Omaha, Nebraska

Timothy R. Donahue, MD
Assistant Professor of Surgery
Department of Molecular and Medical Pharmacology
University of California Los Angeles
Los Angeles, California

Jeffrey A. Drebin, MD, PhD
John Rhea Barton Professor of Surgery and Chairman
Department of Surgery
University of Pennsylvania Perelman School of Medicine
Philadelphia, Pennsylvania

Barish H. Edil, MD
Associate Professor of Surgery
Pancreas and Biliary Surgery Program Director
University of Colorado
Aurora, Colorado

Douglas B. Evans, MD
Professor and Chair
Department of Surgery
Medical College of Wisconsin
Milwaukee, Wisconsin

William E. Fisher, MD
Director of Elkins Pancreas Center
Professor
Michael E. DeBakey Department of Surgery
Baylor College of Medicine
Houston, Texas

Evan L. Fogel, MSc, MD, FRCP(C)
Professor of Clinical Medicine
Digestive and Liver Disorders
Indiana University Health
University Hospital
Indianapolis, Indiana

Jonathan A. Fridell, MD, FACS
Associate Professor of Surgery
Division of Transplant Surgery
Department of Surgery
Indiana University School of Medicine
Indianapolis, Indiana

Benjamin N. Gayed, MD
Resident in General Surgery
Department of Surgery
Indiana University School of Medicine
Indianapolis, Indiana

Michael G. House, MD
Associate Professor
Department of Surgery
Indiana University School of Medicine
Indianapolis, Indiana

Matthew S. Johnson, MD
Professor of Radiology
Department of Radiology
Indiana University School of Medicine
Indianapolis, Indiana

Michael L. Kendrick, MD
Professor of Surgery and Chair
Division of Subspecialty Surgery
Mayo Clinic College of Medicine
Rochester, Minnesota

Robert L. King, MD
Fellow, Interventional Radiology
Department of Radiology
Indiana University School of Medicine
Indianapolis, Indiana

Wesley D. Leung, MD, MS
Fellow, Gastroenterology
Indiana University School of Medicine
Indianapolis, Indiana

Keith D. Lillemoe, MD
Surgeon-in-Chief
Department of Surgery
Massachusetts General Hospital
W. Gerald Austen Professor of Surgery
Harvard Medical School
Boston, Massachusetts

Edward Lin, DO, MBA, FACS
Associate Professor of Surgery
Emory University School of Medicine
Atlanta, Georgia

Jason B. Liu, MD
General Surgery Resident
University of Chicago Pritzker School of Medicine
Chicago, Illinois

Mary A. Maluccio, MD
Associate Professor
Department of Surgery
Indiana University School of Medicine
Indianapolis, Indiana

Richard S. Mangus, MD, FACS
Assistant Professor of Surgery
Division of Transplant Surgery
Department of Surgery
Indiana University School of Medicine
Indianapolis, Indiana

Robert C.G. Martin II, MD, PhD
Sam and Lolita Weakley Endowed Chair in Surgical Oncology
Director of the Division of Surgical Oncology
Director of the Upper GI and HPB Multi-Disciplinary Clinical
Professor of Surgery and Academic Advisory Dean
Division of Surgical Oncology
Department of Surgery
University of Louisville
Louisville, Kentucky

Rebecca M. Minter, MD
Associate Professor of Surgery
Associate Professor of Medical Education
Associate Chair of Education
HPB and Advanced GI Surgery
Department of Surgery
University of Michigan
Ann Arbor, Michigan

Somala Mohammed, MD
Resident in General Surgery
Department of General Surgery
Baylor College of Medicine
Houston, Texas

Katherine A. Morgan, MD, FACS
Associate Professor
Division of Gastrointestinal and Laparoscopic Surgery
Medical University of South Carolina
Charleston, South Carolina

David M. Nagorney, MD
Professor
Section of Hepatobiliary and Pancreatic Surgery
Division of Multispecialty General Surgery
Department of Surgery
Mayo Clinic College of Medicine
Rochester, Minnesota

Attila Nakeeb, MD, FACS
Professor of Surgery
Chief section of HPB Surgery and Surgical Oncology
Indiana University School of Medicine
Indianapolis, Indiana

Alessandro Paniccia, MD
General Surgery Resident
Anschutz Medical Campus
University of Colorado Denver
Denver, Colorado

Timothy M. Pawlik, MD, MPH, PhD, FACS
Professor of Surgery and Oncology
Chief Division of Surgical Oncology
Department of Surgery
Johns Hopkins Hospital
Baltimore, Maryland

Prejesh Philips, MD
Surgical Oncology Fellow
Division of Surgical Oncology
Department of Surgery
University of Louisville
Louisville, Kentucky

Charles H.C. Pilgrim, MBBS (Hons), PhD
Fellow
Department of Surgical Oncology
Medical College of Wisconsin
Milwaukee, Wisconsin

Henry A. Pitt, MD
Chief Quality Officer
Temple University Health System
Associate Vice Dean for Clinical Affairs
Temple University School of Medicine
Philadelphia, Pennsylvania

Howard A. Reber, MD
Professor of Surgery
Department of Surgery
David Geffen School of Medicine at UCLA
Los Angeles, California

Kumaresan Sandrasegaran, MD
Associate Professor of Radiology
Department of Radiology
Indiana University School of Medicine and Clinical Sciences
Indianapolis, Indiana

Juan M. Sarmiento, MD, FACS
Associate Professor of Surgery
Emory University School of Medicine
Atlanta, Georgia

C. Max Schmidt, MD, PhD, MBA, FACS
Associate Professor of Surgery, Biochemistry, and Molecular Biology
Department of Surgery
Indiana University School of Medicine
Indianapolis, Indiana

Shimul A. Shah, MD, MHCM
Associate Professor of Surgery
Director of Liver Transplantation and Hepatobiliary Surgery
Department of Surgery
University of Cincinnati
Cincinnati, Ohio

Steven M. Strasberg, MD
Pruett Professor of Surgery
Washington University in St. Louis
St. Louis, Missouri

Temel Tirkes, MD
Assistant Professor of Radiology
Department of Radiology
Indiana University School of Medicine
Indianapolis, Indiana

Mark J. Truty, MD, MSc
Assistant Professor
Senior Associate Consultant
Section of Hepatobiliary and Pancreatic Surgery
Division of Multispecialty General Surgery
Department of Surgery
Mayo Clinic College of Medicine
Rochester, Minnesota

Ching-Wei D. Tzeng, MD
Hepatopancreatobiliary Surgery Fellow
Department of Surgical Oncology
University of Texas MD Anderson Cancer Center
Houston, Texas

Jean-Nicolas Vauthey, MD
Bessie McGoldrick Professor in Clinical Cancer Research
Chief of Liver Service
Department of Surgical Oncology
The University of Texas MD Anderson Cancer Center
Houston, Texas

Charles M. Vollmer Jr, MD
Associate Professor of Surgery
Department of Surgery
University of Pennsylvania Perelman School of Medicine
Philadelphia, Pennsylvania

Joshua A. Waters, MD
Resident
Department of Surgery
Indiana University School of Medicine
Indianapolis, Indiana

Nicholas J. Zyromski, MD
Associate Professor
Department of Surgery
Indiana University School of Medicine
Indianapolis, Indiana

FOREWORD

Do we really need *another book* on HPB surgery? After all, there are the books by Blumgart and Clavien and all the other abdominal surgery textbooks. Well, the answer for the focused readership of this *Handbook of Hepato-Pancreato-Biliary Surgery* is *yes—definitely*! While many of these other definite treatises certainly address the multitude of problems, questions, controversies, and various intricacies of the world of HPB, most all are long tomes, not immediately and readily readable, and, as always, being the true reference sources, are more than 2 years behind, and are very daunting to the reader looking for a concise, up-to-date "review" of relevant anatomy (not the total Grant's anatomic detail), acute and chronic pancreatitis, the spectrum of pancreatic neoplasms (both benign and malignant), portal hypertension, selected, surgically relevant biliary and hepatic anatomy, benign and malignant hepatic surgical disorders, and transplantation. Several other focused topics include minimally invasive HPB procedures, relevant novel technology being used currently, and even endoscopic treatments of HPB disorders.

What differentiates this working handbook are the following aspects. *First*, the topics/chapters are carefully selected to address relevant, real-world topics. *Second*, the chapters are relatively short, concise and, most importantly, readable for the medical student, resident, fellow, and practicing surgeon. Note that the chapters are a bit more than the classic bare-bones "handbook" and address a topic in enough depth to provide a comprehensive but not exhaustive discussion. My term for this book would be "comprehensive brevity." *Third*, the book focuses on the *surgical* practice of HPB, with an emphasis on diagnosis, treatment, some technique, and complications. *Fourth*, the reference list at the end of each chapter offers "selected" readings rather than an exhaustive library. *Fifth*, the authors are generally younger, enthusiastic, and more engaging than the more typical classic greybeards—but all are active clinical practitioners who understand the problems.

So, do we need another book on HPB surgery? I say yes—it is not a textbook but equally so more than a "pocket handbook" to put out fires that arise; best description is comprehensive brevity. Congratulations to the editors for developing a truly useful, up-to-date, focused, readable review of current HPB surgery.

Michael G. Sarr, MD
James C. Masson Professor of Surgery
Mayo Clinic
Rochester, Minnesota

PREFACE

Over the past decade, hepato-pancreato-biliary (HPB) surgery has emerged as a mature specialty of general surgery. While a significant percentage of HPB surgery problems are malignant, HPB surgeons also treat a large number of benign disease conditions such as acute and chronic pancreatitis, bile duct injury and benign bile duct stricture, primary sclerosing cholangitis, benign liver lesions, cirrhosis, and portal hypertension. Diagnosis, evaluation, and both operative and nonoperative treatment of these patients are often undertaken in a multidisciplinary format. Surgical decision making in these complex patients is challenging and requires excellent judgment that comes from experience. Treatment of many HPB conditions (such as necrotizing pancreatitis, chemotherapy for pancreatic cancer) is an actively evolving process.

Given this entire picture, the goal of this handbook is to provide an in-depth yet concise overview of contemporary treatment of specific HPB surgical conditions. The target audience for the book includes surgical residents in training, HPB surgery fellows, and general surgeons in practice who may not encounter these complex HPB surgical conditions in day-to-day practice. Others who will likely find the text useful include parallel specialty practitioners like gastroenterologists, interventional radiologists, and medical oncologists (i.e. those typically involved in multidisciplinary treatment of HPB patients) who will gain benefit from understanding surgical perspective of these conditions.

The authors have been selected specifically for their expertise in their chapter's specific topics. As a whole, the author block represents substantial academic gravitas in HPB surgery. The depth of their surgical experience is accessible through clear prose and will be beneficial to all those invested in the care of HPB surgery patients.

TABLE OF CONTENTS

SECTION II: LIVER

Pancreas

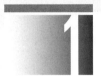

Pancreatic Anatomy and Physiology

Somala Mohammed and William E. Fisher

GROSS ANATOMY

Surgeons must thoroughly understand the anatomy of the pancreas and its surrounding structures in order to minimize inadvertent injury and subsequent complications. In an adult, the pancreas weighs between 75 and 100 g and is about 15 to 20 cm long. However, the shape, size, and texture of the pancreas are quite variable. The pancreas is located in the retroperitoneum and is obliquely oriented with the tail being more superior than the head. The pancreas is covered with a fine connective tissue but lacks a true dorsal surface or capsule. Pain from inflammation of the pancreas is therefore typically described as being located in the midepigastrium and penetrating to the back. The inflammatory process in acute pancreatitis can spread inferiorly through the retroperitoneum down the perinephric and paracolic gutters rather than diffusely throughout the peritoneal cavity.

The pancreas is commonly divided into five regions: the head, uncinate process, neck, body, and tail. The head is the thickest part of the pancreas and lies to the right of the superior mesenteric vessels. It is attached to the second and third portions of the duodenum, and the two organs share a common blood supply from the pancreaticoduodenal arcade. The anterior surface of the pancreatic head is near the first portion of the duodenum and the transverse mesocolon while the posterior surface is close to the hilum and medial border of the right kidney, right ureter, the inferior vena cava, right renal vein and artery, and the right crus of the diaphragm. In the majority of patients, the common bile duct passes through the pancreatic head and is covered by varying amounts of parenchyma before joining with the main duct of Wirsung and emptying into the second portion of the duodenum.

The uncinate process is an extension of the pancreatic head. It passes posterior, inferior, and slightly to the left from the head, staying adjacent to the third and fourth portions of the duodenum. It then continues behind the superior mesenteric vessels. On a sagittal section, the uncinate process can be seen between the aorta and the superior mesenteric artery (SMA). The uncinate process varies in size and shape. It may be absent in some, or it may completely encircle the superior mesenteric vessels in others. Short fragile vessels from the SMA and vein supply the uncinate process and must be divided during resection of the pancreatic head. Pancreatitis or cancer can make the attachments between the uncinate process and surrounding mesenteric vessels difficult to separate intraoperatively.

The neck of the pancreas is defined as the portion of the gland located anterior to the superior mesenteric vein (SMV) and splenoportal confluence. It is the thinnest portion of the gland and is covered anteriorly by the pylorus. The second lumbar vertebra is just posterior to the neck of the pancreas, which can be crushed against this bony structure with blunt anterior–posterior abdominal trauma. The gastroduodenal artery passes superiorly to inferiorly to the right of the pancreatic neck and at the inferior margin of the pancreas gives rise to the right gastroepiploic artery and then terminates as the superior pancreaticoduodenal artery. An ulcer in the posterior duodenal bulb can erode through the posterior wall of the duodenum into the gastroduodenal artery, which must sometimes be oversewn to stop the bleeding. Behind the pancreatic neck at its inferior border, the SMV joins the splenic vein and then continues toward the porta hepatis as the portal vein (PV).

Once the gastrocolic omentum is divided, the body and tail of the pancreas can be seen occupying the floor of the lesser sac, posterior to the stomach. The celiac axis is located superior to the proximal body of the pancreas with the hepatic artery coursing to the right, and the splenic artery coursing to the left along the superior border of the body and tail of the pancreas. The splenic artery is often tortuous and may pass directly through the pancreatic parenchyma or even anterior to the pancreatic tail. The transverse mesocolon attaches to the inferior edge of the body and tail of the pancreas. The body of the pancreas begins to the left of the superior mesenteric vessels. This portion of the pancreas measures approximately 4 to 5 cm in width and 1.5 to 2 cm in thickness. It lies anterior to the aorta at the origin of the SMA and is anterior to the left renal vessels, the left crus of the diaphragm, and the splenic vein. Resection of the pancreatic tail with division at the neck is equivalent to a 60% to 70% resection, while division at the proximal body is equivalent to a 50% to 60% resection.

The tail of the pancreas refers to the portion of the pancreas that is anterior to the left kidney and left adrenal gland. In about 50% of patients, the pancreatic tail extends into the hilum of the spleen and can thus be injured during a splenectomy. The tail of the pancreas is attached to the splenic flexure of the colon. Therefore, the pancreas can also be injured during a left colectomy.

EMBRYOLOGY AND PANCREATIC DUCT ANATOMY

The pancreas is derived as an outpouching of the primitive foregut endoderm and is formed by the fusion of a ventral and dorsal pancreatic bud. The ventral bud develops into the inferior portion of the head and the uncinate process while the dorsal bud develops into the body and tail. The ventral bud rotates behind the duodenum from the right to the left and fuses with the dorsal bud by the 6th to 8th week of gestation. The fusion of the buds results in fusion of the two ductal systems in most individuals. The embryonal ventral duct connects directly with the common bile duct and becomes the main duct of Wirsung. The embryonal dorsal duct arises from the duodenum and becomes the accessory duct of Santorini. With gut rotation, the two ducts fuse in the head of the pancreas such that in most cases, the majority of the pancreas drains through the duct of Wirsung into the common channel formed from the bile duct and pancreatic duct. A "common channel" greater than 10 mm has been termed "pancreaticobiliary maljunction" (PBM). Patients with PBM are felt to have an increased incidence of biliary malignancy. The length of the common channel is variable. The junction of the main duct and the accessory duct occurs at a major bend in the main duct termed the "genu."

Two pancreatic ducts that drain into the duodenum are the main duct of Wirsung and the accessory duct of Santorini. Throughout the tail and body, the main duct runs midway between the superior and inferior borders of the pancreas, slightly closer to the posterior side. After passing into the neck, the main duct travels inferior and posterior before joining the distal common bile duct and entering the second portion of the duodenum. The pancreatic duct is usually only 2 to 4 mm in diameter, with its widest portion in the head. Pancreatic cancer within the head of the pancreas typically obstructs both the bile duct and pancreatic duct resulting in jaundice, and imaging shows dilation of both bile and pancreatic ducts, the "double duct sign." Pancreatic cancer in the body or tail of the gland often obstructs the pancreatic duct only; patients typically present after months of vague abdominal pain radiating to the back.

The normal pancreatic duct contains around 20 secondary branches, which drain the tail, body, head, and uncinate process. These branches enter the main duct at right angles and alternate in location on each side of the duct. The pressure of the pancreatic ductal system is about twice that in the common bile duct, and this pressure differential prevents reflux of bile into the pancreatic duct. The muscle fibers around the ampulla form the sphincter of Oddi, which controls the flow of pancreatic and biliary secretions into the duodenum. The sphincter's contraction and relaxation are regulated by complex neural and hormonal factors including cholecystokinin (CCK) from the duodenal mucosa, which causes sphincter relaxation.

The accessory duct of Santorini drains the superior and anterior portions of the pancreatic head. In 60% of individuals, the accessory duct enters separately into the duodenum via the minor papilla, which is located approximately 2 cm proximal and anterior to the ampulla of Vater. In 30% of individuals, either no minor papilla is present or there is a minor papilla but the terminal portion of the accessory duct is diminutive in size and does not permit the passage of pancreatic fluid. In 10% of patients, no connection is present between the accessory duct and the main duct. In the latter group of patients, contrast medium injected into the main duct would not delineate the anatomy of the minor duct. The normal pancreatic ductal system is quite small. Two to three milliliters of contrast medium can fill the main pancreatic duct and 7 to 10 mL can fill its branches and smaller ducts as well. Injection of contrast material forcefully and at large volumes risks distention of the ducts and postprocedural pancreatitis.

Various congenital anomalies can result from the failure of rotation or fusion of the two pancreatic buds and their associated ducts. Pancreas divisum is the most common congenital variant of the ductal system, occurring in 5% to 15% of the population, and resulting from failure of the dorsal and ventral buds to fuse. Subsequently, the duct of Santorini from the dorsal bud drains most of the pancreas via the minor papilla. In these patients, the inferior portion of the head and uncinate process continues to drain separately through the duct of Wirsung via the major papilla (Fig. 1.1). Most patients with pancreas divisum are asymptomatic. However, in some patients the minor papilla may be inadequate to handle the flow of pancreatic fluid from the majority of the gland. This theoretically leads to outflow obstruction and potentially, pancreatitis.

Annular pancreas (AP) is an uncommon variant characterized by a thin band of normal pancreatic tissue surrounding the second portion of the duodenum. Annular pancreas occurs due to incomplete rotation of the ventral pancreatic bud, so that it remains on the right side of the duodenum. The incidence of AP is approximately 1 out of 20,000 individuals. More than 60% of patients with this anomaly present during the neonatal period with features of gastric outlet obstruction. Many children with annular pancreas have other congenital abnormalities such as Down syndrome and esophageal or duodenal atresias. Children with AP typically present with duodenal obstruction (often diagnosed by prenatal ultrasound). This obstruction is treated by duodenostomy, as dividing the pancreatic annulus may lead to pancreatic fistula from dividing a main pancreatic duct. In contrast to

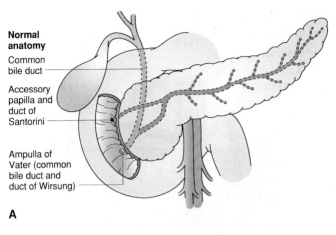

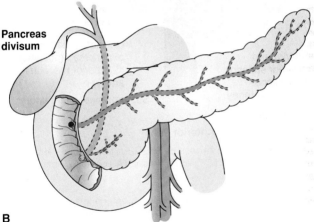

FIGURE 1.1 A. Normal pancreatic ductal anatomy. **B.** Failure of the ventral and dorsal buds to fuse results in pancreas divisum, in which case the majority of the pancreas drains through the duct of Santorini into the minor papilla. In these patients, the inferior portion of the head and the uncinate process continue to drain separately through the duct of Wirsung into the major papilla. (From Mulholland MW, Lillemoe KD, Doherty GM, et al. *Greenfield's surgery: scientific principles and practice*, 4th ed. *Philadelphia, PA*: Lippincott Williams & Wilkins, 2005:1939.)

children, adults presenting with AP often have different and more challenging pancreatobiliary disease such as pancreatitis or biliary obstruction.

ARTERIAL BLOOD SUPPLY

The pancreas has a rich blood supply derived from both the celiac trunk and the SMA (Fig. 1.2). The celiac trunk gives rise to the splenic artery, the left gastric artery, and the common hepatic artery. The common hepatic artery gives rise to the gastroduodenal artery before continuing as the proper hepatic artery. The gastroduodenal artery gives off the right gastric artery

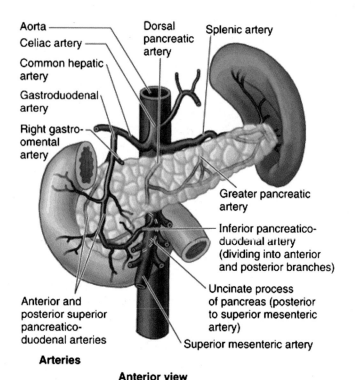

Aorta

Celiac artery

Common hepatic artery

Gastroduodenal artery

Right gastro-omental artery

Dorsal pancreatic artery

Splenic artery

Greater pancreatic artery

Inferior pancreatico-duodenal artery (dividing into anterior and posterior branches)

Uncinate process of pancreas (posterior to superior mesenteric artery)

Superior mesenteric artery

Anterior and posterior superior pancreatico-duodenal arteries

Arteries

Anterior view

FIGURE 1.2 Arterial anatomy of the pancreas. (From Moore KL, Agur AM, Dalley AF. *Clinically oriented anatomy*, 7th ed. Philadelphia, PA: Lippincott Williams & Wilkins, 2013:266.)

superior to the duodenum, travels inferiorly, anterior to the pancreatic neck and posterior to the duodenum, and gives rise to the right gastroepiploic artery at the inferior border of the duodenum, and then continues as the superior pancreaticoduodenal artery. This branches into the anterior and posterior superior pancreaticoduodenal arteries. The SMA gives rise to the inferior pancreaticoduodenal artery, which also divides into anterior and posterior branches. The pancreaticoduodenal arcades are always present and form an extensive network of blood vessels that supply both the pancreatic head and the second and third portions of the duodenum. This shared blood supply renders duodenal-preserving pancreatectomy a complex feat. A rim of pancreatic tissue containing the arcade must be left intact.

Patients with celiac stenosis may derive all hepatic arterial blood flow retrograde from the SMA via collateral pancreaticoduodenal arcades. Therefore, it is prudent to temporarily occlude the gastroduodenal artery prior to dividing this vessel during pancreatic head resection. This maneuver ensures adequate antegrade hepatic arterial flow is present from the celiac artery.

The neck, body, and tail of the pancreas are supplied by many branches from the splenic artery and the SMA. The inferior pancreatic artery usually arises from the SMA and runs to the left along the inferior border of the body and tail of the pancreas, parallel to the splenic artery. Three vessels run perpendicular to the long axis of the pancreatic body and tail and connect the splenic artery and inferior pancreatic artery. They are, from medial to lateral, the dorsal, great, and caudal pancreatic arteries. At the pancreatic neck, the dorsal pancreatic artery arises from the splenic artery and gives off both right and left branches. The right branch supplies the head of the pancreas and usually joins the posterior arcade. The left branch passes through the body and tail of the pancreas, often making connections with branches of the splenic artery or left gastroepiploic artery. These arteries form arcades within the body and tail of the pancreas, and account for the rich blood supply of the organ. Detailed knowledge of the blood supply to the neck, body, and tail of the pancreas is important when performing a distal pancreatectomy with splenic preservation or a central pancreatectomy. Equally important is recognizing the broad arterial variability present.

Preoperative planning for patients with pancreatic cancer includes high-quality computed tomography imaging to evaluate the primary tumor or any sites of distant metastases, assess the patency of nearby vessels, and delineate their relationship to the primary lesion. Tumors can then be classified as resectable, locally advanced, or metastatic. A subset of tumors blurs the distinction between resectable and locally advanced. These tumors of borderline resectability include those that abut the SMA, celiac axis, or hepatic artery (<180 degrees) or display short-segment occlusion of the SMV, portal vein, or confluence of the two vessels with suitable remaining vessels for reconstruction. Locally advanced, surgically unresectable tumors include those that encase the celiac axis, hepatic artery, or SMA (>180 degrees), or that occlude the SMV, portal vein, or its confluence leaving no technical options for reconstruction. Encasement is defined as involvement of greater than 50% of the circumference of the vessel whereas abutment refers to less than 50% involvement.

Preoperative imaging also delineates aberrant vascular anatomy. The most common arterial variant is a replaced right hepatic artery that arises from the SMA instead of the proper hepatic artery. This variant is found in 10% to 15% of patients and usually courses posteriorly and superiorly from the SMA around the posterior side of the portal vein and then up to the porta hepatis on the right side. The artery may be involved by pancreatic head tumors. It must also be differentiated from the inferior pancreaticoduodenal arteries, which also arise from the SMA and take a similar course to the replaced right hepatic. Inadvertent injury or resection of a replaced right hepatic artery can lead to hepatic ischemia or compromise of the biliary enteric anastomosis. A replaced left hepatic artery, present in 10% of the population, typically arises from the left gastric artery and travels along the superior border of the lesser omentum. A replaced left hepatic artery is usually distant from pancreatic head masses but may be involved with tumors of the pancreatic body. Less common arterial variants include accessory left and right hepatic arteries, which are similar to the replaced hepatic arteries but are found in addition to the typical hepatic arterial anatomy.

VENOUS BLOOD SUPPLY

The venous drainage of the pancreas follows the arterial supply. The veins are generally located anterior to the arteries, and both veins and arteries lie posterior to the pancreatic ducts. All pancreatic veins ultimately drain into the portal vein, splenic vein, SMV, or inferior mesenteric vein. Just as an arterial arcade supplies the pancreatic head, a venous arcade of pancreaticoduodenal vessels drains this region as well. The anterior superior pancreaticoduodenal vein joins the right gastroepiploic vein, which also receives the middle colic vein, and drains directly into the SMV. Anterior traction on the transverse colon during colectomy or pancreatectomy can avulse these veins, which then retract behind the pancreas and can be difficult to control.

The posterior superior pancreaticoduodenal vein enters the portal vein above the superior margin of the pancreas. The anterior and posterior inferior pancreaticoduodenal veins enter the SMVs together or separately. Typically, numerous small venous branches drain from the pancreatic parenchyma directly into the lateral posterior aspect of the portal vein. With few exceptions, the veins generally enter along the lateral and posterior sides of the SMV or portal vein and there are usually no anterior venous tributaries. Therefore, a plane can be developed behind the pancreatic neck and the underlying superior mesenteric/portal vein during pancreatic resection, unless the tumor is invading the vein.

Three major venous branches drain the body and tail of the pancreas: the inferior pancreatic vein, the caudal pancreatic vein, and the great pancreatic vein. All these vein branches drain into the splenic vein, which runs in a groove on the dorsal pancreas. Many other unnamed venous branches from the pancreatic parenchyma also drain into the splenic vein, and these branches must be divided when performing a distal pancreatectomy with splenic preservation. The inferior mesenteric vein courses behind the pancreas and usually joins the splenic vein. In some cases (about 15%), the inferior mesenteric vein joins the left side of the SMV or directly with the portal vein at the splenoportal confluence (Fig. 1.3). This variable anatomy has implications for pancreaticoduodenectomy with venous resection. Ideally the splenic vein–portal vein junction should be preserved if possible, especially if the inferior mesenteric vein needs to be ligated and divided or

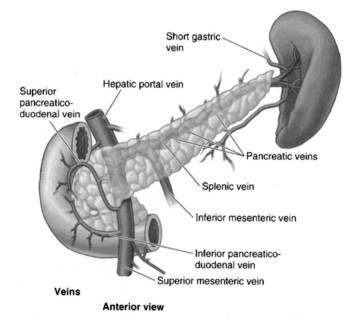

FIGURE 1.3 Venous anatomy of the pancreas. (From Moore KL, Agur AM, Dalley AF. *Clinically oriented anatomy*, 7th ed. Philadelphia, PA: Lippincott Williams & Wilkins, 2013:266.)

if the inferior mesenteric vein enters the SMV. This may require reimplantation of the splenic vein into the interposition graft (usually the jugular vein).

Vascular involvement by tumor no longer represents an absolute contraindication to pancreatectomy. Cancer located at the inferior aspect of the pancreatic head or at the uncinate process may involve either the portal vein or the SMV with or without involvement of one of its two primary branches, the jejunal and ileal veins. The infrapancreatic venous anatomy is variable. The main trunk of the SMV is observed in over 90% of patients, but in the remaining 10% of patients, the jejunal and ileal veins merge at the level of the splenic vein without forming a common trunk. These veins are smaller and more fragile than the main trunk, and either one of them can safely be ligated and resected if the other is of sufficient caliber to allow for collateral venous drainage of the gut. Involvement of the confluence of the two smaller veins along with the main trunk is managed by ligation of the jejunal branch as well as segmental resection and reconstruction of the SMV trunk and proximal ileal branch. Reconstruction of this branch is preferred because the jejunal branch is usually more posterior and technically difficult to access for reconstruction.

LYMPHATIC DRAINAGE

A diffuse and widespread network of lymphatic channels is closely associated with the blood vessels supplying the pancreas. Pancreatic cancer is metastatic to the lymph nodes in 50% to 70% of patients. There are five main groups of lymph nodes for the pancreas: superior, inferior, anterior, posterior, and splenic nodes (Fig. 1.4). The anterior and posterior superior half of the pancreatic head drains to the superior nodes, which are located along the superior border of the pancreas and celiac trunk. The anterior and posterior inferior half of the pancreatic head and body drain to inferior nodes, located near the groove between the pancreas and duodenum. Additional drainage is to nodes along the hepatoduodenal ligament, including those along the portal vein and the hepatic artery.

The anterior portions of the pancreatic head also drain to a group of anteriorly located nodes that ultimately drain to the right of the celiac trunk and SMA, while the posterior portions of the head drain to posteriorly located nodes. The upper part of the pancreatic body drains into the superior pancreatic nodes, while the lower part drains into inferior pancreatic, superior mesenteric, and para-aortic nodes. Tumors of the body and tail may be locally unresectable due to metastases to nodes in the transverse mesocolon or jejunal mesentery. The tail of the pancreas drains to splenic nodes located along the splenic vessels.

INNERVATION OF THE PANCREAS

Pancreatic innervation comes from the sympathetic division of the autonomic nervous system through the splanchnic nerves and from the parasympathetic division through the vagus nerve. These nerves follow the blood vessels and lymphatics. They contain a mixture of motor efferent and sensory afferent nerve fibers from both autonomic systems. The parasympathetic supply begins in the dorsal motor nucleus of the vagus nerve in the medulla of the brain. These fibers travel in the vagus nerve and pass through the celiac plexus. They then travel with arteries that branch from the celiac trunk and ultimately enter the pancreatic parenchyma and synapse with terminal ganglion cells within the gland. The postganglionic fibers terminate at pancreatic islet cells. Almost 90% of the fibers carried by the vagus nerve are sensory in function, related to stretch, chemoreceptors, osmoreceptors, and thermoreceptors.

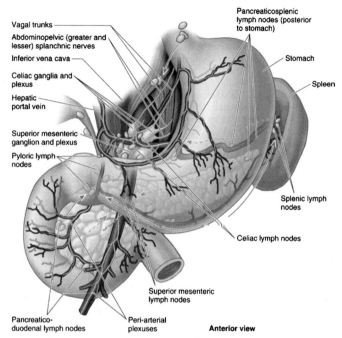

Vagal trunks

Abdominopelvic (greater and lesser) splanchnic nerves

Inferior vena cava

Celiac ganglia and plexus

Hepatic portal vein

Superior mesenteric ganglion and plexus

Pyloric lymph nodes

Pancreaticosplenic lymph nodes (posterior to stomach)

Stomach

Spleen

Splenic lymph nodes

Celiac lymph nodes

Superior mesenteric lymph nodes

Pancreatico-duodenal lymph nodes

Peri-arterial plexuses

Anterior view

FIGURE 1.4 Lymphatic drainage of the pancreas. (From Moore KL, Agur AM, Dalley AF. *Clinically oriented anatomy,* 7th ed. Philadelphia, PA: Lippincott Williams & Wilkins, 2013:243.)

The sympathetic supply begins with ganglia in the thoracic spinal cord. Fibers pass through the sympathetic chain and descend in the greater and lesser splanchnic nerves. The former is composed of preganglionic efferent fibers from the 5th through 9th thoracic segments while the latter is composed of fibers from the 10th and 11th segments. These fibers pass through the diaphragmatic crura and synapse on cell bodies in the celiac or superior mesenteric ganglia. Postganglionic fibers then travel with branches of the arteries to reach the pancreas.

Some afferent fibers cross midline in the celiac plexus. Interconnections between afferent fibers from the pancreas and other sensory fibers from the abdominal wall also exist. This anatomy may explain the referred pain associated with pancreatic diseases. The etiology of pain secondary to pancreatic cancer is poorly understood, however. Explanations include infiltration of nerve sheaths by malignancy, increased ductal pressure, and gland inflammation. Pancreatic pain is generally transmitted through the celiac plexus, located near the emergence of the celiac trunk from the aorta at the level of the first lumbar vertebra. Celiac plexus nerve block can be performed for patients with pain secondary to cancer as well as for patients with chronic pancreatitis.

PHYSIOLOGY

The pancreas is both an endocrine and an exocrine organ. The exocrine component of the pancreas accounts for 80% to 90% of the organ's mass, while the endocrine component accounts for approximately 2%.

The remainder of the pancreas consists of connective tissue, including the extracellular matrix, blood vessels, and the ductal network. The exocrine component secretes the enzymes responsible for digestion while the endocrine component is critical in glucose homeostasis.

The functional unit of the exocrine pancreas is the acinus and its associated ductal system. Acinar cells are large pyramidal cells with their basolateral aspect in contact with nerves, blood vessels, and the connective tissue stroma and their apical aspect facing the central lumen of the acinus. Within the apex are numerous zymogen granules that contain digestive enzymes. Approximately 20 to 40 acinar cells come together to form a functional unit called an acinus. The centroacinar cell, a second type of cell in the acinus, secretes fluid and electrolytes to modify the pH of the pancreatic fluid. The acinus drains into small intercalated ducts, which join to form interlobular ducts and secondary ducts that ultimately drain into the main pancreatic duct. Acute and chronic pancreatitis can cause duct disruption which can lead to a pancreatic pseudocyst. Pancreatic inflammation and subsequent scarring can also lead to duct stricture and dilation, duct and acinar cell destruction, chronic pain, and eventually exocrine pancreatic insufficiency.

The acinar cells secrete enzymes that fall into three major groups: amylases, lipases, and proteases. Enzymatic secretion is stimulated by the hormones secretin and CCK and by the parasympathetic nervous system. Each acinar cell can secrete all types of enzymes, but the ratio of the different enzymes released is adjusted to the composition of digested food. The final product is an alkaline fluid that is colorless, odorless, and isosmotic, containing over 20 enzymes and zymogens. Anywhere between 1 and 2 L of fluid is secreted daily. The pH of this solution is approximately 8.0 and results from the secretion of bicarbonate from centroacinar cells. Water and electrolytes are also secreted by the centroacinar and intercalated cells in response to secretin. Sodium and potassium cations are present in similar concentration as in plasma, but bicarbonate and chloride anions vary in concentration according to their rate of secretion. As the rate increases, bicarbonate concentration increases and chloride concentration decreases. The sum of the two concentrations remains constant, however, and equals that of plasma.

The endocrine function of the pancreas is performed by islets of Langerhans, of which there are nearly 1 million in the normal adult pancreas. The islets consist of 3,000 to 4,000 cells of five major types: alpha cells that secrete glucagon, beta cells that secrete insulin, delta cells that secrete somatostatin, epsilon cells that secrete ghrelin, and PP or F cells that secrete pancreatic polypeptide. The beta cells are located centrally within the islet and constitute 70% of the islet mass whereas the other islet cell types are located at the periphery. The PP, alpha, and delta cells account for 15%, 10%, and 5% of the islet cell mass, respectively. The cellular composition of the islets varies throughout the pancreas. Beta cells and delta cells are present in all islets, whereas alpha cells are almost exclusively present in the tail, body, and superior part of the head of the pancreas. PP cells are almost exclusively present in the head of the pancreas (Table 1.1).

Although patients can live after total pancreatectomy with exogenous digestive enzymes and hormones administration, the loss of islet–acinar cell coordination leads to clinically challenging impairments in digestive function and glucose regulation. Frequent glucose measurement and insulin administration is required to correct for complete absence of insulin production. However, these patients also lack the insulin counterregulatory hormones and often have problems with severe hypoglycemia after insulin administration. Only approximately 20% of the normal pancreas is required

TABLE 1.1 Cells of the endocrine pancreas

	Location Within Islet	% of Islet Mass	Location on Pancreas	Hormone Secreted	Hormone Function
Alpha	Peripheral	10	Tail, body, superior head	Glucagon	↑ Glycogenolysis ↑ Gluconeogenesis
Beta	Central	70	Throughout	Insulin	↑ Glycogen synthesis ↑ Protein synthesis ↑ Lipogenesis
Delta	Peripheral	5	Throughout	Somatostatin	↓ Endocrine/exocrine pancreas secretions ↓ Bile flow, gallbladder contraction ↓ Absorption of glucose, fats, amino acids Many other functions
Epsilon	Peripheral	<1	Throughout	Ghrelin	↑ Hunger, growth hormone secretion ↓ Satiety
PP/F	Peripheral	15	Head	Pancreatic polypeptide	↑ Insulin release

The islets of Langerhans are composed of cells of five major types, depicted above.

to prevent exocrine or endocrine insufficiency after partial pancreatectomy; however, many patients requiring pancreatectomy have diseased pancreas remnant, and endocrine or exocrine insufficiency can develop with removal of even smaller portions of the pancreas.

Suggested Readings

Balachandran A, Darden DL, Tamm EP, et al. Arterial variants in pancreatic adenocarcinoma. *Abdom Imaging* 2008;33(2):214–221.

Bockman DE. Anatomy and fine structure. In Beger HG, Warshaw AL, Buchler MW, et al. (eds.), *The pancreas*, 2nd ed. Massachusetts, United States: Blackwell Publishing, 2008.

Fisher WE, Andersen DK, Bell RH, et al. Pancreas. In Brunicardi FC, Andersen DK, Billiar TR, et al. (eds.), *Schwartz's principles of surgery*, 9th ed. New York, NY: The McGraw-Hill Companies, 2010.

Glasgow RE, Mulvihill SJ. Liver, biliary tract, and pancreas. In: O'Leary JP (ed.), *Physiologic basis of surgery*, 4th ed. Philadelphia, PA: Lippincott Williams & Wilkins, 2008.

Katz MHG, Fleming JB, Pisters PWT, et al. Anatomy of the superior mesenteric vein with special reference to the surgical management of first-order branch involvement at pancreaticoduodenectomy. *Annals Surg* 2008;248(6):1098–1102.

Kooby DA, Loukas M, Skandalakis LJ, et al. Surgical anatomy of the pancreas. In: Fischer JE (ed.), *Fischer's mastery of surgery*, 6th ed. Philadelphia, PA: Lippincott Williams & Wilkins, 2012.

Riall TS. Pancreas anatomy and physiology. In: Mulholland MW, Lillemoe KD, Doherty GM, et al. (eds.), *Greenfield's surgery: scientific principles and practice*, 5th ed. Philadelphia, PA: Lippincott Williams & Wilkins, 2010.

Skandalakis JE, Skandalakis LJ, et al. Pancreas. In: Skandalakis JE, Colborn GL, Weidman TA, et al. (eds.), *Skandalakis' surgical anatomy*, 1st ed. Athens, Greece: Paschalidis Medical Publications, 2004.

Varadhachary GR, Tamm EP, Abbruzzese JL, et al. Borderline resectable pancreatic cancer: definitions, management, and role of preoperative therapy. *Annals Surg Oncol* 2006;13(8):1035–1046.

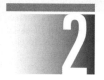

Acute Pancreatitis

Benjamin N. Gayed and Nicholas J. Zyromski

INTRODUCTION

The incidence of acute pancreatitis (AP) in the United States has increased over several decades, and current estimates exceed 40/100,000. This serious medical condition accounts for more than 270,000 inpatient admissions in the United States each year. Approximately 80% of AP cases in the United States are mild and self-limited; the remaining 20% of pancreatitis cases qualify as severe acute pancreatitis (SAP). Persistent organ failure is a defining feature of SAP, which is associated with high morbidity and a mortality rate of 15% to 20%. Patients with SAP have variable necrosis of the pancreatic parenchyma and peripancreatic soft tissue. The natural history of SAP is dynamic. The early phase lasts for the 1st week of AP; the late phase overlaps with the early phase and lasts weeks to months. Up to 20% of people with one episode of AP will go on to have chronic pancreatitis. This chapter discusses the diagnosis and management of AP for surgeons: the majority of the chapter is dedicated to the management of SAP and necrotizing pancreatitis (NP).

PATHOPHYSIOLOGY AND ETIOLOGY

The pathophysiology of pancreatitis is incompletely understood. Increased resistance to pancreatic duct outflow from obstruction (as in gallstone pancreatitis) or decreased radius (as in pancreas divisum) is one of several pathophysiologic theories. Proposed theories all converge with premature enzyme activation in the acinar cells and uninhibited activity of proteases in the parenchyma. Etiologic factors in pancreatitis are better defined, though regional and demographic variation exists. Table 2.1 summarizes common etiologies of AP in the United States.

DIAGNOSIS AND ESTABLISHING SEVERITY

The diagnosis of AP is made clinically and is a diagnosis of exclusion. Historical, biochemical, and radiographic factors support the diagnosis; several of these factors help predict disease severity early in the disease course. The classic presentation of AP involves acute onset of epigastric pain, the intensity of which is usually severe and may radiate either directly to the back or around the patient's side. Patients often describe a "stabbing" "knife-like" pain. Pain from AP is expected to be more centrally located than is the pain of biliary colic, though the length of the pancreas, its position across the retroperitoneum, and its visceral innervation may produce symptoms that localize predominantly on either side of the abdomen. The diagnosis of AP can be made when two of the following three features are present:

TABLE 2.1	Etiology of Acute Pancreatitis

Biliary
Ethanol abuse
Idiopathic
Iatrogenic (post-ERCP most common)
Medication (azathioprine, anti-HIV agents, and others)
Trauma
Hypercalcemia
Congenital
• Pancreas divisum
• Annular pancreas
Toxins
• Jamaican scorpion venom
Hereditary
Hypertriglyceridemia
Tumors
• IPMN (associated with a 25%–30% risk)
• Ductal adenocarcinoma
Other (autoimmune, ischemia, vasculitis)

1. Abdominal pain consistent with the diagnosis
2. Serum amylase or lipase at least three times the upper limit of normal
3. Characteristic imaging findings on contrast-enhanced computed tomography (CECT), magnetic resonance imaging (MRI), or transabdominal ultrasound (U/S)

The onset of AP should be measured from the time that symptoms begin rather than the time of clinical presentation. Elevated serum amylase and lipase are not pathognomonic for AP and may be seen with other gastrointestinal (GI) conditions such as peptic ulcer disease, bowel obstruction, perforation, etc. In chronic pancreatitis patients, these enzymes are less sensitive diagnostic markers and may even be within normal range during an acute flare. Once a diagnosis of AP has been established, it is appropriate to consider the severity of disease.

Severity of AP
Identifying the severity of AP informs the need for closer monitoring, more aggressive resuscitation, and identifying patients appropriate for transfer to tertiary care centers. The evolution of AP severity must be anticipated after diagnosis of AP. Careful and repeated examination is important early in the disease course to determine clinical trajectory.

Multiple systems have been used to predict AP severity. Examples of these scoring systems include Ranson's criteria (Table 2.2), modified Glasgow score, Acute Physiologic and Chronic Health Evaluation (APACHE II) score, the Sequential Organ Failure Assessment (SOFA) score, the Marshall score, and the Balthazar score. No one scoring system is universally accepted and applied in clinical practice. Recent evidence-based guidelines suggest that measurement of the systemic inflammatory response syndrome (SIRS) at admission and at 48 hours may be the easiest and most practical marker of AP severity.

Various biochemical compounds have been studied as potential markers of AP severity (Table 2.3). Serum C-reactive protein (CRP) is the

TABLE 2.2	Ranson's Criteria

On Admission	Within 48 h
Age > 55 y	Calcium < 8.0 mg/dL
WBC > 16,000 cells/mm^3	Hematocrit fall of ≥10%
Blood glucose > 200 mg/dL	PO$_2$ < 60 mm Hg
Serum AST > 250 IU/L	BUN increase ≥5 mg/dL after fluid resuscitation
Serum LDH > 350 IU/L	Base deficit >4 mEq/L
	Fluid sequestration >6 L

Total score (30-d mortality):
0–2 (2%)
3–4 (15%)
5–6 (40%)
7–8 (100%)

most widely used; levels greater than 150 predict severe AP. Serum amylase is not predictive of disease severity regardless of degree of elevation or duration of elevation. Circulating amylase above 1,000 mg/dL supports the diagnosis of a biliary etiology. Urinary trypsin activating peptide (TAP) and interleukins (IL)-2 and 6 increase within 24 hours of AP onset, but clinical utility is limited by the fact that these are typically send-out labs.

The presence and persistence of organ failure may be the single most important predictor of outcome in SAP patients.

The Atlanta classification (developed in 1992 and revised in 2012) identifies three grades of severity based on the presence and timing of complications: mild, moderately severe, and severe. The revised Atlanta criteria are summarized in Table 2.4. A new international "determinant-based" classification has been proposed based on local and systemic determinants of severity—that is, presence of (peri)pancreatic necrosis, presence of infection in necrosis, and presence and persistence of organ failure.

Imaging
Imaging in AP is used (1) to support the diagnosis, (2) to identify the presence of suspected complications, (3) to monitor disease progression (i.e., peripancreatic fluid collections), and (4) for operative planning.

Ultrasound
Transabdominal ultrasound is most useful to identify gallstones with AP. It can be used in place of computed tomography (CT) to support the diagnosis in the setting of normal amylase/lipase levels or with atypical

TABLE 2.3	Biochemical Markers of Acute Pancreatitis Severity

Serum CRP
Interleukin-2
Interleukin-6
Procalcitonin
Polymorphonuclear elastase
Urinary trypsin activating peptide

TABLE 2.4	Revised Atlanta Criteria (2012)

Disease Severity	Clinical Features
Mild acute pancreatitis	• No organ failure • No local or systemic complications
Moderately severe acute pancreatitis	• Transient organ failure (resolves within 48 h) • Local or systemic complications without persistent organ failure
Severe acute pancreatitis	• Persistent organ failure (>48 h) of one or more organs

symptoms. Endoscopic ultrasound (EUS) can differentiate solid and cystic components of retroperitoneal collections. Differentiating a true pseudocyst from walled-off pancreatic necrosis (WOPN) determines whether a drainage procedure or debridement is indicated in a symptomatic or "smoldering" patient (Fig. 2.1). EUS can also be used in cases of idiopathic pancreatitis to better evaluate pancreatic parenchyma and ductal anatomy. Intraoperative ultrasound is very helpful localizing peripancreatic collections, especially those that are predominantly solid.

Computed Tomography
CT is widely available and quite reproducible; as such, CT is the imaging modality of choice in AP. Ideally, CT should be delayed 48 hours to provide time for adequate resuscitation (to minimize nephrotoxicity) and because early in the disease course, radiologic changes of AP are minimal. CECT identifies the presence and extent of (peri)pancreatic fluid collections and necrosis, hemorrhage and pseudoaneurysms (PSAs) (when timed for visceral arteriography), signs of infected necrosis (i.e., air in the retroperitoneal collection), and venous thrombosis. CT is useful for monitoring the disease progression as well, particularly for monitoring the size of fluid collections, pseudocysts, and the extent of necrosis.

No prescribed timing exists to obtain follow-up CT imaging through the course of severe AP, though many experienced practitioners follow serial cross-sectional images on roughly a weekly basis until the

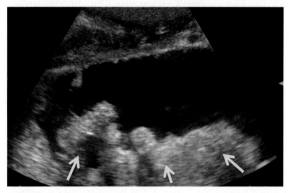

FIGURE 2.1 Ultrasound demonstrating WOPN—collection containing both fluid and solid (*arrows*) necrosis.

patient's clinical condition stabilizes. Acute changes in clinical condition consistent with sepsis should prompt the provider to consider CT imaging to evaluate for signs of infected pancreatic necrosis. Similarly, clinical changes suggesting hemorrhage should prompt consideration of arteriography.

Magnetic Resonance Imaging

MRI can be used in place of CT for diagnosis or surveillance. This modality is particularly useful for patients with allergies to iodinated radiocontrast or concerns about cumulative radiation dose. MRI is also perhaps the most accurate cross-sectional imaging technique with which to distinguish solid and cystic components of retroperitoneal fluid collections (Fig. 2.2). MRI may also be combined with cholangiopancreatography (MRCP) to evaluate the presence of bile duct stones and pancreatic duct integrity. The presence of parenchymal necrosis or a peripancreatic fluid collection obscures MRCP evaluation of pancreatic duct architecture.

MANAGEMENT

Mild AP

Aggressive fluid resuscitation is the mainstay of therapy for mild AP. The degree of resuscitation needed secondary to significant retroperitoneal third spacing is often underappreciated; resuscitation should be guided by evidence of end-organ perfusion (i.e., urine output). Pain is frequently severe enough to warrant narcotic analgesics. Prophylactic antibiotic administration is not indicated mild AP. Nasogastric (NG) decompression may be used to relieve nausea and vomiting, but routine NG decompression does not alter disease course. Gastric antisecretory medication (i.e., histamine receptor-2 blockers, proton pump inhibitors) should be administered routinely. Reintroduction of oral diet is appropriate when pain diminishes. Up to 15% of patients may experience "refeeding pancreatitis" after oral feeding is started; withholding oral diet for a short time is generally successful therapy in these patients.

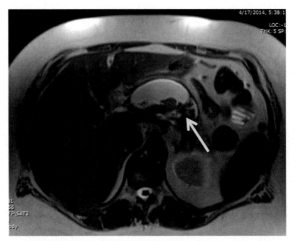

FIGURE 2.2 Magnetic resonance image of the same patient as Figure 2.1; fluid and solid (*arrow*) necrosis.

Cholecystectomy is indicated in all cases of biliary pancreatitis and should be considered in patients with idiopathic AP, or those with recurrent pancreatitis initially attributed to another etiology. The biliary tree should be interrogated by ERCP, MRCP, or intraoperative cholangiography in ALL patients with AP. Removing the gallbladder more than 6 weeks after an initial case of mild biliary pancreatitis leads to recurrent pancreatitis in over one-third of patients. Because of this risk, cholecystectomy should be completed at the earliest opportunity after pancreatitis resolution, ideally prior to hospital discharge. Alternate arrangements for interval cholecystectomy shortly following hospital discharge may be appropriate for responsible patients on a case-by-case basis. In patients with NP, cholecystectomy may be deferred until treatment of the necrotic collections becomes apparent. Should debridement be necessary, cholecystectomy may be performed at the same setting.

Recurrence of AP is very low (3%) following endoscopic sphincterotomy (ES); however, other biliary symptoms (common bile duct stones, cholecystitis, cholangitis) will occur in 10% to 15% of these patients. Therefore, ES may be "definitive" treatment to prevent recurrent AP in patients who are too infirm to tolerate cholecystectomy.

Severe Acute Pancreatitis and Necrotizing Pancreatitis

Natural History

The presence and persistence of organ failure and (peri)pancreatic necrosis define SAP and NP. The mortality of patients with SAP/NP is approximately 20%—this is a serious medical problem. Patients with SAP/NP often require long (>4- to 6-week) hospitalization, as well as some sort of intervention to treat infected necrosis or local complications. Patients and families should be counseled accordingly to expect long hospitalizations, "bumps in the road" and perhaps up to several months of recuperation. Once necrosis becomes established, one of three outcomes is possible (Fig. 2.3). In a small number of patients, the necrosis will reabsorb with no further consequence. In a second group, the necrosis becomes infected, which typically demands treatment. The third group of patients has persistent (presumptively sterile) necrosis. If asymptomatic, these patients do not need further

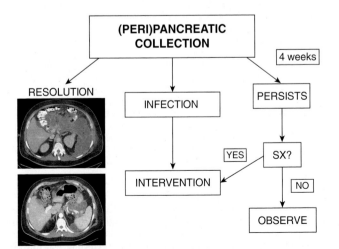

FIGURE 2.3 Outcomes after development of pancreatic necrosis.

treatment directed to the necrotic collection. Symptomatic patients, on the other hand, typically require intervention (these are the "persistently unwell" patients who have nausea, epigastric or upper abdominal pain, low-grade fevers, weight loss, etc.). It is noteworthy that up to 42% of patients with presumed sterile necrosis will be found to have infected necrosis at the time of pancreatic debridement.

The natural history of SAP occurs in two phases: early and late. Each phase demonstrates a mortality peak. The early phase ends 1 to 2 weeks after disease onset and is characterized by the release of proinflammatory mediators and the resultant SIRS. The proinflammatory cascade and systemic release of proteases both likely contribute to distant organ failure; renal and pulmonary systems are particularly vulnerable. SIRS, severe shock, and organ failure may occur without necrosis or infection. Mortality in the early phase from multisystem organ dysfunction and circulatory collapse may be as high as 50% in patients with multisystem organ failure. The late phase is less clearly defined and may persist for months after resolution of the inflammatory cascade. The late phase involves the evolution, progression, and treatment of local complications of SAP. Mortality in the late phase is primarily a result of sepsis-related organ dysfunction either from infected necrosis or from infection in other organ systems of the debilitated patient.

Volume Resuscitation/ICU Monitoring

Fluid resuscitation is the most important component of therapy for the early phase of SAP. Resuscitation should be guided primarily by end-organ perfusion (i.e., urine output) as with mild AP. Lactated Ringer solution is the isotonic crystalloid fluid of choice for resuscitation. Patients with evidence of severe disease require closer monitoring in an intensive care setting. Central venous and arterial catheters are helpful guides for following hemodynamic and volume status in these critically ill patients. Abdominal compartment syndrome is a concern in SAP patients; in our robust clinical experience, this condition is rarely seen.

Antibiotics

The second peak of mortality in SAP patients is almost ubiquitously due to infection. The practice of prophylactic antibiotic administration emerged in hopes of attenuating this second mortality peak. To date, 14 prospective randomized trials have compared antibiotic prophylaxis versus none in SAP. Though all of these studies are underpowered and all suffer some methodologic limitations, NO STUDY to date has definitively shown that prophylactic antibiotic treatment affects SAP mortality. Therefore, broad-spectrum antibiotic *prophylaxis* is not indicated with SAP.

Documented infections (bloodstream, urinary, pulmonary, etc.) should be treated with discrete end point of antibiotic therapy. When infection is documented in (peri)pancreatic necrosis, broad-spectrum antibiotic treatment should be administered to provide coverage of GI flora. Carbapenems are recommended for initial broad-spectrum coverage, but therapy should be tailored according to local resistance patterns and individual culture and susceptibility data.

Nutrition

Nutritional support should be initiated as soon as the patient is resuscitated and hemodynamically stable. Enteral administration is preferable when possible. Prospective data support oral or nasogastric feeding, though many SAP patients will manifest gastric ileus and will tolerate post-Treitz ligament feedings more comfortably. Parenteral nutrition is often necessary to supplement caloric needs. Feeding gastrojejunostomy or jejunostomy tube placement is appropriate if more than 30 days of nutritional support are expected. Reinitiation of oral feeding is appropriate when abdominal pain improves, and many patients in the "holding pattern" of the second phase of SAP will derive nutrition from some combination of oral, enteral, and parenteral nutrition. It is important to remember that all SAP patients will remain catabolic until the inflammatory focus has resolved.

Indications for ERCP
Recent meta-analysis of seven prospective, randomized trials found that routine ERCP does not affect outcome in AP. Therefore, ERCP should be reserved for those patients with biliary obstruction or cholangitis. Early consultation with endoscopists is appropriate for patients with SAP.

Venous Thromboembolism
Venous thromboembolism incidence is remarkably common (>50%) in AP patients, commonly affecting splanchnic vessels (splenic vein, superior mesenteric vein, and portal vein) in addition to extremity veins. Venous thrombosis may be associated with vascular catheterization. In general, we do not routinely anticoagulate patients with splanchnic thrombosis (these will usually not resolve until the underlying inflammatory focus and mass effect from adjacent collections have resolved). Peripheral deep vein thrombosis, however, should be treated with anticoagulation. In addition, screening for peripheral DVT seems warranted in all patients with SAP/NP.

Bleeding
Bleeding severe AP/NP may be due to disruption of retroperitoneal veins (which is almost always self-limiting) or from visceral arterial pseudoaneurysm (PSA). In NP patients, PSA may present with sudden increase of abdominal pain, GI hemorrhage, or blood in a surgical or percutaneously placed drain. CT angiography is an excellent first-line test with which to diagnose (or exclude the presence of) PSA. Treatment of PSA is by transarterial embolization, which is successful in virtually all patients.

Ischemic Viscera—Colon and Gallbladder
Ischemia of the colon or gallbladder should be considered in any patient with SAP who suddenly decompensates. Colon ischemia may occur in up to 8% of SAP patients; the mechanism of colonic ischemia is likely related to venous occlusion with subsequent tissue congestion. Unfortunately, the only method to securely diagnose (or rule out) colon ischemia is by laparotomy. Ischemic cholecystitis may be treated initially with tube cholecystostomy; however, these patients should be followed very closely with a low threshold for operative exploration in those who do not demonstrate rapid improvement after cholecystostomy tube placement.

Fine Needle Aspiration
Fine needle aspiration (FNA) may diagnose infected (peri)pancreatic necrosis; however, no indication currently exists for routine FNA. Clinicians should be aware of the significant (12% to 25%) false-negative rate associated with FNA.

Intervention in Necrotizing Pancreatitis
Infected pancreatic necrosis is nearly always mandates intervention to achieve source control. The management of sterile necrosis is more controversial. Clearly, some patients with symptomatic sterile necrosis will benefit

from debridement. In addition, a number of patients with presumed sterile necrosis will harbor occult infection. Experience has shown that definitive intervention should not be undertaken earlier than 4 weeks from the disease onset. This time frame allows (peri)pancreatic collections to mature and wall off, making debridement safer and easier to achieve at a single setting. Earlier operation results in incomplete debridement of immature necrosis. In addition, early operation is fraught with hazard and potentially catastrophic bleeding complication.

The goals of treating NP include (1) safe debridement of all solid necrotic material, (2) drainage of any pancreatic fistula (externally or if possible internally), (3) gaining access to the alimentary tract, and (4) cholecystectomy (if technically possible and safe) in patients with biliary etiology. The classic approach to treating NP has been open operative debridement. Recently, enthusiasm for minimally invasive approaches to NP patients has grown. These minimally invasive approaches include percutaneous drainage, endoscopic debridement, a combination of percutaneous/endoscopic approach, retroperitoneal debridement (sinus tract necrosectomy or videoscopic assisted retroperitoneal debridement), laparoscopic transabdominal debridement, and transgastric debridement (open or laparoscopic). Regardless of the approach chosen, one physician must be willing to accept responsibility for the duration of the NP patient's care in what is commonly a long-term (months to even years) recuperation.

Patient Selection for Intervention

NP is a very heterogeneous disease. It is critical for the practitioner to realize that one approach does NOT fit all patients. Individual patients must be approached on a case-by-case basis, ideally in the context of an interested multidisciplinary group that includes pancreatic surgeons, therapeutic endoscopists, and interventional radiologists. The appropriate intervention in SAP/NP depends principally upon the location of the peripancreatic collections and the volume of solid necrosis present. An important consideration is the presence of pancreatic parenchymal necrosis, particularly when this is associated with a major pancreatic duct disruption (Fig. 2.4). This common finding will lead to the so-called disconnected pancreatic duct syndrome (DPDS), which will predictably result in persistent pancreatic fistula when drained externally. Figure 2.5 depicts common patterns of necrosis.

Antibiotic Treatment Alone

Several small and one moderately larger series have shown efficacy of antibiotic treatment alone in highly select patients with pancreatic necrosis. This treatment strategy must be reserved for *highly* select patients, who should be kept under very close follow-up. Mechanical intervention should be applied for any sign of clinical deterioration.

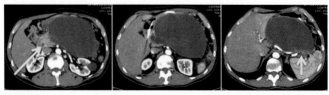

FIGURE 2.4 CT of a patient with DPDS. Viable head (**left panel**, *arrow*) and tail (**right panel**, *arrow*) are present; neck and body are necrotic, and subsequent drainage from the tail is consolidated into a large lesser sac collection.

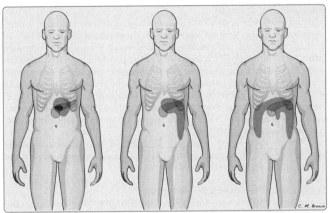

© IUSM 2010 Office of Visual Media

FIGURE 2.5 Patterns of necrosis. **Left** image (collection confined to lesser sac) may be most amenable to transgastric approach. **Middle** image (collection extending down left para-colic gutter) may be most amenable to retroperitoneal debridement. **Right** image (necrosis involving left paracolic gutter, pancreatic head, and/or root of the small bowel mesentery) is a very challenging situation and may be best approached by open debridement.

Percutaneous Drainage

Recent reports suggest that as many as one-third of all NP patients may be successfully treated with percutaneous drainage alone. Importantly, this treatment strategy mandates frequent (72-hour) repeat cross-sectional imaging with drain upsizing and/or additional drain placement. Patients with DPDS, pancreatic head necrosis, or necrosis that extends down the root of the small bowel mesentery are not good candidates for the per-cutaneous approach. Patients who develop infected necrosis prior to the 4-week time point should have percutaneous drains placed. Percutaneous drainage in the setting of early infection often successfully temporizes the clinical situation until safe (i.e., 4 weeks) definitive debridement may be undertaken. If a patient does not rapidly improve after percutaneous drain-age, the surgeon should consider laparotomy to exclude ischemic viscera as a source of deterioration.

Endoscopic Necrosectomy

Transgastric endoscopic debridement of NP was first described in 1996. This approach is attractive for its minimally invasive nature, as well as for the concept of providing durable internal drainage for patients with DPDS. Endoscopic debridement requires a dedicated endoscopist with advanced procedural skills. Patients treated with this approach commonly require multiple (4+) endoscopy sessions, each under general anesthetic.

Combined Endoscopic and Percutaneous Approach

The Virginia Mason group in Seattle has championed a combination pro-cedure including endoscopic transgastric and percutaneous drainage. This approach permits irrigation of the percutaneous drain, which may facilitate mechanical egress of solid material into the alimentary tract. Dedicated cli-nicians (both endoscopists and interventional radiologists) must follow the patient treated with this combined approach, as they also require multiple interventions.

Retroperitoneal Approach

Select patients with appropriate anatomy may be debrided through the retroperitoneum. The "step-up" approach of percutaneous drainage followed at short interval by retroperitoneal debridement if necessary compared favorably to direct open necrosectomy in the Dutch prospective, randomized PANTER trial. A multicenter North American study and another larger series from Liverpool have also shown the efficacy of this approach in select patients. Of particular interest is the finding that nearly one-third of patients treated by the "step-up" approach resolved symptoms with percutaneous drainage alone. Further investigation is focusing on defining specific factors predicting success.

The etiology of AP must not be overlooked—minimally invasive approaches such as percutaneous, endoscopic, and retroperitoneal do not provide direct access for cholecystectomy.

Laparoscopic Transabdominal Debridement

Several small reports have documented the feasibility of laparoscopic (and hand-assisted laparoscopic) debridement of peripancreatic and pancreatic necrosis, again in very select patients. Basic principles of pancreatic debridement—that is, proper timing, thorough debridement, wide pancreatic drainage, and addressing underlying etiology (gallbladder) must be followed in this approach. The totally laparoscopic approach is challenging due to lack of haptic feedback. General advantages of minimally invasive surgery (i.e., shorter hospital stay, earlier return to work, etc.) may be difficult to realize in this challenging group of patients.

Transgastric Debridement

Transgastric debridement can be accomplished endoscopically or surgically and is ideal for collections that are confined to the lesser sac and for those patients with DPDS. Surgical transgastric debridement may be approached laparoscopically or through a short upper midline incision. Intraoperative ultrasound localizes the retrogastric collection; ultrasound is particularly helpful in patients with predominantly solid necrosis. Anterior gastrotomy is created, posterior gastrotomy is placed with ultrasound guidance, and blunt necrosectomy performed through the back wall of the stomach. Many NP patients have splenic vein thrombosis with left-sided (sinistral) portal hypertension; gastric varices potentiate significant hemorrhage in this situation. Long posterior gastrotomy is incorporated into what essentially amounts to cyst-gastrostomy. Feeding tube placement and cholecystectomy may be performed at the same setting, if indicated.

Several reports of surgical transgastric debridement have been published recently. This approach appears to be an excellent choice for select patients with necrosis confined to the lesser sac but may not be as useful for those with necrosis extending down the paracolic gutters or the small bowel mesentery root. Long-term follow-up is accruing; patients should be counseled regarding the potential for reaccumulation of retroperitoneal collections or the potential for recurrent AP.

Open Debridement

Open pancreatic debridement represents the time-tested standard as a safe, effective method to achieve thorough debridement of necrotic tissue, wide drainage of the pancreas and debridement bed, access to the alimentary tract, and cholecystectomy (if indicated by biliary etiology). Contemporary outcomes of open debridement at experienced centers document improved morbidity and mortality rates compared to earlier eras, despite the fact that open surgical debridement is being reserved for those patients with the most severe pathology.

Generous exposure should be obtained; the inflammatory response is generally quite dense and mild venous oozing seen during mobilization of tissue is usually self-limited. Intraoperative ultrasound complements preoperative imaging as a surgical "road map" to ensure thorough debridement. Collections in the paracolic gutters provide a safe route by which to access contiguous lesser sac collections. Special care should be taken debriding necrosis around the pancreatic head; catastrophic hemorrhage may accompany inadvertent injury to the superior mesenteric or portal veins. The vascular walls are commonly weakened by the surrounding inflammatory mass, and proximal/distal vascular control is extremely challenging in this densely inflamed operative field. Gentle debridement should only take tissue that is easily dislodged from the retroperitoneum. Wide drainage of the necrosis bed is important to control pancreatic fistula externally. In patients with biliary AP, the decision to perform simultaneous cholecystectomy should be based on the patient's clinical condition; if cholecystectomy is deferred, it should be performed in the near future (as the patient recuperates) to avoid recurrent biliary problems or recurrent pancreatitis. Enteral access is routine in patients requiring open pancreatic debridement; our preference is to place a gastrojejunostomy feeding tube.

OUTCOMES

Most patients with mild AP will recuperate without major clinical consequence. Up to 20% of patients with a first episode of AP will have recurrent AP, some of whom will progress to chronic pancreatitis. Patients with NP, particularly those requiring debridement, often take several months to return to baseline quality of life. Few data exist to document the true incidence of long-term NP complications, which in addition to recurrent AP may include exocrine and endocrine insufficiency, biliary stricture, duodenal stricture (particularly in patients with head necrosis), disconnected pancreatic duct with pancreatic fistula, pseudocyst, or recurrent retroperitoneal collections/abscess. A pragmatic approach to long-term care includes educating the patient as well as their primary care providers to the possibility of long-term complication.

CONCLUSION

AP is a common, serious medical condition causing significant morbidity and mortality. Surgeons caring for AP patients should be prepared to lead a multidisciplinary team and be prepared to care for these patients over the long term of their illness. The challenges of caring for this complex disease process are rewarded by seeing the patients return to good life quality after this debilitating, potentially fatal illness. Research efforts are focused on understanding the disease biology in order to identify specific treatment.

Suggested Readings

Balthazar EJ, Robinson DL, Megibow AJ, et al. Acute pancreatitis: value of CT in establishing prognosis. *Radiology* 1990;174:331–336.

Banks PA, Bollen TL, Dervenis C, et al.,; Acute Pancreatitis Classification Working Group. Classification of acute pancreatitis—2012: revision of the Atlanta classification and definitions by international consensus. *Gut* 2013;62(1):102–111.

Banks PA, Gerzof SG, Langevin RE, et al. CT-guided aspiration of suspected pancreatic infection: bacteriology and clinical outcome. *Int J Pancreatol* 1995;18:265–270.

Büchler MW, Gloor B, Müller CA, et al. Acute necrotizing pancreatitis: treatment strategy according to the status of infection. *Ann Surg* 2000;232:619–626.

Dellinger EP, Forsmark CE, Layer P, et al. Determinant-based classification of acute pancreatitis severity. An international multidisciplinary consultation. *Ann Surg* 2012;256:875–880.

Petrov MS, Shanbhag S, Chakraborty M, et al. Organ failure and infection of pancreatic necrosis as determinants of mortality in patients with acute pancreatitis. *Gastroenterology* 2010;139:813–820.

van Santvoort HC, Besselink MG, Bakker OJ, et al. A step-up approach or open necrosectomy for necrotizing pancreatitis (PANTER trial). *N Engl J Med* 2010;362:1491–1502.

Chronic Pancreatitis

Katherine A. Morgan

Adventures are all very well in their place, but there's a lot to be said for regular meals and freedom from pain

Neil Gaiman

INTRODUCTION

Chronic pancreatitis (CP) is a vexing disorder, marked clinically by intractable debilitating abdominal pain and attendant nutritional failure. CP is complex in its pathogenesis, clinical management, and psychosocial implications. Thus, management challenges arise on all levels in the endeavor to understand and treat this difficult disease.

EPIDEMIOLOGY

CP is a significant public health care concern. The incidence and prevalence of CP in the United States have been estimated to be 4/100,000 and 41/100,000, respectively. Mortality from CP is increased up to 3.5 times the average population, with a 10-year survival approximating 50%. US health care costs for pancreatitis were estimated at $3.7 billion in 2009.

PATHOGENESIS

The etiology and pathophysiology underlying CP are poorly understood. Pancreatitis is likely a heterogenous grouping of different diseases, manifesting as a similar end histologic result of pancreatic inflammation and fibrosis. Risk factors, most evidently excessive alcohol consumption, have been implicated in disease pathogenesis. More likely, however, an intricate interplay of environmental factors, genetic susceptibility, and host immunologic response results in disease development.

Several theories on the etiology of CP have been put forth. The necrosis–fibrosis hypothesis holds that repeated bouts of acute pancreatitis result in organ injury, resulting in fibrosis and CP. A similar model is the sentinel acute pancreatitis event hypothesis, where an environmental stress in a susceptible host leads to an inflammatory response (acute pancreatitis), which then incites a host-specific immune response resulting in fibrosis (CP).

Alcohol causes oxidative stress and mitochondrial damage, and it lowers the threshold for trypsinogen activation. It also shifts cell death from apoptosis to necrosis and stimulates immune-related inflammatory fibrosis. While excessive alcohol consumption is liable in alcoholic pancreatitis, it is not a lone causative agent, as evidenced by the fact that most alcoholics do not develop pancreatitis. Clearly, there is an underlying host susceptibility factor involved. Similarly, tobacco is implicated as a risk factor for CP, with increasingly recognized importance.

TABLE 3.1	Genes Implicated in Chronic Pancreatitis

Gene	Mechanism
Cationic trypsinogen gene (PRSS1)	Inappropriate activation of trypsin
Serum protease inhibitor, Kazal type 1 (SPINK 1)	Failed inhibition of activated trypsin
Cystic fibrosis transmembrane regulator (CFTR)	Decreased pH and flow of pancreatic juice
Chymotrypsin C (CTRC)	Failed inhibition of prematurely activated trypsin
Calcium sensing receptor (CaSR)	Failed intraductal calcium homeostasis

The past two decades have brought revolutionary understanding to the paradigm of pancreatitis pathophysiology with the discovery of the cationic trypsinogen gene (PRSS1) and the delineation of hereditary pancreatitis in 1996. This important revelation clearly demonstrates the phenotypic result of alterations in the trypsinogen pathway, with an autosomal dominant disorder resulting in potentially severe disease with increased susceptibility for cancer development. It has become a milestone model in the genetic basis of pancreatic disease. Since then, several other genes have been implicated in the pathogenesis of pancreatitis, all involving the trypsinogen pathway, including SPINK 1 (serum protease inhibitor, Kazal type 1), CFTR (cystic fibrosis transmembrane regulator), CTRC (chymotrypsin C), and CaSR (calcium-sensing receptor) (Table 3.1).

Important immunologic discoveries including correlations with variations in human leukocyte antigen antigens have come about in the past decade. On a cellular level, pancreatic stellate cells are identified in their important role of extracellular matrix formation and fibrosis development. The understanding of the contribution of substance P, nerve growth factor, brain-derived growth factor, and other cell signaling molecules to disease pathogenesis is evolving. Elucidation of the mechanism of disease development on the genetic and cellular level explicates the concept of individual susceptibility in the face of environmental stressors.

CLINICAL PRESENTATION

Patients may present with complications of pancreatitis such as obstruction (biliary, duodenal, mesenteric vascular thrombosis), perforation (pseudocyst, pancreatic fistula, pancreatic ascites), or bleeding (visceral arterial pseudoaneurysm). The clinical hallmark of CP, however, is intractable, debilitating abdominal pain. Pain is reported by 80% to 94% of patients with CP. It is typically described as sharp and burning, located in the epigastrium and radiating around to the back. Nausea, emesis, and food intolerance often accompany the pain. Patients may not have objective findings associated with pain exacerbation episodes, such as serum amylase elevation, thus leading to challenges for health care workers and patients alike. Commonly, patients with severe disease are challenged in their relationships with family and health care workers and may develop maladaptive behaviors and associated social marginalization.

Endocrine and exocrine organ failure develops with progressive disease. Approximately 60% of CP patients will develop insulin-dependent diabetes. Greater than 90% loss of exocrine function must occur to result in malabsorption, with absorption of fat more significantly affected than protein.

DIAGNOSIS

The diagnosis of CP entails a consistent clinical history, notable for pancreatic-type abdominal pain, along with radiographic evidence of disease. The most relevant imaging modalities include contrast-enhanced computed tomography (CT), secretin-stimulated magnetic resonance pancreatography (MRP), endoscopic retrograde pancreatography (ERP), and endoscopic ultrasound (EUS).

Abdominal CT may show calcifications, parenchymal thickening or atrophy, or pancreatic ductal dilation evidencing disease. Alterations in parenchymal enhancement, decreased response to secretin stimulation, and pancreatic ductal pathology such as strictures or dilation may be better delineated by MRP. ERP can show ductal changes and historically has been the gold standard of objective disease diagnosis, although MRP is quickly replacing ERP for diagnostic purposes at many centers. The ERP-derived Cambridge classification system is the standard disease grading system derived from an international consensus (Table 3.2). EUS is touted as the most sensitive of the imaging modalities, although its utility is limited by interobserver variability. It, too, has a disease grading system based on the identification of objective features of CP (Table 3.3).

MANAGEMENT

In CP patients with debilitating pain who have failed medical management to include alcohol and tobacco abstinence, pain control, nutritional optimization, and behavioral therapies, intervention is indicated for pain relief.

ENDOSCOPIC MANAGEMENT

Therapeutic ERP interventions for CP are undertaken with the goal of relieving an obstructive process. Maneuvers include sphincterotomy, stone extraction, stricture dilation, and stenting. In practice, the endoscopic approach is exhausted prior to surgery, given the perceived advantages of a less invasive procedure, despite two randomized controlled trials demonstrating improved outcomes with surgery in patients with obstructive pancreatopathy. In the first trial by Dite and colleagues from the Czech Republic, 72 patients were randomized to endoscopic or

TABLE 3.2	Cambridge Classification System for Severity of Chronic Pancreatitis by ERCP Imaging	
Grade	**Severity of Pancreatitis**	**ERCP Findings**
1	Normal	No abnormal features
2	Equivocal	Less than 3 abnormal branches
3	Mild	More than 3 abnormal branches
4	Moderate	Abnormal main duct and branches
5	Marked	As above with one or more of: Large cavities (>10 mm) Gross gland enlargement (>2× normal) Intraductal filling defects or calculi Duct obstruction, structure or gross irregularity Contiguous organ invasion

ERCP, endoscopic retrograde cholangiopancreatography
From Sarner M, Cotton PB. Classification of pancreatitis. *Gut* 1984;25:756–759.

	Conventional EUS Criteria for Chronic Pancreatitis

Parenchymal Criteria	Duct Criteria
Hyperechoic foci	Irregular duct contour
Hyperechoic strands	Visible side branches
Hyperechoic lobules, foci, or areas	Hyperechoic duct margin
Cyst	Dilated main duct
Normal (low probability)	0–2 criteria present
Indeterminate (intermediate probability)	3–4 criteria present
High probability	5–9 criteria present

EUS, endoscopic ultrasound
From Wallace MB, Hawes RH, Durkalski V, et al. The reliability of EUS for the diagnosis for chronic pancreatitis: interobserver agreement among experienced endosonographers. *Gastrointest Endosc* 2001;53:294–299.

surgical intervention for pancreatic duct obstruction and associated pain. Endoscopic therapy consisted of 52% sphincterotomy and stenting and 23% stone removal. Operative management included 20% drainage procedures and 80% resections. At 5-year follow-up, the surgical group had a greater proportion of patients who were pain free (34% vs. 15%), while the rate of partial pain relief was equivalent between the groups (52% surgery, 46% endoscopy). In another trial by Cahen and colleagues from the Netherlands, 39 patients were randomized to endoscopic or surgical intervention for dilated duct pancreatitis and pain. Endoscopic therapy included sphincterotomy and stent, while operative therapy was with a longitudinal pancreaticojejunostomy (LR-LPJ). At 5-year follow-up, pain relief was achieved in 80% of the surgical group versus 38% of the endoscopic group ($p = 0.001$). The surgical group also had larger improvements in quality of life and underwent fewer procedures. Equivalent morbidity, length of stay, and pancreatic function were seen in the two groups.

SURGICAL MANAGEMENT

The primary indication for surgical intervention in CP is intractable pain, unresponsive to medical therapies. Forty percent to sixty-seven percent of patients with CP will meet these criteria for surgery. The goals of surgery are to effectively and durably relieve pain while minimizing morbidity including preserving pancreatic parenchyma when possible. The etiology of pancreatic pain is poorly understood and likely multifactorial. Thus, operative decision making can be challenging. The pancreatic ductal anatomy is the primary determinant in surgical planning. Generally speaking, patients with a large main pancreatic duct (> 6–7 mm in diameter) are presumed to have an obstructive component to their disease and are thus well served by a drainage procedure. In patients with small duct disease, resection of damaged and poorly drained parenchyma is typically effective. In patients with head-predominant or tail-centered disease, a directed resection is optimal. In patients with a small pancreatic duct and diffuse organ involvement, a total pancreatectomy (TP) with islet autotransplantation (IAT) may be indicated.

The heterogenous nature of CP anatomical changes mandates the surgeon's familiarity with several operative approaches—no one operation is suitable for every patient.

Longitudinal Pancreaticojejunostomy

Operative pancreatic drainage for pancreatitis was described in a small series of patients by Puestow and Gillesby in 1957. A modification of this original drainage procedure that more closely resembles modern day technique was reported by Partington and Rochelle in 1960. The classic operation for pancreatic drainage, the lateral pancreaticojejunostomy (LPJ), entails opening the pancreatic duct anteriorly along its length within a fibrotic gland, medially to the level of the gastroduodenal artery. The opened pancreatic duct is then anastomosed to a Roux-en-Y jejunal limb (Fig. 3.1).

Potential significant procedure-specific complications include intraoperative hemorrhage due to splenic vein or gastroduodenal artery injury, postoperative hemorrhage typically from the gastroduodenal artery, and anastomotic leak seen in 10% of cases.

Multiple retrospective case series have been reported evaluating outcomes with LPJ, with pain relief rates of 48% to 91%. Morbidity rates are low (20% on average) and endocrine and exocrine function is often preserved. LPJ is an effective and safe procedure for pain relief in many patients with dilated duct pancreatitis. A secondary failure rate does exist with LPJ, often attributed to disease burden in the head of the pancreas. Intraductal stone disease in the head of the pancreas can be cleared with intraoperative pancreatoscopy and lithotripsy, which has been shown to improve outcomes (reduced readmissions, increased pain relief rates). Patients with significant burden of inflammatory fibrosis in the head of the pancreas may be better served with a localized pancreatic head resection along with a pancreaticojejunostomy.

Local Resection of the Pancreatic Head with Longitudinal Pancreaticojejunostomy

In the mid-1980s, Frey and colleagues described adding a localized resection of the head of the pancreas along with an LR-LPJ. This procedure addresses the inflammatory disease burden often found in the head of the pancreas in patients with dilated duct pancreatitis. In addition, LR-LPJ has the advantage of duodenal preservation. In modern series, pain relief rates of 62% to 88% are reported, with morbidity of 20% to 30% (Fig. 3.2).

Pancreatoduodenectomy

In 1946, Dr. Whipple described pancreatoduodenectomy (PD) for CP. Patients with an inflammatory mass in the head of the pancreas and those with diffuse small duct disease with the head as the suspected pacemaker of disease may benefit from PD. Pain relief rates of 70% to 89%, morbidity of 16% to 53%, and mortality of less than 5% are reported. Procedure-specific significant complications include intraoperative hemorrhage from portal vein injury, postoperative biliary leak, postoperative pancreatic fistula (POPF), postoperative hemorrhage from the ligated gastroduodenal artery, and delayed gastric emptying, the latter two often associated with postoperative pancreatic leak. Grading of POPF is according to clinical significance (Table 3.4).

The pylorus-preserving pancreatoduodenectomy (PPPD) was popularized in the 1970s by Traverso and Longmire and has been embraced by many pancreatic surgeons. Pylorus preservation is intended to improve nutritional outcomes, although studies have not confirmed this proposed advantage. Pain relief rates and endocrine outcomes are similar between the classic PD (with antrectomy) and PPPD, although improved professional rehabilitation and improved quality of life after PPPD have been touted. Technical conduct of PD (and distal pancreatectomy [DP]) is detailed in Chapter 7.

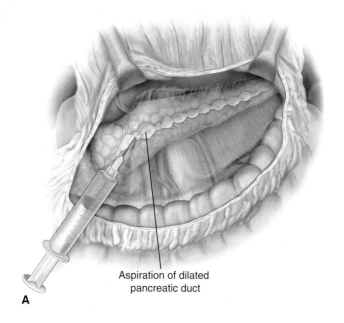

Aspiration of dilated
pancreatic duct

A

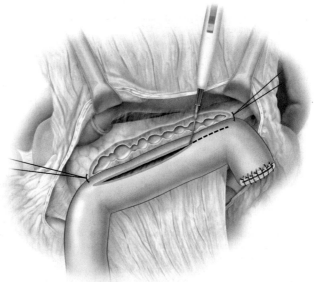

B

FIGURE 3.1 **A.** After exposure of the full length of the pancreas, the pancreatic duct is identified by aspiration using a 21-gauge needle on a 5-mL syringe. **B.** The Roux-en-Y limb is brought
alongside the pancreas in an isoperistaltic fashion. The longitudinal pancreatic ductotomy is visible. Two corner stitches are placed between the jejunum and the apices of the ductotomy. An
enterotomy is then made lengthwise along the jejunum, in parallel to the pancreatic ductotomy.

(*Continued*)

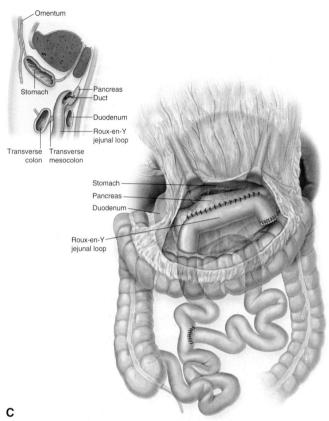

C

FIGURE 3.1 **(Continued)** **C.** A completed Roux-en-Y lateral pancreatojejunostomy. (From Lillemoe K, Jarnigan W, eds. *Master techniques in surgery: hepatobiliary and pancreatic surgery*. Philadelphia, PA: Lippincott Williams & Wilkins, 2013.)

Duodenum-Preserving Pancreatic Head Resection

In the 1970s, Beger described the technique of duodenum-preserving pancreatic head resection. In this procedure, the inflamed and fibrotic pancreatic head tissue is resected, leaving the duodenum and terminal bile duct intact. The intent is to minimize surgical morbidity, including the long-term morbidity of duodenal resection. Pain relief after this procedure has been reported in 77% to 88% of patients with professional rehabilitation in 63% to 69% and morbidity of 29%. Several variations of duodenum-preserving pancreatic head resection have evolved at various centers, primarily in Europe (Fig. 3.3).

Multiple randomized controlled trials comparing the different approaches to pancreatic head resection have been undertaken and are summarized in Table 3.5. While the advantage of any single procedure has not been demonstrated, this effort in outcome research has been important in moving the field of pancreatic surgery forward.

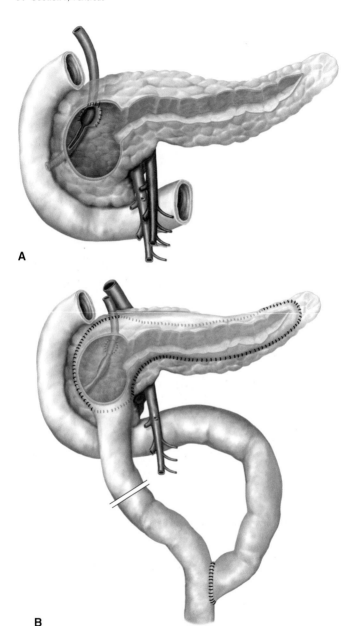

A

B

FIGURE 3.2 Frey procedure. **A.** The Frey procedure combines a circumscript excision in the pancreatic head with longitudinal opening of the pancreatic duct toward the tail. **B.** Reconstruction is performed with an anastomosis with a Roux-en-Y jejunal loop. Compared to the Beger procedure, the extent of resection of the pancreatic head is smaller; however, reconstruction is easier as it only requires one anastomosis to the pancreas. (From Lillemoe K, Jarnigan W, eds. *Master techniques in surgery: hepatobiliary and pancreatic surgery.* Philadelphia, PA: Lippincott Williams & Wilkins, 2013.)

Grade	A	B	C
Clinical condition	Well	Often well	Ill appearing/bad
Specific treatment	No	Yes/no	Yes
US/CT (if obtained)	Negative	Negative/positive	Positive
Persistent drainage (after 3 wk)	No	Usually yes	Yes
Reoperation	No	No	Yes
Death related to POPF	No	No	Possibly yes
Signs of infection	No	Yes/no	Yes
Sepsis	No	No	Yes
Readmission	No	Yes/no	Yes/no

US, ultrasound; CT, computed tomography; POPF, postoperative pancreatic fistula.
From Bassi C, Dervenis C, Butturini G, et al. Postoperative pancreatic fistula: an international study group (ISGPF) definition. *Surgery* 2005;138:8–13.

Distal Pancreatectomy

In CP patients with a midpancreatic body ductal stricture or those with disease localized to the body and tail of the pancreas, a DP can be beneficial. Pain relief rates of 57% to 84% are reported with return to work in 29% to 73% and morbidity rates of 15% to 32%. POPF is the most important potential procedure-specific complication and occurs in up to 30% of cases.

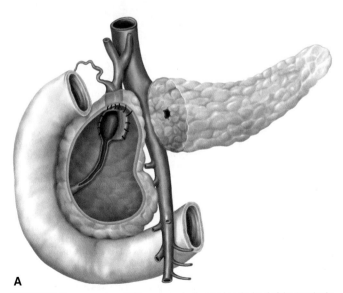

A

FIGURE 3.3 Beger procedure. **A.** The pancreas is dissected on the level of the portal vein. The pancreatic head is excavated and the duodenum is preserved with a thin layer of pancreatic tissue. If the bile duct is obstructed, it can be opened and an internal anastomosis with the excavated pancreatic head can be performed as shown.

(*Continued*)

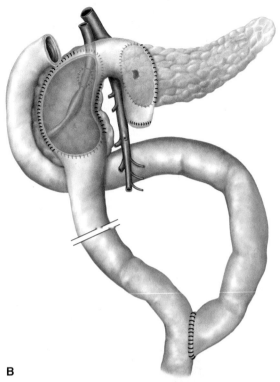

B

FIGURE 3.3 (Continued) B. The reconstruction is performed with two anastomoses, of the pancreatic tail remnant and of the excavated pancreatic head with a Roux-en-Y jejunal loop. (From Lillemoe K, Jarnigan W, eds. *Master techniques in surgery: hepatobiliary and pancreatic surgery*. Philadelphia, PA: Lippincott Williams & Wilkins, 2013.)

Total Pancreatectomy with Islet Autotransplantation

An early description of TP for CP comes from Dr. Clagett in 1944. Tellingly, his patient died 10 weeks postoperatively from a hypoglycemic event. In some patients with debilitating pain from CP, TP can be an effective means of pain relief. Candidates for TP include patients with diffuse small duct pancreatitis, those that have failed lesser procedures, and those with hereditary pancreatitis.

Parenchymal preserving procedures are always considered preferentially to TP when possible to minimize morbidity. The obligatory incipient pancreatogenic diabetes that results from TP can be prohibitively morbid, even with current diabetes management tools including the insulin pump. The largest recent series of patients undergoing TP is from the Mayo Clinic in 2005. In that series, 26% of long-term survivors were rehospitalized for glycemic control, and diabetes-related quality of life was poor.

In the 1970s, IAT was developed at the University of Minnesota, where islets are harvested from the resected pancreas immediately after resection and returned to the patient through the portal vein into the liver. The first successful procedure was described by Dr. Sutherland in 1978. Over the

	Comparative Randomized Controlled Trials of Pancreatic Head Resection				

Study	Comparison	N	Morbidity	Mortality	Pain Relief, %
Klempa et al. 1995	PD	21	51	0	70
	DPPHR	22	54	5	82
Buchler et al. 1995	PPPD	20	20	0	67
	DPPHR	20	15	0	94
Farkas et al. 2006	PPPD	20	40	0	90
	DPPHR	20	0	0	85
Izbicki et al. 1995	DPPHR	20	20	0	95
	LR-LPJ	22	9	0	89
Izbicki et al. 1998	LR-LPJ	31	19	3	90
	PPPD	30	53	0	71
Strate et al. 2005	DPPHR	38	NR	NR	82
	LR-LPJ	36	NR	NR	81

PD, pancreatoduodenectomy; DPPHR, duodenum-preserving pancreatic head resection; PPPD, pylorus-preserving pancreatic head resection; LR-LPJ, local resection pancreatic head with longitudinal pancreaticojejunostomy.

past decade, interest in this technique has grown, with now several centers offering TP–IAT for CP.

Morbidity rates of 48% to 56% and 0% to 2% mortality are reported in TP–IAT. Pain relief is described in 80% to 85% patients after TP–IAT. Statistically significant improvements in both physical and mental health–related quality of life are noted as early as 6 months postoperatively and appear durable in 3-year follow-up. Insulin independence is described in 25% to 40% patients in short-term follow-up up to 3 years. Longer-term follow-up demonstrates decline in islet function over time; however, C-peptide production has been documented up to 13 years postoperatively. Longer-term follow-up is needed for this relatively radical procedure.

Minimally Invasive Pancreatic Surgery

Laparoscopic pancreatic resection originated in the 1990s with the explosion of laparoscopy and the associated development of laparoscopic tools including the endoscopic stapler. Laparoscopic distal pancreatectomy (LDP) is the most commonly performed laparoscopic pancreas resection. A large multi-institutional study evaluated 667 DPs, 159 (24%) of which were laparoscopic. Of these, only 14 (9%) of these LDPs were for CP. While LDP is most commonly performed for benign or low-grade neoplasms, it is also applied to patients with CP. The inflammatory distortion of anatomy, loss of normal tissue planes, and frequent coexistence of sinistral (left-sided) portal hypertension in CP make these cases extremely challenging.

Laparoscopic PD is being performed at many centers now throughout the world. The largest single-center series is from India by Palanivelu with 75 patients, with mean operative time of 357 minutes, blood loss 74 mL, hospital stay 8.2 days, morbidity 26.7%, and mortality 1.3%. At the Mayo Clinic, Kendrick has reported on 65 patients, with outcomes similarly comparable to open resection, and has additionally reported on 11 patients safely undergoing major venous reconstruction via a totally laparoscopic route. The limitations of laparoscopic PD in the CP patient are similar to those encountered for DP.

CONCLUSIONS

CP remains a challenging disorder in the current era. In basic science, progress is occurring in the understanding of underlying genetic and cellular mechanisms of disease, with hopes for smart pharmacologic interventions including enzyme pathway inhibition. On the surgical front, sophisticated therapies are evolving including minimally invasive techniques and TP with IAT. In addition, in neuroscience, the recognition of neuroplasticity and maladaptive central pain pathways as an important factor in CP pain management holds promise for continued progress in the management of this difficult disease.

Suggested Readings

Bachem MG, Zhou Z, Zhou S, et al. Role of stellate cells in pancreatic fibrogenesis associated with acute and chronic pancreatitis. *J Gastroenterol Hepatol* 2006;21:S92–S96.

Beger HG, Krautzberger W, Bittner R, et al. Duodenum preserving resection of the head of the pancreas in severe chronic pancreatitis. *Surgery* 1985;97:465–475.

Buchler MW, Friess H, Muller MW, et al. Randomized trial of duodenum preserving pancreatic head resection versus pylorus preserving whipple in chronic pancreatitis. *Am J Surg* 1995;169:65–69.

Cahen DL, Gouma DJ, Laramee P, et al. Long-term outcomes of endoscopic vs surgical drainage of the pancreatic duct in patients with chronic pancreatitis. *Gastroenterology* 2011;141:1690–1695.

Demir IE, Teiftrunk E, Maak M, et al. Pain mechanisms in chronic pancreatitis: of a master and his fire. *Langenbecks Arch Surg* 2011;396:151–160.

DiMagno EP, Go VL, Summerskill WH. Relations between pancreatic enzyme outputs and malabsorption in severe pancreatic insufficiency. *N Engl J Med* 1973;288:813–815.

Farkas G, Leindler L, Daroczi M, Farkas G. Prospective randomized comparison of organ preserving pancreatic head resection with pylorus preserving pancreatoduodenectomy. *Langenbecks Arch Surg* 2006;391:338–342.

Frey CF, Smith GJ. Description and rationale of a new operation for chronic pancreatitis. *Pancreas* 1987;2:701–707.

Gorry MC, Gabbaizedah D, Furey W, et al. Mutations in the cationic trypsinogen gene are associated with recurrent acute and chronic pancreatitis. *Gastroenterology* 1997;113:1063–1068.

Izbicki JR, Bloechle C, Broering DC, et al. Extended drainage versus resection in surgery for chronic pancreatitis: A prospective randomized trial comparing the longitudinal pancreaticojejunostomy combined with local pancreatic head excision with the pylorus preserving pancreatoduodenectomy. *Ann Surg* 1998;228:771–779.

Izbicki JR, Bloechle C, Knoefel WT, et al. Duodenum preserving resection of head of the pancreas in chronic pancreatitis. A prospective randomized trial. *Ann Surg* 1995;221:350–358.

Kendrick ML, Cusati D. Total laparoscopic pancreaticoduodenectomy: feasibility and outcome in an early experience. *Arch Surg* 2010;145:19–23.

Klempa I, Spatny M, Menzel J, et al. Pancreatic function and quality of life after resection of the head of the pancreas in chronic pancreatitis. A prospective, randomized comparative study after duodenal preserving resection of the head of the pancreas versus Whipple's operation. *Chirurg* 1995;66:350–359.

Morgan K, Owczarski SM, Borckardt J, et al. Pain control and quality of life after pancreatectomy with islet autotransplantation for chronic pancreatitis. *J Gastrointest Surg* 2012;16:129–134.

Nealon WH, Thompson JC. Progressive loss of pancreatic function in chronic pancreatitis is delayed by main pancreatic duct decompression. A longitudinal prospective analysis of the modified Puestow procedure. *Ann Surg* 1993;217:458–468.

Schnelldorfer T, Mauldin PD, Lewin DN, et al. Distal pancreatectomy for chronic pancreatitis. Risk factors for postoperative pancreatic fistula. *J Gastrointest Surg* 2007;11:991–997.

Strate T, Taherpour Z, Bloechle C, et al. Long term follow up of a randomized trial comparing the Beger and Frey procedures for patients suffering from chronic pancreatitis. *Ann Surg* 2005;241:591–598.

Yadav D, Timmons L, Benson JT, et al. Incidence, prevalence, and survival of chronic pancreatitis: a population based study. *Am J Gastroenterol* 2011;106:2192–2199.

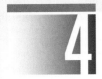

4   Pancreatic Adenocarcinoma

Jashodeep Datta, Jeffrey A. Drebin,
and Charles M. Vollmer Jr

EPIDEMIOLOGY

Cancer of the exocrine pancreas, commonly referred to as pancreatic ductal adenocarcinoma (PDAC), affects over 44,000 people a year and is the fourth leading cause of cancer-related deaths in the United States with approximately 37,000 annual mortalities. Approximately 11 new cases of PDAC are diagnosed per 100,000 of the population annually. At diagnosis, most patients are advanced (metastatic), with only 15% to 20% of patients being candidates for a potentially curative surgical resection. Resection offers the best possibility for cure (particularly when margin negative and node negative), with 5-year survival rates around 20% when performed at specialized high-volume centers. Nevertheless, median survival after resection is only about 2 years and, for all stages, 5-year survival is an abysmal 3%.

PATHOLOGY

Solid Epithelial Neoplasms of the Exocrine Pancreas

The most common solid exocrine pancreatic tumors are *pancreatic ductal adenocarcinoma* and its variants, *acinar cell carcinoma* and *pancreatoblastoma*. PDAC accounts for greater than 90% of all exocrine tumors of the pancreas and represents the vast majority of cases referred for surgical consultation. Thus, the rest of the discussion in this chapter will focus on the management of PDAC. Histologically, the neoplastic cells in PDAC show ductal differentiation, induce an intense and characteristic desmoplastic stromal reaction, and display an infiltrative growth pattern. PDAC is thought to develop from benign proliferative precursor lesions, termed pancreatic intraepithelial neoplasia (PanIN), as a result of the progressive accumulation of tumorigenic mutations. Variants of PDAC include giant cell, adenosquamous, mucinous (noncystic), and anaplastic carcinomas. *Acinar cell carcinomas* tend to form larger tumors than PDAC, form acini which display an eosinophilic and granular cytoplasm, and have a slightly better prognosis than PDAC. *Pancreatoblastomas* occur in children 1 to 15 years old, contain both epithelial and mesenchymal components, are usually larger than 10 cm, and have a more favorable prognosis than PDAC.

ETIOLOGY

Risk Factors for Pancreatic Ductal Adenocarcinoma

The risk of developing PDAC is related to demographic, acquired, and host factors. Overall, any given person has a 0.5% risk of developing PDAC by age 70.

(a) *Demographic Factors*: The peak incidence of PDAC is in the seventh to eighth decades, with more than 80% of cases occurring between 60 and 80 years. PDAC is more common in men compared to females, with a relative risk of 1.35. Compared with Whites, both the incidence and mortality rates for PDAC are higher in African Americans of both genders. Other demographic characteristics associated with PDAC include lower socio-economic status, migrant status, and Ashkenazi Jewish heritage.

(b) *Acquired or Environmental Factors:* Tobacco smoke exposure is the most consistently observed environmental risk factor for the development of PDAC, while the contributory role of alcohol or various dietary substances is more equivocal. PDAC risk increases in obese patients—a large cohort study showed a 1.72 relative risk of PDAC in patients with body mass index (BMI) ≥ 30 kg/m^2 compared to individuals with BMI ≤ 23 kg/m^2. Moreover, moderate physical activity was associated with decreased PDAC rates. An association between diabetes mellitus (DM) and PDAC has also been posited due to the observation that approximately 80% of PDAC patients have impaired glucose metabolism, impaired glucose tolerance, or DM. Type 2 DM of at least 5 years' duration has been demonstrated to increase the risk of PDAC twofold. However, among newly diagnosed diabetics, only 0.85% developed PDAC within 3 years. Additionally, chronic pancreatitis, cystic fibrosis, benign endocrine tumors, and pernicious anemia have also been implicated in elevating PDAC risk.

(c) *Host Factors:* Only around 2% of PDAC can be considered "inherited." This consists of two distinct cohorts: (i) familial lineage of PDAC (genetics as yet undetermined) and (ii) genetic syndromes caused by recognized germ line mutations. These are as follows: (i) *hereditary pancreatitis (50-fold risk):* autosomal dominant, *PRSSI* mutation on gene 7q35, and recurrent pancreatitis from a young age; (ii) *hereditary nonpolyposis colorectal cancer (HNPCC type II) (eightfold risk):* autosomal dominant, *MSH2/MLH1* mutation, and colonic, endometrial, and gastric cancers; (iii) *Peutz-Jeghers syndrome (32-fold risk):* autosomal dominant, *STK11/ LKB1* mutation on 19p13, and gastrointestinal hamartomatous polyps and mucocutaneous pigmentation; (iv) *familial atypical multiple mole melanoma (FAMMM) syndrome (12- to 20-fold risk):* autosomal dominant, *p16* mutation on 9p21, and multiple atypical nevi and melanoma; (v) *hereditary breast and ovarian cancer (5- to 10-fold risk):* autosomal dominant, *BRCA2* mutation on 13q12–13, and breast and ovarian cancers; and (vi) *ataxia–telangiectasia:* autosomal recessive, *ATM* mutation on 11q22–23, and ataxia, telangiectasia, and hematologic malignancies. In addition, analysis of kindreds enrolled in the National Familial Pancreas Tumor Registry revealed an 18-fold increased risk of PDAC in familial PDAC kindreds compared to sporadic PDAC groups. The germ line mutation(s) responsible for the familial predisposition to PDAC is/ are yet to be elaborated. Elevated risk begins with at least two affected first-degree relatives and escalates significantly with each additional family member. There is *no* known established relationship between a family history of pancreatic cancer and the development of pancreatic cystic neoplasms that devolve into PDAC.

Molecular Genetics

Significant advances have been made in understanding the molecular genetics associated with PDAC in recent years. The pathogenesis of PDAC involves alterations in the following: (i) *tumor suppressor genes: p16, p53, MADH4/DPC4,* and *BRCA2* are found to be inactivated in up to 90%, 75%, 55%, and 7% of sporadic PDAC cases, respectively; (ii) *oncogenes:* activating point mutations in *K-ras*—a guanine nucleotide–binding protein involved in growth factor signal transduction—are seen in between 80% and 100% of PDAC cases. In spite of being widely investigated as a potential diagnostic or prognosticative marker in PDAC, *K-ras* cannot be recommended for

PDAC detection based on the available data. Other oncogenes implicated in PDAC pathogenesis are *BRAF, AKT2,* and *MYB*; and (iii) *DNA mismatch repair genes*: approximately 4% of PDAC appears related to dysregulation of DNA mismatch repair genes—*MSH2, MLH1, PMS1, PMS2, MSH6/GTBP,* and *MSH3.* It is postulated that these mutations occur in a cumulative fashion over the life span of a developing PDAC.

DIAGNOSIS

Clinical Presentation

The nonspecific symptoms associated with early PDAC—anorexia, nausea, and weight loss—typically preclude its diagnosis at an early stage in most cases. The majority of patients with right-sided PDAC present with jaundice secondary to obstruction of the intrapancreatic portion of the common bile duct and subsequently develop dark urine, light-colored stools, and pruritus. These tumors can also cause mechanical obstruction of the duodenal C-loop, leading to weight loss, gastric outlet obstruction and, ultimately, vomiting. Left-sided tumors generally do not cause jaundice and may present with epigastric/back pain from celiac axis lymphovascular infiltration or focal, segmental pancreatic duct obstruction or, sometimes, duodenal obstruction at the ligament of Treitz. More subtle presentations may be encountered in elderly patients with new-onset DM or with episodes of acute pancreatitis in the absence of cholelithiasis or ethanol abuse. The most consistent physical finding in PDAC is jaundice, seen in up to 87% in head-based tumors but just 13% of distal (usually body) tumors. Hepatomegaly, palpable gallbladder (Courvoisier sign), and malnutrition may be observed. Signs of advanced disease include ascites, cachexia, liver nodularity, left supraclavicular adenopathy (Virchow node), periumbilical adenopathy (Sister Mary Joseph node), and pelvic drop metastasis (Blumer shelf).

Laboratory Analysis

Workup usually reveals an elevated total and conjugated serum bilirubin, alkaline phosphatase, and γ-glutamyl transferase reflective of biliary obstruction. Transaminases, amylase, and lipase may be normal. In patients with jaundice, malabsorption of fat-soluble vitamins decreases the hepatic production of vitamin K–dependent clotting factors and results in the prolongation of prothrombin time. This coagulopathy can be normalized by the administration of parenteral or subcutaneous vitamin K. Normocytic anemia and hypoalbuminemia may reflect the chronic nutritional sequelae of the neoplastic disease process.

The most extensively studied serum tumor marker in PDAC is the Lewis blood group–related mucin glycoprotein, CA 19-9. The use of CA 19-9 as a diagnostic or screening marker for PDAC is limited by several factors. CA 19-9 is only moderately accurate (sensitivity 81%) in identifying PDAC when using the normal cutoff value of 37 units/mL. In addition, up to 15% of individuals do not secrete CA 19-9 because of their Lewis antigen status. Moreover, patients with small-diameter or early tumors—who would derive the greatest survival benefit from surgical resection—often have normal CA 19-9 levels. Lastly, elevated CA 19-9 levels can be seen in benign pancreatic or biliary disease, and CA 19-9 is spuriously elevated in the setting of jaundice. Nevertheless, CA 19-9 may complement other diagnostic modalities, such as computed tomography (CT), endoscopic retrograde cholangiopancreatography (ERCP), or endoscopic ultrasound (EUS), such that the combined diagnostic accuracy for PDAC nearly approaches 100%. Severely elevated preoperative CA 19-9 levels (>1,000 units/mL) suggest advanced or unresectable disease. In such instances, many authorities recommend staging laparoscopy even when high-fidelity imaging suggests a resectable tumor. Finally, CA 19-9 finds its best utility in postoperative surveillance. Increasing CA 19-9 levels after surgical resection typically indicate recurrence or disease progression, whereas stable or declining levels postoperatively indicate absence of recurrence and improved overall prognosis. CEA has little to no additive value in securing a diagnosis of PDAC.

Investigational Diagnostic Markers

The limited diagnostic utility of CA 19-9 has prompted a search for novel tumor biomarkers to facilitate the earlier detection of PDAC. These can be classified as (i) *serum markers* : CA 242, CEA, TPA, TPS, M2-pyruvate kinase, Mic-1, IGFBP-1a, haptoglobin, serum amyloid A, etc. and (ii) *tissue markers*: K-ras, p53, mucins (MUC1/2/5), microRNAs, *p21*, *SMAD4*, *Bcl-2*, etc. The first four listed tissue markers have shown promise in early studies, but none are superior to CA 19-9 nor widely available for use in clinical practice.

Diagnostic Imaging

Imaging has assumed a crucial role in the diagnosis and stratification of PDAC patients to stage-appropriate therapy. The goals of imaging are identification of the primary tumor, assessment of regional invasion and vascular or lymph node involvement, evaluation of distant metastasis, and determination of resectability. Common imaging modalities in PDAC are the following:

(a) *Transabdominal Ultrasonography (TAUS):* TAUS has an operator-dependent sensitivity of 60% to 70% in detecting PDAC, which typically appears as a hypoechoic mass. This modality has largely been replaced by axial imaging.

(b) *Computed Tomography (CT):* Multidetector-row CT (MDCT) with three-dimensional reconstruction is the *preferred* noninvasive imaging modality for the diagnosis and staging of PDAC. MDCT utilizes dual-phase imaging in the arterial and venous phases of enhancement, acquiring sub-3-mm slices during one 20-second breath hold. PDAC typically appears as a hypodense mass—although it can appear isodense—in the parenchyma and is best seen on the portal venous phase of enhancement. MDCT also provides a comprehensive view of tumor abutment or encasement of the major peripancreatic vascular structures (celiac axis, superior mesenteric artery [SMA] and superior mesenteric vein [SMV], splenic artery, and portal vein [PV]) as well as peripancreatic lymphadenopathy and hepatic or omental metastasis. Finally, it provides the best spatial road map for the anatomic relationships between the primary tumor and the local vasculature.

(c) *Magnetic Resonance Imaging (MRI):* Several technical improvements in MRI technology have improved its ability to diagnose and stage pancreatic cancer. A majority of PDACs have low-signal intensity on T1-weighted fat-suppressed images. Upon dynamic imaging after gadolinium contrast injection, PDAC enhances relatively less than surrounding parenchyma and reveals progressive enhancement on subsequent phases. MR cholangiopancreatography (MRCP) can optimally assess the biliary and pancreatic ductal anatomy as well as the postresection pancreatic remnant. Although some authorities consider MRI comparable to MDCT in detecting PDAC, obtaining *both* studies offers no significant advantage in assessing patients with radiographically resectable disease. MRCP is more useful for evaluating cystic masses of the pancreas.

(d) *Positron Emission Tomography (PET):* In this functional imaging technique, a positron-emitting tracer—fluorine-18—is labeled to fluorodeoxyglucose (FDG), which is rapidly taken up by tumor cells. Although unenhanced PET/CT has a limited role in the local staging of PDAC due to its poor depiction of primary tumor and its relationship to adjacent vasculature, intravenous contrast-enhanced PET/CT has been shown to have improved accuracy for PDAC detection in recent studies. However, since FDG also localizes at sites of inflammation and infection, PET imaging is largely used as an adjunct modality to detect disseminated disease. Furthermore, its reimbursement is currently limited for PDAC, as opposed to its acceptance for other established solid malignancies.

(e) *Endoscopic Ultrasound (EUS):* EUS has gained popularity in recent years as a minimally invasive modality for the local staging of PDAC. Its particular benefit is realized in the clarification of small (< 2 cm) lesions in the setting of negative or equivocal CT findings, evaluation of malignant lymphadenopathy, detection of vascular involvement, and the ability to obtain a tissue diagnosis when combined with fine needle aspiration (FNA). Combined with FNA, EUS has a sensitivity of 93% and 88% for T- and N-stage disease, respectively. However, unless protocol-based neoadjuvant therapy is planned or the patient is a poor operative candidate, a tissue diagnosis is *not* required in acceptable-risk patients with resectable lesions on noninvasive axial imaging (CT or MRI). Moreover, EUS is invasive, operator dependent, and cannot assess liver or distant metastasis, thereby limiting its utility.

(f) *Endoscopic Retrograde Cholangiopancreatography:* Although its sensitivity for the diagnosis of PDAC approaches 90%, the routine use of *diagnostic* ERCP for suspected PDAC is unsupported. With the current advances in CT/MRI technology, diagnostic ERCP should be reserved for select groups of patients: (i) those with obstructive jaundice but without a detectable mass on CT or MRI; (ii) symptomatic but nonjaundiced patients with equivocal findings on CT or MRI; and (iii) suspected pancreatic cancer in the setting of chronic pancreatitis. Even in these circumstances, many authorities advocate for noninvasive alternatives, such as MRCP. Nevertheless, ERCP is often utilized prior to surgical consultation for relief of jaundice.

Clinicopathologic Staging

The American Joint Committee on Cancer (AJCC) staging for pancreatic cancer is based on the TNM classification, incorporating extent of primary tumor (T), presence of regional lymph node involvement (N), and presence of distant metastasis (M) (Table 4.1).

MANAGEMENT

Preoperative Considerations
Assessing Surgical Resectability

Although the TNM classification is used for pathologic staging and clinical description, the crucial step for the surgeon in the preoperative workup of PDAC patients is to determine operability—an option available to fewer than a quarter of all patients at diagnosis. PDAC of the pancreatic head, neck, or uncinate process is stratified into the following: (a) *resectable*, defined as no radiographic evidence of extrapancreatic disease, a patent SMV–PV confluence, and no evidence of tumor extension to the celiac axis or SMA; (b) *borderline resectable*, defined as nonmetastatic tumor with SMA abutment (≤180 degrees), abutment or encasement of

	AJCC Staging of Pancreatic Ductal Adenocarcinoma (seventh edition)

Tumor (T)
Tx: Primary tumor cannot be assessed
T0: No evidence of primary tumor
Tis: Carcinoma in situ
T1: Tumor limited to the pancreas, 2 cm or less in greatest dimension
T2: Tumor limited to the pancreas, more than 2 cm in greatest dimension
T3: Tumor extends beyond the pancreas but without involvement of the celiac axis or the superior mesenteric artery
T4: Tumor involves the celiac axis or the superior mesenteric artery (unresectable primary tumor)
Regional Lymph Nodes (N)
Nx: Regional lymph nodes cannot be assessed
N0: No regional lymph node metastasis
N1: Regional lymph node metastasis
Distant Metastasis (M)
Mx: Distant metastasis cannot be assessed
M0: No distant metastasis
M1: Distant metastasis

Stage	T	N	M	5-Year Survival (%)
IA	T1	N0	M0	20–30
IB	T2	N0	M0	20–30
IIA	T3	N0	M0	10–25
IIB	T1, T2, T3	N1	M0	10–15
III	T4	Any N	M0	0–5
IV	Any T	Any N	M1	—

the gastroduodenal artery (GDA) up to or around a short, reconstructable segment of the common hepatic artery (CHA), or complete occlusion of the SMV–PV confluence, with suitable, uninvolved vein above and below to allow venous reconstruction (as a general rule, tumors encasing up to 2 cm of the SMV and/or PV for up to a 180-degree circumference are considered technically possible); (c) *locally advanced*, defined as encasement (>180 degrees) of the celiac axis or SMA or occlusion of SMV–PV confluence without an option for venous resection and reconstruction; and (d) *metastatic*, defined as distant metastatic spread to the liver, peritoneum, or rarely the lung. It is important to realize that, for this disease, *operability ≠ resectability*. Up to 85% (but certainly not 100%) of radiographically amenable lesions are resectable intraoperatively, whereas fewer than 20% of locally advanced lesions are ultimately amenable to resection.

Role of Diagnostic Laparoscopy

The use of diagnostic laparoscopy in PDAC staging remains controversial. Although the combination of laparoscopy with laparoscopic ultrasound can improve the accuracy of determining peritoneal and/or hepatic dissemination to almost 98%, we do *not* recommend the *routine* application of diagnostic laparoscopy in PDAC due to its questionable cost-effectiveness as well as the impressive accuracy of modern high-fidelity axial imaging. Moreover, even in potentially unresectable disease, laparoscopy is unnecessary if the patient were to benefit most from surgical palliation (see below). Alternatively, a more selective use of diagnostic laparoscopy is justified in those patients with a high risk of occult metastatic disease in whom nonsurgical palliation would be durable. This scenario includes the following: (a) lesions in the pancreatic body or tail; (b) larger (> 3 cm) primary tumors; (c) equivocal radiographic findings suggestive of occult metastasis such as low-volume ascites, peritoneal carcinomatosis, or small hepatic lesions not amenable to percutaneous biopsy; and (d) markedly elevated CA 19-9 or hypoalbuminemia suggestive of advanced disease. In addition, diagnostic laparoscopy may be considered in certain cases of borderline resectable and/or locally advanced disease—understanding that evidence of metastatic spread might alter whether radiation therapy would be used in conjunction with chemotherapy.

Role of Preoperative Biliary Drainage for Obstructive Jaundice
In the past, a majority of patients with resectable PDAC who presented with obstructive jaundice underwent either endoscopic or percutaneous transhepatic preoperative biliary drainage (PBD) before surgical referral. Recently, however, the *routine* use of PBD in *resectable* PDAC has been discouraged in the light of convincing evidence that PBD increases the rate of postoperative complications and offers little benefit compared with early surgery for resectable tumors. In a recent randomized multicenter trial, van der Gaag et al. showed that PBD was associated with significantly higher rates of serious perioperative complications compared with early surgery, while mortality and length of hospital stay did not differ significantly between the groups. However, the role of biliary drainage as temporary palliation in patients with borderline resectable tumors undergoing neoadjuvant therapy is clinically relevant. In such situations, authorities advocate the use of self-expandable metal stents over plastic stents given their improved durability should the tumor be ultimately deemed unresectable.

Role of Neoadjuvant Therapy for PDAC
There is growing enthusiasm for the use of neoadjuvant chemoradiation in PDAC that relies on the following theoretical principles: (a) increased efficacy of chemoradiation in well-oxygenated tissue not devascularized by surgery; (b) potential for downstaging, thereby improving R0 resection and decreasing locoregional recurrence rates; and (c) identifying patients with rapidly progressive disease who might not derive a survival advantage from surgery. Several groups have utilized neoadjuvant regimens involving gemcitabine, 5-FU, or paclitaxel plus radiation for resectable PDAC. Current data suggest that while neoadjuvant chemotherapy is well tolerated and does not delay surgical intervention, there is *no* clear survival benefit to this strategy compared with standard postoperative adjuvant therapy. A 2009 AHPBA-SSO-SSAT consensus panel indicated that neoadjuvant therapy for *resectable* PDAC should be considered investigational and offered within the context of clinical trials or multidisciplinary treatment programs.

However, there may be an emerging role for neoadjuvant strategies in *borderline resectable* tumors. Investigators from the University of Virginia demonstrated that 46% of patients with borderline resectable PDAC underwent surgical resection after completing neoadjuvant capecitabine-based chemoradiation. This group had favorable overall survival (OS)—median 23 months—similar to that of a historical cohort of patients with resectable PDAC. In a recent report from the M.D. Anderson Cancer Center, 66% of borderline resectable PDAC patients underwent resection after neoadjuvant therapy (chemoradiation alone or gemcitabine-based chemotherapy followed by chemoradiation), of which an R0 resection was achieved in 95%. Median OS in this cohort was up to 33 months following their uniquely highly standardized protocol. These data solidify the role for induction therapy in borderline resectable PDAC, with attempted resection offered to patients without evidence of cancer progression on presurgical restaging studies. Several challenges remain: (a) adherence to and application of the consensus definition of "borderline resectable" tumors across institutions; (b) what the most effective neoadjuvant modality is (chemotherapy alone, chemoradiation, or a combination); and (c) need for a multi-institutional trial to validate these optimistic early reports. As is the case for resectable tumors, it remains a fact that there has been *no* direct clinical comparison of the two techniques that would clearly advocate one over the other.

Surgical Resection and Related Controversies

Resection of PDAC can be broadly categorized into two types: (i) *pancreaticoduodenectomy* for tumors situated in the head, neck, or uncinate process or (ii) *distal pancreatectomy* for tumors of the body and tail. While technical details of these operations can be found in Chapter 7 by Pilgrim et al., a discussion of the global conduct of these operations and select lingering controversies in the operative management of PDAC follows.

Pancreaticoduodenectomy (Whipple Procedure)

The preliminary steps of a PD or Whipple procedure involve assessment of resectability. The liver, peritoneal surfaces, celiac axis level lymph nodes, and remainder of the abdomen are inspected for metastatic disease. As noted earlier, this assessment may be performed laparoscopically in select circumstances. A Kocher maneuver is performed to assess for retroperitoneal, SMV, SMA, or celiac takeoff involvement. The SMV is identified in the plane anterior to the third portion of the duodenum between the transverse mesocolon and the uncinate process by opening the lesser sac through the gastrocolic omentum. The porta hepatis is examined by mobilizing the gallbladder and tracing the cystic duct to its junction with the common hepatic duct. Once the tumor is considered resectable on both of these fronts, early division of the extrahepatic biliary tree allows caudal retraction of the distal common bile duct and visualization of the anterior aspect of the PV. In a pylorus-preserving PD, division of bowel occurs 2 cm distal to the pylorus and 20 cm distal to the ligament of Treitz. The divided proximal jejunum is delivered posterior to the superior mesenteric vessels to facilitate dissection of the pancreas off the right lateral aspect of the SMV. Vein resection may be required and ranges from primary repair to patch reconstruction to interposition grafting. The pancreatic neck overlying the SMV–PV is divided, and the pancreatic head is meticulously dissected off the right lateral aspects of the SMV–PV. Dissection of the retroperitoneal "mesopancreas" ensues with the aim of removing the tissue up to the adventitial layer of the SMA along the right side of its course. Reconstruction involves a pancreaticoenteric anastomosis—most commonly pancreaticojejunostomy (PJ)—in an end-to-end or end-to-side fashion using either a duct-to-mucosa or invagination technique. Alternatively, a pancreaticogastrostomy (PG) can be used. The biliary–enteric anastomosis is typically performed in an end-to-side fashion approximately 10 cm distal to the PJ on the pancreaticobiliary limb of the jejunum. The duodenojejunostomy (DJ) is placed, in a majority of cases, in an antecolic orientation 50 to 60 cm downstream to the biliary–enteric anastomosis. Enteric feeding tubes (gastrostomy or jejunostomy) can be used selectively in those patients who the surgeon expects may not thrive postoperatively.

Distal Pancreatectomy

Fewer resections are performed for tumors of the body and tail of the pancreas due to a higher incidence of advanced disease at initial presentation. Resection of these tumors is achieved with a distal pancreatectomy accompanied by, in a vast majority of cases, splenectomy. As with PD, initial exploration is geared to rule out hepatic or peritoneal metastasis, and laparoscopy has a higher yield than with proximal tumors. If metastasis is not present, the lesser sac is entered and involvement of the SMV is adjudicated. If resection is attempted, the spleen and distal pancreas are mobilized in a retrograde fashion. The pancreas is then transected to the left of the SMV–PV trunk and the main pancreatic duct ligated. This is usually performed with a stapling device, although suturing the duct is acceptable—evidence does not support any particular technique. However, due to limitations in the posterior extent of resection and the ability to achieve a complete N1 nodal dissection with the classic distal pancreatosplenectomy, Strasberg et al. proposed the radical antegrade modular pancreatosplenectomy (RAMPS) procedure in 2003. This approach, which relies on medial to lateral dissection, improves visibility, enables an N1 nodal dissection, enhances the ability to achieve microscopically negative tangential margins, and permits adjustment of the depth of the posterior extent of resection coupled with early rather than late control of the vasculature. Long-term results revealed R0 resection rates of up to 81%, negative tangential margins in 89%, and median survival of 26 months.

Surgical Palliation

PDAC patients found to have unresectable disease at laparotomy, or those with tumor-related symptoms poorly alleviated by nonoperative methods, are appropriate candidates for surgical palliation. It involves biliary bypass, gastroenteric bypass, chemical splanchnicectomy, or combinations thereof. Hepatico- or choledochojejunostomy, using a Roux-en-Y conduit, is the preferred method of biliary bypass and results in a decreased risk of recurrent jaundice compared with choledochoduodenostomy or cholecystojejunostomy. Some patients undergoing biliary bypass alone ultimately require gastroenteric bypass for eventual duodenal obstruction. A prospective trial evaluating the role of prophylactic gastrojejunostomy (GJ) in unresectable PDAC found that 19% of patients randomized to no GJ developed late gastric outlet obstruction requiring intervention compared with 0% in the GJ group ($p < 0.01$), although mean OS between the groups was similar. Finally, chemical splanchnicectomy—injection of 50% alcohol at the celiac nerve plexus—significantly reduces mean pain scores in patients with unresectable right-sided PDAC. This should be reserved for unresectable patients who present with significant pain prior to laparotomy.

Controversies in Pancreatic Resection for PDAC

(a) *Role for Extended Lymphadenectomy:* Four randomized trials have attempted to answer if there is benefit to extended lymph node dissection in PDAC. The data, substantiated by numerous strong meta-analyses, suggest that extended lymphadenectomy increases the morbidity without significantly improving median or 5-year survival.

(b) *Classical Versus Pylorus-Preserving PD:* Most surgeons prefer the pylorus-preserving PD because it reduces operative time and blood loss, retains the entire gastric reservoir, and does not compromise oncologic outcomes (negative margin rate or OS) compared with the classical variant. Furthermore, no appreciable difference is observed in gastric physiology or nutrition postoperatively.

(c) *Vascular Resection and Reconstruction:* The data examining vascular resection and reconstruction after PD for PDAC are nonstandardized. Several single-center experiences suggest that, in the absence of other contraindications for resection, a controlled venous resection and reconstruction when the tumor cannot be separated from the SMV, PV or SMV–PV confluence is safe and feasible. Recently, however, a large retrospective analysis of the ACS NSQIP database revealed that vascular resection after PD is associated with a significantly higher overall morbidity and 30-day postoperative mortality. Arterial resection is not advised with the exception of a short segment of hepatic artery for those tumors invading the GDA takeoff. Most experienced pancreatic surgeons avoid concomitant arterial and venous resection.

(d) *Margin Status:* Current margin nomenclature is poorly defined and the value of intraoperative frozen section analysis has not been studied extensively. Controversy exists over the proper techniques for specimen analysis by pathologists. Achieving an R0 resection and a negative SMA/uncinate margin correlates most strongly with positive long-term outcomes. Patients with R1 resections should be strongly considered for adjuvant multimodal therapy.

(e) *Minimally Invasive PD:* Although minimally invasive distal pancreatic resections are being increasingly employed for cancer, minimally invasive PD (MIPD) for PDAC continues to lack widespread acceptance because matched comparative trials and long-term outcomes comparing MIPD to the open approach are lacking. Recently, comparisons between the two suggest that MIPD is associated with reduced length of stay and blood loss without compromising standard oncologic principles. Although long-term follow-up is lacking, short-term results suggest equivalent, but not better, rates of recurrence and survival when highly skilled specialists apply MIPD techniques.

Postoperative Considerations

Postoperative Complications

The overall complication rate after PDAC resection, especially PD, continues to approach 40%. The most common immediate complications are postoperative pancreatic fistula (approximately 15%), delayed gastric emptying (approximately 5%), hemorrhage (approximately 5%), and wound infection (approximately 20%). Long-term effects of parenchymal resection may manifest in pancreatic insufficiency. These include diabetes and steatorrhea—both of which occur in approximately 25% of all patients.

(a) *Postoperative Pancreatic Fistula (POPF):* A gradation of POPF—A (biochemical, with no clinical impact) through C (rendering a life-threatening, major deviation from clinical recovery)—was developed by a consensus panel (ISGPF) in 2005. There is *no* unequivocal evidence to suggest that anastomotic route (PJ vs. PG), anastomotic technique (duct-to-mucosa vs. invagination vs. single-layer end-to-side PJ), pancreatic duct stenting, or use of long-acting somatostatin analogs alters the incidence of POPF formation.

(b) *Delayed Gastric Emptying (DGE):* The severity of DGE after pylorus-preserving PD—grades A through C—relates to the need for nasogastric decompression, volume of gastric effluent, and inability to tolerate oral intake postoperatively. The pathogenesis of DGE remains unclear, although putative mechanisms include antral ischemia, absence of duodenal motilin, gastric atony from a vagotomized stomach, and gastric dysrhythmia secondary to POPF or edema from fluid overload. There is convincing randomized evidence that (i) an antecolic compared with a retrocolic reconstruction and (ii) postoperative administration of erythromycin (motilin agonist) significantly reduce the incidence of DGE after pylorus-preserving PD.

Postoperative Adjuvant Therapy

Adjuvant therapy, supported by a large body of evidence, is a critical part of the postoperative management of PDAC. The Gastrointestinal Tumor Study

Group (GISTG, 1985) originally showed that 5-FU–based chemoradiation followed by maintenance chemotherapy had a significant median OS benefit compared with observation alone (20 months vs. 11 months, p = 0.03). Despite limited accrual, the GITSG trial was the first to show a potential benefit for adjuvant therapy after resection of pancreatic cancer. The European Organization for Research and Treatment of Cancer (EORTC, 1999) study was similar and randomized resected patients to concurrent chemoradiation *without* subsequent chemotherapy versus observation alone. Median OS was not significantly different (24.5 months vs. 19 months, p = 0.208). The European Study Group for Pancreatic Cancer (ESPAC-1, 2004) study was conducted with a 2 × 2 factorial design. The four arms included surgery alone, 5-FU–based chemotherapy alone, 5-FU–based chemoradiation alone, and both modalities. Patients receiving chemotherapy (chemotherapy alone or chemoradiation followed by chemotherapy) had a significantly improved median OS compared with the no-chemotherapy arm (chemoradiation alone or surgery alone; 19.7 months vs. 14 months, p = 0.0005). Interestingly, patients who received radiation (chemoradiation alone or chemoradiation followed by chemotherapy) had worse median OS compared with those not receiving radiation (chemotherapy alone and surgery alone; 15.9 months vs. 17.9 months, p = 0.05).

With gemcitabine emerging as a viable alternative to 5-FU chemotherapy, the CONKO-001 study demonstrated that resected patients receiving adjuvant gemcitabine had significantly improved median OS compared with observation alone (22.8 months vs. 20.2 months, p = 0.005). The ESPAC-3 trial, a head-to-head comparison between adjuvant gemcitabine versus 5-FU alone, found a nonsignificant difference in median OS (23.6 months vs. 23.0 months). Of note, there was a greater incidence of high-grade, treatment-related toxicities in the 5-FU arm. The Radiation Therapy Oncology Group (RTOG-9704), which compared adjuvant gemcitabine + 5-FU–based chemoradiation and 5-FU + 5-FU–based chemoradiation, found a nonstatistically significant survival benefit with gemcitabine (20.5 months vs. 16.9 months, p = 0.09). Although both 5-FU and gemcitabine have been validated as viable adjuvant options, gemcitabine has largely replaced 5-FU in the Unites States due its greater tolerability and improved quality-of-life outcomes.

The Debate Surrounding Adjuvant Radiotherapy
Although the benefit of adjuvant chemotherapy is unequivocally agreed upon, the concurrent use of radiation therapy remains contentious. In the United States, the use of adjuvant chemoradiation is still largely standard practice. Proponents for this approach cite the survival benefit seen in the GISTG trial and the design flaws underlying the conclusions of the ESPAC-1 trial. In Europe, adjuvant chemotherapy alone is preferred, presumably from different interpretations of the same data presented above.

Future Directions in Adjuvant Therapy
Adjuvant trials with erlotinib, FOLFIRINOX, maintenance capecitabine, and a therapeutic vaccine GI-4000 are underway and are described elsewhere.

OUTCOMES AND FOLLOW-UP

Historically, after PDAC resection, the perioperative mortality rate was 20% to 40% and 5-year survival approximately 3%. These statistics have changed dramatically, with current operative mortality rates having declined to well under 5% and 5-year survival regularly eclipsing 20% in recent studies from high-volume pancreatic surgery centers. This improvement is likely multifactorial and is related to advances in preoperative imaging, improvements in surgical technique and perioperative care, and availability of broader adjuvant therapy options. Recently, a contemporary analysis of 424 PDAC resections from the University of Pennsylvania and Beth Israel Deaconess Medical Center demonstrated median, 1-year, and 5-year survivals of 21.3 months, 76%, and 23%, respectively. The 30-day mortality was only 0.7%. Seventy-six percent of patients received adjuvant therapy. Patients with major complications (Clavien grade IIIb–IV) survived similarly to those without complications. In general, predictors of survival include patients with R0/N0/M0 characteristics, tumor diameters less than 3 cm, negative resection margins, and well or moderate tumor differentiation and those who receive adjuvant chemoradiation.

CONCLUSION

Overall, the prognosis of PDAC continues to be disappointing. However, survival in resectable PDAC has increased dramatically over the last few decades, in part due to significant improvements in surgical expertise and adjuvant multimodal therapy. Correspondingly, the therapeutic boundaries in PDAC care are being pushed with respect to expanding indications for PDAC resection and aggressive neoadjuvant strategies in borderline resectable tumors. Continuing refinement in our surgical techniques, combined with emerging chemo- and radiotherapeutic options, provides cautious optimism for the future of this often frustrating disease.

Suggested Readings

Bardeesy N, DePinho RA. Pancreatic cancer biology and genetics. *Nat Rev Cancer* 2002;2(12):897–909.

Castleberry AW, White RR, De La Fuente SG, et al. The impact of vascular resection on early postoperative outcomes after pancreaticoduodenectomy: an analysis of the American College of Surgeons National Surgical Quality Improvement Program database. *Ann Surg Oncol* 2012;19(13):4068–4077.

Diener MK, Knaebel HP, Heukaufer C, et al. A systematic review and meta-analysis of pylorus-preserving versus classical pancreaticoduodenectomy for surgical treatment of periampullary and pancreatic carcinoma. *Ann Surg* 2007;245(2):187–200.

Hruban RH, Brune K, Klein A, et al. Familial pancreatic cancer. In: Von Hoff DD, Evans DB, Hruban RH (eds.), *Pancreatic cancer*. Boston, MA: Jones and Bartlett, 2004.

Katz MH, Fleming JB, Bhosale P, et al. Response of borderline resectable pancreatic cancer to neoadjuvant therapy is not reflected by radiographic indicators. *Cancer* 2012;118(23):5749–5756.

Kawai M, Yamaue H. Analysis of clinical trials evaluating complications after pancreaticoduodenectomy: a new era of pancreatic surgery. *Surg Today* 2010;40(11):1011–1017.

Kendrick ML. Laparoscopic and robotic resection for pancreatic cancer. *Cancer J* 2012;18(6):571–576.

Lewis R, Drebin JA, Callery MP, et al. A contemporary analysis of survival for resected pancreatic ductal adenocarcinoma. *HPB (Oxford)* 2013;15(1):49–60.

Mitchem JB, Hamilton N, Gao F, et al. Long-term results of resection of adenocarcinoma of the body and tail of the pancreas using radical antegrade modular pancreatosplenectomy procedure. *J Am Coll Surg* 2012;214(1):46–52.

Smaglo BG, Pishvaian MJ. Postresection chemotherapy for pancreatic cancer. *Cancer J* 2012;18(6):614–623.

Stokes JB, Nolan NJ, Stelow EB, et al. Preoperative capecitabine and concurrent radiation for borderline resectable pancreatic cancer. *Ann Surg Oncol* 2011;18:619–627.

Van der Gaag NA, Rauws EA, van Eijck CH, et al. Preoperative biliary drainage for cancer of the head of the pancreas. *N Engl J Med* 2010;362:129–137.

Zamboni GA, Kruskal JB, Vollmer CM, et al. Pancreatic adenocarcinoma: value of multidetector CT angiography in preoperative evaluation. *Radiology* 2007;245(3):770–778.

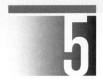

Pancreatic Cysts Including Intraductal Pancreatic Mucinous Neoplasm (IPMN)

Joshua A. Waters and C. Max Schmidt

ETIOLOGY

Few entities within the practice of pancreatic surgery have garnered more interest and discussion in the last decade than pancreatic cystic lesions. Cystic lesions of the pancreas can be divided broadly into inflammatory and neoplastic categories. Inflammatory cysts of the pancreas, primarily comprised of pseudocysts, will be discussed elsewhere in this handbook. The objective of this chapter is to characterize pancreatic cystic lesions that arise of neoplastic etiology.

Cystic lesions of the pancreas, though once believed to be rare, may be present in up to 25% of patients based on autopsy studies and up to 15% of patients based on cross-sectional imaging studies. Although there are numerous ways to subdivide pancreatic cystic lesions, the most clinically relevant way to further categorize cystic pancreatic lesions is based on their malignant potential. Three broad categories commonly used to describe pancreatic cysts lesions are benign, premalignant, or malignant.

Benign

Although benign from an oncologic standpoint, benign cysts may grow to cause local compressive symptoms or other complications of mass effect. They are also important to recognize because they may mimic premalignant or malignant lesions of the pancreas.

Serous cystic neoplasms (SCNs), also known historically as serous cystadenomas (SCA), are the most common benign cystic neoplasm of the pancreas. These lesions are lined by glycogen-rich cuboidal epithelium. These lesions are most common in women (70%) and usually occur sporadically. In some patients, they can be multifocal, but this multifocality is most common in association with the autosomal dominant von Hippel-Lindau syndrome. SCN may be macrocystic (Fig. 5.1) or microcystic with multiple small septations. Microcystic SCN often have a characteristic honeycomb appearance allowing them to be more readily recognized on cross-sectional and endoscopic ultrasound (EUS) imaging. Importantly, however, tightly packed multifocal branch duct intraductal papillary mucinous neoplasm (IPMN) can mimic microcystic SCN, making it sometimes indistinguishable. Although less common, the macrocystic variety of SCN can notoriously mimic mucinous cystic lesions (both mucinous cystic neoplasms [MCN] and IPMN). *Lymphoepithelial cysts* are much rarer than their benign counterparts and more commonly occur in men. These lesions are lined with keratinized squamous epithelium and have a characteristic exophytic appearance on cross-sectional imaging (Fig. 5.2). They have been known to erode into surrounding structures, which often renders these cysts symptomatic, and they may sometimes appear malignant in nature. Finally, *simple pancreatic cysts* are unilocular and invariably benign. These cysts may have some association with polycystic disease of other organs (kidney, liver), but do not demonstrate a gender or age predilection.

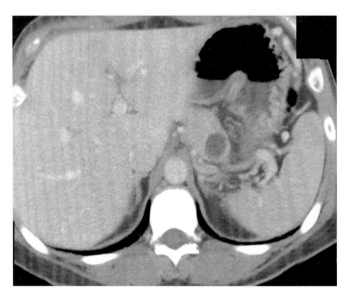

FIGURE 5.1 CT scan demonstrating a macrocystic serous cystic neoplasm (SCN) within the body of the pancreas.

Premalignant and Malignant

The clinical importance of identification of premalignant/malignant pancreatic cysts cannot be overstated. Their identification represents an opportunity to intervene prior to the development of invasive pancreatic malignancy. That said, the majority of premalignant pancreatic cysts will

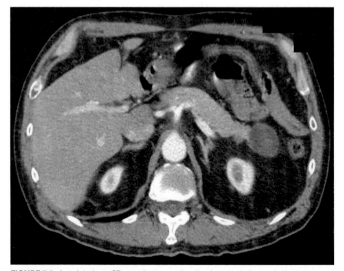

FIGURE 5.2 Arterial-phase CT scan demonstrating the characteristic exophytic appearance of a pancreatic lymphoepithelial cyst.

not transform into pancreatic cancer in a given patient's lifetime, so surveillance is often recommended. Pancreatic cysts in the premalignant/malignant category include mucinous cysts (MCN and IPMN), cystic neuroendocrine tumors, and solid pseudopapillary neoplasm (SPN).

Mucinous cystic neoplasms (MCNs) occur primarily in female patients in the fifth to sixth decade of life. These are mucin-filled lesions without any connection to the pancreatic ductal system. They are unifocal and macrocytic with histology demonstrating ovarian-type stroma. They may demonstrate calcifications. When MCN transform, they become mucinous cystadenocarcinoma, which may represent up to 10% to 20% of MCN. Early in their course, mucinous cystadenocarcinoma may represent a more indolent form of cancer when compared to pancreatic adenocarcinoma. These lesions may stain positive for human chronic gonadotropic or estrogen receptors. *Intraductal papillary mucinous neoplasm* (IPMN) represents a spectrum of lesions with several common features including pancreatic ductal connection, mucin-producing epithelium, and papillary histology (Fig. 5.3). These cystic lesions may be unifocal, multifocal, or multicentric and occur most commonly in older patients (sixth to seventh decade). Anatomically, IPMN may involve the main or branch pancreatic ducts or both. Invasive IPMN is the malignant endpoint in the IPMN oncologic spectrum. Malignant lesions may represent around 25% of all resected IPMN specimens and fall into two distinct histologic subtypes. The tubular subtype imitates the appearance and behavior of pancreatic ductal adenocarcinoma, whereas the colloid subtype is characterized by large pools of extracellular mucin and follows a relatively more indolent course. *Cystic pancreatic neuroendocrine tumors* (pNETs) are rare variants of typical pNET and may occur anywhere on the spectrum from benign to malignant behavior. These lesions occur more commonly in women and are typically sporadic, though they may exist as part of a multiple endocrine neoplasia syndrome. *Solid and cystic pseudopapillary neoplasms* (SPNs) are rare heterogenous solid and cystic lesions that occur almost exclusively in younger

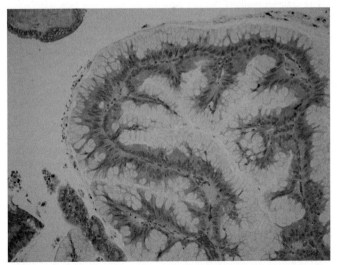

FIGURE 5.3 Hematoxylin and eosin stain histologic operative specimen demonstrating the prominent mucin-laden papillary epithelial architecture consistent with IPMN.

women. These lesions represent a spectrum from premalignant to malignant (about 10%), but generally have an indolent course.

DIAGNOSIS

The explosion in interest surrounding cystic lesions of the pancreas is due in part to their increased recognition through improved resolution and broader use of contemporary cross-sectional imaging. In addition, there is an increased awareness of the importance of pancreatic cyst identification and characterization to promote early detection, prevention, and potential cure of pancreatic cancer. A comprehensive approach to evaluation and characterization of these lesions is critical to determine: first, the type of cystic lesion and, second, the relative oncologic risk of the lesion. Diagnosis relies on clinical, serologic, radiologic, cytopathologic, and cyst fluid (biochemical and DNA) evaluation.

Clinical

Obtaining a detailed clinical history and physical examination plays an important role in the diagnosis and differentiation of pancreatic cystic lesions. As highlighted above, the epidemiologic patterns of these cysts with regard to age and sex may aid in the development of the initial differential diagnosis (e.g., MCN occurring primarily in females). Symptoms attributable to any of these lesions may be subtle. In observational studies, the most commonly reported symptoms include epigastric pain or fullness, early satiety, and sometimes nausea. Evaluation for symptoms related to pancreatic exocrine and endocrine dysfunction is also important. Compression or occlusion of the pancreatic ductal system secondary to a cystic lesion may result in a spectrum of exocrine pancreatic dysfunction and ultimately failure. Symptoms of exocrine insufficiency may initially present as bloating and flatulence, but ultimately may progress to steatorrhea, malabsorption, and weight loss. Pancreatic duct obstruction may also precipitate pancreatitis. Derangements in insulin production may lead to new-onset or worsening diabetes mellitus in some patients. As with most pancreatobiliary malignancies, the presence of jaundice and cachexia is an ominous sign, which may indicate advanced malignancy. Physical examination will typically be somewhat low yield in these lesions. These patients rarely present with reproducible epigastric tenderness on exam, but a palpable abdominal mass may be present in the setting of larger lesions.

Serologic

The use of laboratory studies in the diagnosis and workup for cystic lesions of the pancreas may be of some adjunctive value. Assay for the development of new or worsening diabetes (serum hemoglobin A_{1c}, fasting serum glucose) as well as pancreatic enzymes (serum amylase and lipase) to assess for pancreatitis in the setting of epigastric pain and nausea should be performed. Additionally, serum tumor markers for pancreaticobiliary malignancy, particularly cancer antigen (CA) 19-9, should be checked, as this has been shown to correlate with presence of invasive disease in the setting of IPMN. Elevation of serum alkaline phosphatase has been correlated with malignancy in pancreatic head cysts well prior to elevation of bilirubin. As of yet, there are no other viable serologic biomarkers for diagnosis or determination of malignant potential of pancreatic cystic lesions.

Radiologic

Cross-sectional imaging is the workhorse for the initial diagnosis and characterization of pancreatic cysts. Although debate exists as to their relative value, computed tomography (CT) and magnetic resonance imaging/magnetic resonance cholangiopancreatography (MRI/MRCP) are the two primary noninvasive imaging modalities utilized for characterization these lesions.

Regardless of the modality utilized, certain radiologic characteristics of pancreatic cystic lesions may suggest a particular etiology. Two elements, with rare exception, that are predictive of IPMN are ductal connection and multifocality. These two features are extremely rare in other cystic lesions. A central stellate scar is a classic finding for SCN, and mural calcifications may often be present in (but are not pathognomonic of) MCN (Fig. 5.4). Finally, in the setting of malignant degeneration, cystic lesions of the pancreas on cross-sectional imaging may demonstrate features of invasion into extrapancreatic organs, vascular structures, or the biliary tree. Peritoneal and hematogenous metastases may also be detected in this setting.

Dual-phase intravenous contrast-enhanced *computed tomography* (CT) scan is the mainstay for initial diagnosis and characterization of pancreatic cysts. Many pancreatic cysts (up to 30%) will actually be identified as incidentally detected lesions on CT scan performed for other indications. Current high-resolution CT scan technology allows for very accurate characterization of these lesions. Most cystic lesions will appear hypodense with respect to the surrounding pancreatic parenchyma on CT. It is critical to obtain thin (1 mm) cuts through the pancreas as smaller lesions are easily overlooked with less detailed imaging.

Magnetic resonance cholangiopancreatography (MRCP) is another noninvasive imaging modality that has gained wide acceptance as important adjunct in characterizing pancreatic cysts. The ability to obtain a detailed pancreatic ductogram (Fig. 5.5) may provide the clinician with information regarding ductal connection (MRI is two to three times more sensitive than CT scan alone) and may be more accurate in delineating subtle main pancreatic duct (MPD) involvement. Some authors suggest that MRCP is superior in defining IPMN type and extent and routinely employ this technique in preoperative planning and surveillance strategies.

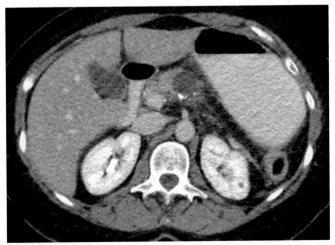

FIGURE 5.4 MCN of the pancreas with the associated mural calcification seen on CT.

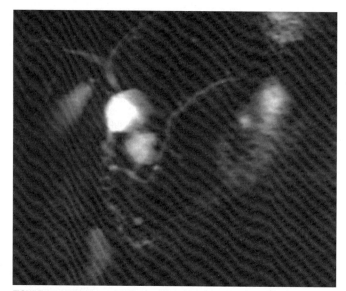

FIGURE 5.5 MRCP illustrating the grapelike morphology of a branch-type IPMN with an obvious ductal connection.

Positron emission tomography (PET) scan has been examined as an adjunctive imaging study to determine the presence of [18]fludeoxyglucose (FDG) avid foci within IPMN particularly as a marker for invasive malignancy. Currently, PET scanning is used to help with clinical decision making in cases where there is a high index of suspicion for malignancy concomitant with a moderate to high risk of surgical intervention. The sensitivity of PET scan for high-grade dysplastic lesions and small foci of invasive cancer is limited, resulting in a significant false-negative rate.

Although noninvasive imaging techniques are the frontline in the diagnosis of pancreatic cystic lesions, *endoscopic ultrasound* (EUS) has become very important in the detailed evaluation for many pancreatic cysts. Although EUS is highly operator dependent, this technique allows for detailed characterization of cyst size, number, relationship with vascular and ductal structures, and presence of an associated mass or mural nodule. The presence of mural nodule or associated mass (Fig. 5.6) in the setting of IPMN in particular has been reproducibly demonstrated as a strong predictor of underlying malignancy, and EUS is the most accurate method of identifying and characterizing these features. Additionally, this modality provides the surgeon or gastroenterologist with the ability to perform fine needle or core biopsy with assay of cyst wall or fluid. Limitations of EUS include difficulty in fully assessing the pancreatic uncinate process, the invasive nature of the test, and the aforementioned operator dependence. In addition, this modality is not generally available outside of the larger centers.

Endoscopic retrograde cholangiopancreatography (ERCP) was at one time commonly used in the diagnosis of IPMN. It has very little role in the workup of other cystic pancreatic lesions, as it can only evaluate cysts that are contiguous with the MPD. Interestingly, ERCP was noted to have a false-negative rate in the evaluation of IPMN, particularly in branch-type

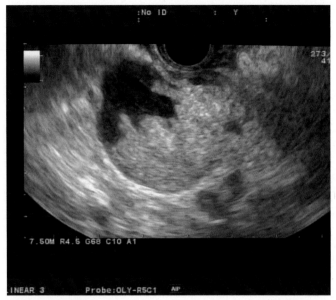

FIGURE 5.6 EUS illustrating mural nodularity within a branch-type IPMN. This feature alone is highly suggestive of malignancy.

lesions, where mucin plugging may preclude a full and accurate ductogram. Additionally, there is limited ability to sample non–main duct–involved IPMN. For these reasons, ERCP has been largely supplanted by EUS and cross-sectional imaging techniques, especially MRI/MRCP.

Cytopathologic

Cytopathology, typically derived from fine needle aspiration (FNA) obtained via EUS guidance, has very high specificity (95% to 100%) but limited sensitivity (50% to 60%) for underlying malignancy in the setting of mucinous cystic lesions (MCN and IPMN). Thus, a cytopathologic finding of high-grade atypia is almost always indicative of an underlying malignant lesion. Cytopathology is highly accurate (nearly 100%) in the characterization of cystic pNET and nearly as accurate for identifying SPN. Limitations of EUS–FNA cytopathology include difficulty in accessing the pancreatic uncinate and the need for transgastric passage of the biopsy needle, which may result in false-positive assays for mucin.

Cyst Fluid Analysis

One of the best ways to differentiate pancreatic cysts is via cyst fluid analysis. The most useful biochemical marker is carcinoembryonic antigen (CEA). A high CEA level at a threshold of greater than 192 ng/mL is 80% accurate in differentiating mucinous (IPMN, MCN) from nonmucinous (SCN) lesions. The higher the CEA, the more certain the lesion is to be mucinous. This is important, as nonmucinous lesions less commonly represent malignant risk. Absolute CEA level is not an accurate indicator of malignancy. Cyst epithelial DNA shed into the cyst fluid allows for genetic characterization of these lesions. A commercial test (PathFinder TG) assesses the quantity and quality of DNA within the specimen as well as the presence

T A B L E 5.1	DNA Markers in Cyst Fluid and/or Cyst Epithelium According to Pancreatic Cyst Type				
Type	KRAS	GNAS	RNF43	CTNNB1	VHL
IPMN	+	+	+		
MCN	+		+		
SPN				+	
SCN					+

KRAS, Kirsten rat sarcoma oncogene; GNAS, guanine nucleotide–binding protein alpha-stimulating, complex locus; RNF43, ring finger protein 43; CTNNB1, beta-catenin gene; VHL, von Hippel-Lindau.

and copy number of Kirsten rat sarcoma viral oncogene homolog (Kras) mutations, guanine nucleotide protein GSα (GNAS) mutations, and microsatellite instability to predict loss of heterozygosity at specific loci (e.g., 17q). This test is strongly correlated with malignancy in mucinous cystic lesions, particularly in recent multi-institutional molecular registry studies. Future pancreatic cyst characterization in cases undiagnosed by cytopathology will likely be largely dictated by cyst fluid analysis. Table 5.1 indicates a number of DNA and biochemical markers, respectively, at various stages of commercial development in the characterization of pancreatic cysts. Importantly, CA19-9 and amylase have not been found to be accurate indicators of malignancy or ductal connectivity.

MANAGEMENT

Nearly all decisions regarding the management of pancreatic cysts hinge on either the presence of symptoms or the risk of existing or future progression to malignancy. This highlights the critical role of clinical history, preoperative imaging, and cytopathologic analysis in the evaluation and management of these lesions. Although algorithms for preoperative evaluation and operative decision making exist, the approach to each patient should be individualized based on symptoms, anticipated malignant potential, extent of disease, and patient fitness.

Operative Indications and Technical Tips

The indications for resection of cystic pancreatic lesions are typically approached based on two primary considerations, symptoms and oncologic risk. When dealing with lesions on the low end of the malignant risk spectrum (e.g., SCN), the decision to embark on pancreatic resection is driven by the goal to alleviate present and future symptoms. For example, some authorities have suggested that SCN should be considered for resection when they reach a diameter of 4 cm or greater, as these lesions may have a greater propensity for future growth and worsening symptoms. This preemptive approach is not endorsed by all pancreatic surgeons, however; so patients should be carefully considered for operative versus expectant management.

A much more clear set of indications are apparent in those patients with evidence of invasive malignancy. These patients should be approached with resection criteria similar to those utilized in pancreatic ductal adenocarcinoma. Importantly, invasive pancreatic cystic lesions have demonstrated a lower rate of vascular and lymphatic invasion than "garden variety" pancreatic cancer, so are in general more amenable to resection.

The most controversial (and most studied) set of indications regarding resection for cystic pancreatic lesions are for IPMN. Numerous retrospective series have demonstrated MPD involvement as an independent predictor of malignancy in IPMN (up to 60% at the time of resection). For this reason, all fit patients with main duct involvement should be considered for pancreatic resection. Typically, the degree of oncologic risk in main duct IPMN is defined based on the maximal segmental cystic dilation of the MPD. An MPD ≥ 5 mm is worrisome, and if ≥ 10 mm, it is considered a high-risk stigmata of malignancy according to the international consensus guidelines (2012). The decision to resect cystic lesions not involving the main duct is more complex. In surgical series, branch duct IPMN malignant risk has been reported to occur in 5% to 20% of (mostly symptomatic) patients. The incidence of malignancy in MCN is similar to that in IPMN. The presence of high-risk stigmata (i.e., mural nodularity), concerning cytopathology or multiple mutations on molecular profiling, should strengthen the case for resection. The relationship between cyst size and malignancy has been a debated topic in the literature, with most current series demonstrating no correlation, though some demonstrate positive relationship. Current international consensus guidelines no longer dictate a size cutoff recommendation for operative resection.

Preoperative Considerations
When considering pancreatic resection in the management of cystic neoplasms of the pancreas, the primary goal is to perform segmental pancreatic resection to encompass all evident disease. In dealing with the unifocal cystic lesions of the pancreas, this approach is usually straightforward. For lesions of the pancreatic head and uncinate process, pancreaticoduodenectomy is the most common approach, whereas for lesions of the body/tail, distal (left-sided) pancreatectomy is typically appropriate. In distal pancreatectomy, splenic preservation is preferred unless there is a significant chance invasive disease is present or the lesion is intimately associated with the splenic hilum or vessels. Patients with larger (> 2.5 cm) cystic pNET may also benefit from splenectomy for optimal lymph node retrieval. Some authors have advocated enucleation in select cases and demonstrated reduced operative morbidity and potential mortality. Enucleation should only be considered if the preoperative likelihood of invasive malignancy is expected to be low and the lesion is not in close proximity to or involving the MPD. Tail lesions as they approach the spleen may be less optimal for enucleation. This is in part due to minimal parenchyma spared with enucleation and an elevated chance for MPD injury due to the small size of the MPD and the difficulty of intraoperative ultrasound to accurately discriminate relationship of the cyst to the MPD. Multifocal cystic lesions, that is, IPMN, may require substantially more complex preoperative planning. It is not uncommon to have radiologic evidence of branch duct IPMN in multiple anatomic distributions, which would not be encompassed by a single segmental pancreatic resection. The use of total pancreatectomy carries an unbalanced and generally unacceptable risk of morbidity and mortality in the setting of often premalignant and indolent disease. Thus, the approach (except in unusual cases) is to perform segmental resection to include the most oncologically concerning lesion(s) (i.e., mural nodularity, high-grade atypia, main duct involvement), with subsequent surveillance of the residual gland/cysts.

Intraoperative Considerations
Several important technical points should be considered when conducting pancreatic resection for cystic lesions of the pancreas. Although cross-sectional imaging may provide an excellent roadmap to guide the extent of pancreatic resection, these lesions may be difficult to identify intraoperatively. Therefore, liberal use of intraoperative ultrasound to identify the cyst or cysts should be considered, particularly when planning enucleation,

as this may aid in defining the anatomic relationship with the MPD. Additionally, when undertaking resection for IPMN, particularly main duct involved, frozen section should be obtained to ensure that no high-grade dysplasia or invasive IPMN is present at the resection margin. Additional margins should be taken when feasible in the setting of high-grade dysplasia or frank invasion. If the main duct margin is positive for low- to moderate-grade dysplasia but the gross lesion appears to be removed, further resection is dictated based upon preoperative discussions of future symptom management, malignant risk, patient preoperative pancreatic functional reserve, and patient fitness.

Postoperative Management and Complications

The postoperative management of a patient undergoing segmental pancreatic resection for any cystic lesion of the pancreas is largely similar to a patient undergoing pancreatectomy for other indications. Patients with pancreatic cystic lesions typically have softer pancreatic parenchyma (unless they have a history of significant pancreatitis). The MPD diameter is also typically small, as there is rarely an obstructing mass. Given these factors, the rate of pancreatic fistula has been reported to be elevated when compared to fistula rates after resection for other indications. Additionally, although enucleation may represent a less morbid approach to certain cystic lesions, some authors have suggested an elevated risk of pancreatic fistula development compared to segmental resection. Early recognition and percutaneous drainage (if necessary) of pancreatic fistulas not controlled by operatively placed drains (if present) is imperative to reduce major complication such as systemic inflammatory response or sepsis, vascular pseudoaneurysm, breakdown of enteric or biliary reconstruction, and wound infection/dehiscence.

OUTCOMES AND FOLLOW-UP

Cystic neoplasms of the pancreas represent a unique opportunity for the clinician to intervene prior to the development of pancreatic malignancy. When resected in the premalignant or in situ setting, the disease-specific survival for IPMN or MCN may approach 95% to 100% at 5 years. Even in the setting of invasive IPMN, the overall survival and stage-matched survival is favorable when compared to patients undergoing resection for typical ductal adenocarcinoma.

Patients undergoing resection for cystic lesions should undergo routine postoperative follow-up with clinical exam and cross-sectional imaging as appropriate. For invasive cystic lesions, this will likely entail every a 6-month exam and imaging surveillance unless dictated differently by medical oncology treatment or trial protocol. For nonmalignant pNET and SPN, this may entail interval exam and surveillance imaging for a period of at least 5 years. For SCN or noninvasive MCN, as long as margins were clear, surveillance imaging is not required. On the other hand, IPMN requires a more involved postoperative surveillance strategy. As mentioned previously, because of its multicentric/multifocal nature, operative management of IPMN often requires segmental resection of the most concerning lesion, thereby leaving low-risk disease in the remnant gland. The risk profile of the residual disease has been demonstrated to be related to the histologic grade of the resected disease. Those patients with low- to moderate-grade IPMN on initial resection have an exceedingly small risk of progression to malignancy in the remnant gland, whereas patients with high-grade disease in the resected specimen (even with negative margins) are at higher risk of cancer progression in the remnant gland and should be considered for a more intensive surveillance approach. Even patients without evidence of residual disease in the remnant gland are at risk of de novo development of IPMN or progression of disease that was radiologically occult at the time of resection. For these reasons, surveillance with cross-sectional imaging should be undertaken at routine intervals. Finally, numerous reports have described an elevated risk of concomitant gastrointestinal malignancy in patients with MCN or IPMN of the pancreas. These patients should be vigilant with the American Cancer Society recommendations about screening for prostate, colon, breast, and lung cancer. The clinician should maintain a high index of suspicion for nonpancreatic neoplasia in these patients.

CONCLUSIONS

Cystic neoplasms of the pancreas are an increasingly recognized entity with important clinical implications. The accurate diagnosis and characterization of these lesions with clinical history, cross-sectional imaging (CT, MRCP, EUS), as well as cytopathologic sampling are critical in oncologic risk stratification and subsequent clinical decision making. The subset of cysts with little to no malignant potential should only be considered for resection in the setting of substantial size, mass effect, or refractory symptoms. Cysts with malignant features or high malignant potential should be considered for operative resection in fit patients. Primary surveillance strategies may be acceptable for low-risk lesions, as pancreatic resection carries substantial morbidity. Surveillance of the pancreatic remnant after resection is dictated based on cyst diagnosis and dysplastic grade. In the setting of IPMN, surveillance should be conducted indefinitely as these lesions are commonly multicentric and may recur or develop de novo in the remnant gland.

Suggested Readings

Cauley CE, Waters JA, Dumas RP. Outcomes of primary surveillance for intraductal papillary mucinous neoplasm. *J Gastrointest Surg* 2012;16(2):258–267; discussion 266.

D'Angelica M, Brennan MF, Suriawinata AA, et al. Intraductal papillary mucinous neoplasms of the pancreas: an analysis of clinicopathologic features and outcome. *Ann Surg* 2004;239:400.

Katabi N, Klimstra DS. Intraductal papillary mucinous neoplasms of the pancreas: clinical and pathologic features and diagnostic approach. *J Clin Pathol* 2008;61;1303–1313.

Schmidt CM, White PB, Waters JA, et al. Intraductal papillary mucinous neoplasms: predictors of malignant and invasive pathology. *Ann Surg* 2007;246(4):644–654.

Sohn TA, Yeo CJ, Cameron JL, et al. Intraductal papillary mucinous neoplasms of the pancreas: an updated experience. *Ann Surg* 2004;239:788–797.

Tanaka M, Fernández-del Castillo C, Adsay V, et al. International Consensus Guidelines 2012 for the Management of IPMN and MCN of the Pancreas. *Pancreatology* 2012;12(3):183–197.

Wargo JA, Fernandez-del-Castillo C, Warshaw AL. Management of pancreatic serous cystadenomas. *Adv Surg* 2009;43:23–34.

Waters JA, Schmidt CM. Intraductal papillary mucinous neoplasm—when to resect? *Adv Surg* 2008;42:87–108.

6 Pancreatic Neuroendocrine Neoplasms

Rebecca A. Busch and Clifford S. Cho

INTRODUCTION

Pancreatic neuroendocrine neoplasms are relatively rare. The incidence of clinically detected cases is approximately 4 cases per million people per year in the United States. Like the more common exocrine pancreatic adenocarcinoma, they are capable of regional and distant metastatic dissemination. But, they can also be relatively indolent. Indeed, autopsy studies suggest that the actual incidence of pancreatic neuroendocrine neoplasms may be as high as 1.5%. This combination of relative rarity and indolence has challenged the ability of investigators to definitively characterize the natural history and optimal treatment of this disease. However, recent studies to be outlined in this chapter have yielded important new insights for the hepato-pancreatico-biliary surgeon.

ETIOLOGY

Initially believed to arise from the endocrine islets of Langerhans, recent studies suggest that these neoplasms originate from pluripotent cells within pancreatic ductules. As a result, previous descriptors like "islet cell tumors" and "islet cell carcinomas" have been dropped in favor of "pancreatic neuroendocrine neoplasms." Pancreatic neuroendocrine neoplasms have been categorized into "functioning" variants (those that overproduce pancreatic endocrine hormones capable of inducing specific clinical signs and symptoms) and "nonfunctioning" variants (those that exhibit no clear pattern of symptomatic hormonal overproduction).

Pancreatic neuroendocrine neoplasms can occur sporadically or as a component of inherited genetic syndromes. Genetic and epigenetic alterations of the p16/MTS1 tumor suppressor gene have been implicated in the development of sporadic pancreatic neuroendocrine neoplasms. Whereas loss of heterozygosity at chromosome 11q appears to be associated with functional lesions, loss of heterozygosity at chromosome 6q has been associated with nonfunctional neoplasms. The inherited genetic syndrome most commonly associated with pancreatic neuroendocrine neoplasms is multiple neuroendocrine neoplasia type 1 (MEN 1), an autosomal dominant trait associated with mutations of the presumed tumor suppressor gene menin. In addition, von Hippel-Lindau disease and neurofibromatosis type 1 are also associated with pancreatic neuroendocrine neoplasms.

DIAGNOSIS

Clinical Presentation

Historically, it was believed that functioning variants comprised the majority of pancreatic neuroendocrine neoplasms; however, as more diagnoses are being made by imaging and not by symptoms, most contemporary series suggest that nonfunctioning neoplasms comprise the large majority. Nevertheless, the often bizarre and characteristic behavior of functional neoplasms warrants discussion of their various subtypes (Table 6.1).

	TABLE 6.1 Summary of Functioning Pancreatic Neuroendocrine Neoplasms

Neoplasm	Common Clinical Characteristics	Secretory Product	Symptoms	Diagnostic Criteria
Insulinoma	Small (< 2 cm) 90% solitary Evenly distributed throughout pancreas 90% benign Seen in 5%–8% of MEN1	Insulin (promotes hypoglycemia)	Whipple triad: 1. Hypoglycemic symptoms during monitored fast 2. Blood glucose <50 mg/dL with symptoms 3. Symptom relief after administration of glucose	During 72-hour fast: Glucose <50 mg/dL Insulin >5 µ/mL Insulin: glucose ratio >0.4 Elevated C-peptide, proinsulin
Gastrinoma	Sporadic form: solitary MEN1: multifocal 90% within gastrinoma triangle 50% malignant 30% present with metastases 15%–35% associated with MEN1	Gastrin (promotes gastric acid production)	Zollinger-Ellison syndrome: 90% gastroduodenal ulcerations 75% epigastric pain 75% diarrhea	Gastrin >10× upper limit normal Gastrin increase >200 pg/mL after secretin stimulation
Glucagonoma	Large Solitary Body/tail of the pancreas 75% malignant	Glucagon (promotes hyperglycemia, amino acid metabolism)	"4 Ds": Diabetes Dermatitis (necrolytic migratory erythema) Deep venous thrombosis Depression	Fasting glucagon >1,000 pg/mL Skin biopsy of necrolytic migratory erythema

(Continued)

TABLE 6.1 Summary of Functioning Pancreatic Neuroendocrine Neoplasms (*Continued*)

Neoplasm	Common Clinical Characteristics	Secretory Product	Symptoms	Diagnostic Criteria
VIPoma	Large Solitary Body/tail of the pancreas Malignant 50% present with metastases	Vasoactive intestinal polypeptide (VIP) (promotes intestinal secretion and motility and inhibits intestinal absorption)	Verner-Morrison/WDHA syndrome: Watery diarrhea Hypokalemia Achlorhydria/hypochlorhydria	Fasting VIP >500 pg/mL
Somatostatinoma	Large Solitary Head of the pancreas Malignant Commonly present with metastases Associated with von Recklinghausen disease (NF type 1)	Somatostatin (inhibits pancreatic endocrine and exocrine secretion and gallbladder contractility)	Diabetes Malabsorption Cholelithiasis	Fasting somatostatin >100 pg/mL

Insulinomas are the most common type of functional pancreatic neuroendocrine neoplasm. They tend to be small (<2 cm), solitary, benign lesions that can arise anywhere within the pancreas and can be associated with MEN1 (although less commonly than gastrinomas). The diagnosis of insulinoma can be made by the classic *Whipple triad* of clinical findings: (1) symptoms of hypoglycemia during monitored fasting or exercise; (2) blood glucose levels of less than 50 mg/dL during these symptomatic episodes; and (3) relief of these symptoms following administration of glucose. To detect the Whipple triad, patients with suspected insulinoma are closely monitored during a 72-hour inpatient fast. Following measurement of baseline serum glucose and insulin levels, blood glucose levels are measured every 2 hours, and insulin levels are measured at the onset of hypoglycemic symptoms or when blood glucose levels become lower than 50 mg/dL. Nearly all patients with insulinoma will have inappropriately elevated plasma insulin levels (>5 μU/mL) in the setting of hypoglycemia. Elevated levels of C peptide and proinsulin are also typically present and help to differentiate insulinoma from factitious hypoglycemia; the onset of symptoms during fasting helps to differentiate insulinoma from postprandial reactive hypoglycemia.

Gastrinomas are the second most common type of functional pancreatic neuroendocrine neoplasm. Unlike insulinomas, 90% of gastrinomas are found within the *gastrinoma triangle*: an anatomical region defined by the cystic and common bile ducts superiorly, the second and third portions of the duodenum inferiorly, and the pancreatic neck and body medially (Fig. 6.1). Two-thirds of gastrinomas are located within the pancreas, and a third may be found within the duodenum. In sporadic, noninherited forms of gastrinoma, tumors tend to be solitary. However, gastrinomas arising in the context of MEN1 are multifocal and highly prone to recurrence. Because of the ability of gastrin to induce gastric acid secretion, gastrinomas typically present with the classic and often refractory signs and symptoms of *Zollinger-Ellison syndrome*, consisting of gastroduodenal ulcerations (90%), epigastric pain (75%), diarrhea associated with the large-volume gastric acid secretion (75%), and malabsorption leading to weight loss. The incidence of gastrinoma among patients presenting with peptic ulcer disease has been estimated to be approximately 1%, and this diagnosis should be entertained in patients presenting with advanced or refractory peptic ulcer disease. Unlike insulinomas, gastrinomas are often malignant, with about 50% of patients presenting with evidence of hepatic metastases.

Patients with suspected gastrinoma should undergo serum gastrin measurement. The upper limit of normal gastrin level is approximately 100 pg/mL; serum gastrin levels ten times greater than the upper limit of normal in the presence of gastric pH less than 5.0 are diagnostic of gastrinoma. However, patients with gastrinoma often present with more subtle degrees of hypergastrinemia. The differential diagnosis for moderate hypergastrinemia includes achlorhydria (as can occur with proton pump inhibitor therapy), retained antrum following partial gastrectomy, gastric outlet obstruction, and renal insufficiency. The secretin stimulation test is a means of increasing the sensitivity of detecting gastrinoma. Following intravenous administration of 2 μg/kg secretin, a paradoxical rise in serum gastrin by greater than 200 pg/mL is considered positive for gastrinoma. Similarly, a paradoxical rise in serum gastrin of greater than 50% following infusion of calcium gluconate is also indicative of gastrinoma.

Unlike insulinomas and gastrinomas, *glucagonomas* are characteristically larger lesions that tend to be localized along the body and tail of the pancreas. Like gastrinomas, they exhibit a proclivity for aggressive behavior,

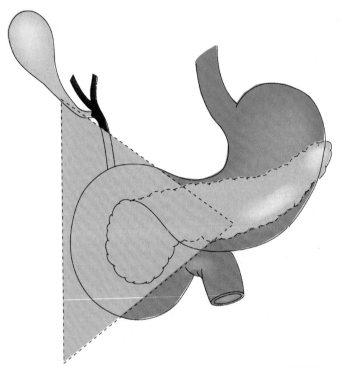

FIGURE 6.1 Most gastrinomas are found within the gastrinoma triangle. (From: Mulholland MW, Lillemoe KD, Doherty GM, et al. *Greenfield's surgery: scientific principles & practice*, 5th ed. Philadelphia, PA: Lippincott Williams & Wilkins, 2011.)

with approximately 50% of cases harboring evidence of distant metastatic disease. The ability of glucagon to promote gluconeogenesis and amino acid oxidation explains the characteristic clinical findings of diabetes (resulting from hyperglycemia) and dermatitis (resulting from amino acid deficiency). Skin manifestations of dermatitis include necrolytic migratory erythema, characterized by painful blistering plaques along the face, abdomen, lower extremities, and mucous membranes. Interestingly, up to a third of patients with glucagonoma develop deep venous thrombosis, warranting consideration of anticoagulation therapy.

Serum glucagon levels greater than 1,000 pg/mL can be diagnostic for glucagonoma. However, as with gastrinoma, more subtle elevations can be seen in patients with glucagonoma. Unlike gastrinoma, provocative testing is not available to help distinguish glucagonoma from potentially confounding conditions that can induce hyperglucagonemia such as pancreatitis, sepsis, Cushing syndrome, fasting, renal insufficiency, and hepatic failure.

Like glucagonomas, *VIPomas* often present as large, solitary lesions localized to the pancreatic body and tail and often present with evidence of metastatic disease. Rare extrapancreatic VIPomas have been observed in the colon, bronchus, liver, adrenal glands, and para-aortic ganglia. Vasoactive intestinal polypeptide (VIP) promotes intestinal secretion and motility while inhibiting intestinal absorption of water and electrolytes. As a result, the classic *Verner-Morrison syndrome* of VIPomas is also referred to by the acronymic *WDHA syndrome* (consisting of massive watery diarrhea, hypokalemia, and achlorhydria). In patients presenting with profuse secretory diarrhea, the diagnosis of VIPoma can be made by measuring elevated fasting serum VIP levels (typically > 500 pg/mL).

In contrast to glucagonomas and VIPomas, the majority of *somatostatinomas* are found within the pancreatic head. Like gastrinomas and VIPomas, somatostatinomas can present outside of the pancreas (most commonly in the duodenum and ampulla). Duodenal somatostatinomas are a common manifestation of von Recklinghausen disease (neurofibromatosis type 1). Pancreatic somatostatinomas tend to present as larger tumors with metastatic disease. Somatostatin inhibits secretion of pancreatic insulin and exocrine enzymes and inhibits gallbladder contractility; as a result, somatostatinomas often present with symptoms of diabetes, malabsorption, and cholelithiasis. The diagnosis of somatostatinoma among patients presenting with these symptoms is supported by elevated serum levels of somatostatin greater than 100 pg/mL.

Nonfunctioning pancreatic neuroendocrine neoplasms tend to present evenly throughout all regions of the pancreas. Taken as a whole, they were previously characterized as generally rarer, larger, and more aggressive than functioning pancreatic neuroendocrine neoplasms. However, these characterizations may have been historical artifacts of diagnosis. As more and more pancreatic neuroendocrine neoplasms are being diagnosed incidentally with imaging evaluations rather than by symptoms referable to hormonal production or tumor mass, the prevalence of small, asymptomatic, nonfunctioning pancreatic neuroendocrine neoplasms appears to be increasing. Thus, the extent to which functioning and nonfunctioning pancreatic neuroendocrine neoplasms differ in terms of inherent tumor biology and behavior is unclear. Nonfunctioning lesions can occasionally secrete measurable levels of proteins that do not induce significant symptomatology, but often do not express any known hormones. As a result, elevated serum levels of proteins like pancreatic polypeptide, neuron-specific enolase, and neurotensin can have high specificity but very poor sensitivity in the diagnosis of nonfunctioning pancreatic neuroendocrine neoplasms.

Imaging and Localizing Studies

Diagnostic imaging for pancreatic neuroendocrine neoplasms takes advantage of some of their unique biologic characteristics. The majority of pancreatic neuroendocrine neoplasms are markedly well vascularized. As a result, contrast-enhanced imaging by computed tomography (CT) or magnetic resonance imaging (MRI) should employ both early arterial and delayed portal-phase imaging sequences, as they tend to appear very bright during early arterial-phase administration of contrast (Fig. 6.2) or on portal-phase imaging (Fig. 6.3). Radiographic diagnosis can be further enhanced with MRI, as pancreatic neuroendocrine neoplasms tend to exhibit low signal intensity on T1-weighted imaging and high signal intensity on T2-weighted imaging (Fig. 6.4). These imaging characteristics can also be used in the detection of extrapancreatic metastases.

Another relevant biologic characteristic of pancreatic neuroendocrine neoplasms is that they tend to grow as rounded, well-circumscribed lesions. The ability of endoscopic ultrasonography (EUS) to clearly recognize these morphologic characteristics (Fig. 6.5) may explain its heightened sensitivity in the detection of smaller lesions as compared with cross-sectional CT and MRI. Intraoperative ultrasonography with direct probe application on

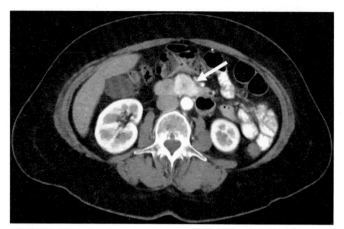

FIGURE 6.2 CT imaging of neuroendocrine neoplasm arising from the uncinate process demonstrates brisk uptake of contrast on early arterial-phase imaging (*white arrow*).

the surface of the pancreas or duodenum can be especially useful in the detection of occult and multifocal lesions (as can be seen with insulinomas or with duodenal or pancreatic gastrinomas arising in a setting of MEN1).

Somatostatin receptor scintigraphy (octreotide scanning) takes advantage of the fact that many pancreatic neuroendocrine neoplasms

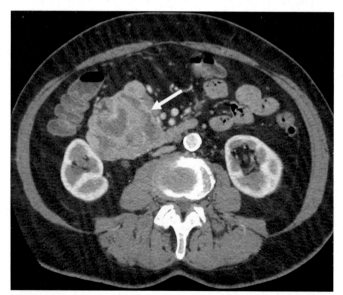

FIGURE 6.3 CT imaging of neuroendocrine neoplasm arising from the pancreatic head demonstrates contrast enhancement on portal-phase imaging with areas of central necrosis (*white arrow*).

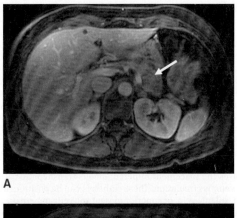

A

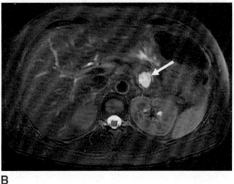

B

FIGURE 6.4 A. MRI imaging of neuroendocrine neoplasm arising from the pancreatic body demonstrates a rounded lesion of low signal intensity on T1-weighted sequences (*white arrow*). **B.** MRI imaging of the same neuroendocrine neoplasm arising from the pancreatic body demonstrates high signal intensity on T2-weighted sequences (*white arrow*).

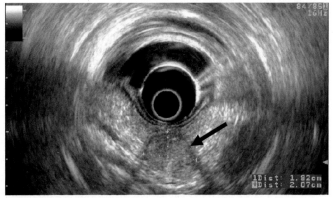

FIGURE 6.5 EUS imaging of the neuroendocrine neoplasm arising from the pancreatic tail demonstrates a rounded and well-circumscribed lesion (*black arrow*).

overexpress somatostatin receptor proteins. Octreotide is a somatostatin analogue (and somatostatin receptor ligand) that can be radiolabeled with ^{111}In and administered intravenously. Scintigraphic localization of radiolabeled octreotide uptake, especially when used in conjunction with single-photon emission computed tomography, can identify both primary pancreatic neuroendocrine neoplasms and foci of metastatic disease with high sensitivity. Recent analyses, however, suggest that they rarely yield additional information beyond that which can be obtained with traditional cross-sectional imaging studies alone. Of note, insulinomas typically do not overexpress somatostatin receptor and are thus poorly visualized with somatostatin receptor scintigraphy.

Venous sampling is a means of tumor localization that takes advantage of pancreatic neuroendocrine neoplasm's ability to secrete hormones into the portal venous circulation. Now largely of historic interest, venous sampling involves the placement of percutaneous transhepatic catheters into the portal venous circulation. These catheters can be positioned within the portal vein, splenic vein, or superior mesenteric vein and are used to collect venous blood samples for insulin or gastrin measurement. Identifying the venous basin in which hormone levels are elevated may facilitate the localization of radiographically occult insulinomas and gastrinomas. The utility of this technique is enhanced with the addition of *selective arterial stimulation*. In this approach, a percutaneous transarterial catheter is positioned within the common hepatic artery, splenic artery, or gastroduodenal artery and used for selective infusion of either secretin or calcium. The ability of these agents to stimulate hormonal production can then be used to localize tumors to various locations (e.g., pancreatic tail or body vs. pancreatic head or neck, hepatic metastases) based on their arterial supply.

MANAGEMENT

Until recently, safe and effective chemotherapeutic agents were not available for the treatment of pancreatic neuroendocrine neoplasms. As a result, surgical resection has been the mainstay of therapy for this disease. Complete surgical resection remains the only potentially curative intervention for pancreatic neuroendocrine neoplasms. However, because the course of this disease can be gradual and indolent, operative intervention has also been employed in the attempt to palliate symptoms and possibly prolong survival for patients with metastatic disease.

Localized Disease

Surgical resection is the standard treatment intervention for patients with localized and resectable pancreatic neuroendocrine neoplasm. The specific type of resection is tailored to the location and distribution of disease and to the patient's ability to tolerate a major pancreatic resection. The standard operative approach for resection of tumors within the pancreatic head or uncinate process is pancreaticoduodenectomy, whereas left or distal pancreatectomy is reserved for tumors within the pancreatic body or tail. Total pancreatectomy is typically reserved for large or multifocal tumors involving the pancreatic head, neck, and body. Central pancreatectomy has been advocated as a means of preserving functional pancreatic parenchyma for patients with tumors localized to the pancreatic neck or body; however, any potential advantage in endocrine function must be counterbalanced by the risk of fistula at the site of the pancreaticojejunostomy or pancreaticogastrostomy that must be constructed to drain the pancreatic tail remnant. For small tumors in locations not involving the main pancreatic duct, enucleation has been advocated as an alternative and potentially less invasive means of tumor extirpation. In this technique, dissection proceeds along the peritumoral plane, and only the tumor is removed. Because of the limited extent of resection (as compared with partial or total pancreatectomy), enucleation carries a higher risk of positive resection margins and does not permit pathologic assessment of peripancreatic lymph nodes. Therefore, although enucleation has been shown to be associated with lower operative morbidity, this potential advantage must be counterbalanced by the risk of oncologically incomplete tumor clearance. Surgical margins and nodal metastases have been shown to be prognostically significant variables for patients with resected pancreatic neuroendocrine neoplasms; therefore, enucleation is typically reserved for patients with tumors that are very likely to be benign (e.g., insulinomas) or for patients who may not tolerate radical resection. In this context, retrospective studies have not consistently identified measurable survival differences between patients treated with enucleation versus radical resection.

Gastrinoma Arising in a Setting of MEN1

One circumstance that deserves special attention is that of gastrinoma arising in the setting of MEN1. These patients harbor a genetic predisposition toward the development of multifocal gastrinoma, as manifested by their very high rates of local and distant disease recurrence following surgical intervention. In fact, the goal of surgical intervention in these patients is often directed more at control of refractory peptic ulcer disease–related symptoms than at cure. Indeed, whether and how to undertake operative therapy for patients with gastrinoma and MEN1 remains an area of controversy and debate. Preoperatively, every effort is expended to define the extent of disease within the pancreas and peripancreatic tissues using cross-sectional CT and/or MRI modalities as well as EUS, as utilization of multiple techniques maximizes the sensitivity of multifocal tumor detection. However, because of finite limits in the sensitivity of even these preoperative maneuvers, additional maneuvers are undertaken at the time of operative exploration in order to maximally define the extent of disease. In addition to performing intraoperative US of the pancreas and peripancreatic tissues, many surgeons advocate performing a duodenotomy to more fully evaluate for small tumors possibly residing within the duodenal wall. Digital palpation and transillumination of the entire duodenal wall have been suggested as effective adjuncts to enhance the detection of small tumor foci. Operative resection should then be tailored toward the distribution of disease that is present, and often necessitates a distal pancreatectomy with resection of any duodenal wall tumors that may be present. On occasion, a total pancreatectomy may be necessary. Because of the high likelihood of nodal metastases, a regional peripancreatic lymphadenectomy should also be undertaken.

Metastatic Disease

Like other gastroenteropancreatic malignancies, neuroendocrine neoplasms have a tendency to metastasize to the liver. Treatment directed at hepatic neuroendocrine metastases has been advocated as a means of mitigating tumor burden–mediated symptoms and, possibly, as a way to prolong survival.

In well-selected cases, surgical resection of hepatic neuroendocrine metastases has been associated with favorable control of symptoms and with durable survival outcomes. However, these analyses have been limited to noncontrolled, retrospective studies, some of which have suboptimally compared patients undergoing surgical resection to patients who were not candidates for operative intervention. Analyses that have included large patient numbers and durable follow-up suggest that the likelihood of eventual disease recurrence following surgical metastasectomy is very high. Given the relative rarity and the relatively indolent disease course of even metastatic neuroendocrine neoplasms, the extent to which hepatic metastasectomy may prolong survival remains unclear.

Hepatic neuroendocrine metastases are commonly multifocal and are often not amenable to complete operative resection. In many cases, operative resection is combined with intraoperative microwave or radiofrequency ablation in an effort to preserve hepatic parenchyma. Some investigators have suggested that even subtotal cytoreduction can offer palliation of symptoms and prolongation of survival for patients with extensive hepatic neuroendocrine metastases. For many patients with extensive multifocal disease, liver-directed therapy relies on *transarterial chemoembolization* or *radioembolization*. These techniques take advantage of the fact that hepatic metastases derive the majority of their blood supply from the hepatic arterial circulation (as opposed to the portal venous circulation). Selective administration of chemotherapy (most commonly doxorubicin and cisplatin) or radioactive microspheres is followed by arterial embolization. Transarterial embolization therapy has been shown to be capable of controlling symptoms and inducing tumoral regression, but prospective randomized demonstration of survival benefit is not yet available.

Systemic Therapy

Until recently, systemic therapy for patients with pancreatic neuroendocrine neoplasms was restricted to *somatostatin analogs* and *cytotoxic chemotherapy*. Unfortunately, neither approach offered significant efficacy. Somatostatin analogs like *octreotide* or the long-acting variant *lanreotide* are able to inhibit hormonal secretion. In addition, they have been shown to inhibit proliferation of an insulinoma cell line in vitro. However, they do not appear to have any direct cytotoxic effect. Consequently, somatostatin analogue therapy has been shown to be effective in ameliorating hormonal symptoms in 60% to 90% of patients; however, patients typically develop resistance to this therapy after about 1 year, and actual induction of tumoral regression is rare (5% to 15%). Cytotoxic chemotherapy using 5-fluorouracil, streptozocin, and doxorubicin has been shown to have a response rate of 39%. A combination of cisplatin and etoposide has been shown to be associated with a response rate of 42% among patients with poorly differentiated tumors. However, both these regimens are associated with significant risks of adverse effects that often limit their utility.

Very recently, targeted therapies used in the treatment of other malignancies have been shown to have efficacy against pancreatic neuroendocrine neoplasms. Moreover, these agents are associated with comparatively minimal side effects. Two of these agents, *sunitinib* and *everolimus*, have recently received U.S. FDA approval for use in the treatment of pancreatic neuroendocrine neoplasms. Sunitinib is a tyrosine kinase inhibitor that targets a number of angiogenic and mitogenic proteins including vascular endothelial growth factor receptor and platelet-derived growth factor receptors. In a recent phase 3 randomized clinical trial, treatment with sunitinib promoted significant prolongation of median progression-free survival (11.4 months vs. 5.5 months) and significantly higher objective response rates (9% vs. 0%) as compared with placebo for patients with well-differentiated pancreatic neuroendocrine neoplasms. Everolimus is an inhibitor of the protein mammalian target of rapamycin. By inhibiting the cellular proliferation and angiogenic events mediated through mTOR signaling, everolimus can inhibit the growth and survival of pancreatic neuroendocrine neoplasm cell lines in vitro. In a recent multicenter randomized clinical trial, everolimus induced significant prolongation of progression-free survival (11 months vs. 5.4 months) and significantly higher objective response rates (5% vs. 2%) compared with placebo for patients with well-differentiated pancreatic neuroendocrine neoplasms. Importantly, both sunitinib and everolimus were found to have acceptable side effect profiles. Current investigations are examining newer targeted therapy agents as well as combination therapies.

OUTCOMES

Retrospective reports of patients undergoing complete resection of pancreatic neuroendocrine neoplasms are relatively heterogenous in terms of their treatment approaches and patient characteristics. However, review of representative studies with reasonable patient numbers and follow-up durations suggests that survival outcomes after resection may be generally favorable, with 5-year survival estimates ranging between 60% and 90% (Table 6.2). Prediction of individual patient outcomes relies on the identification of prognostically informative clinical variables, and optimal classification of pancreatic neuroendocrine neoplasms, which remains an area of persistent controversy. The seventh edition of the American Joint Commission on Cancer (AJCC) Cancer Staging Manual outlines a staging system for pancreatic neuroendocrine neoplasms that follows a conventional tumor–node–metastasis (TNM) schema (Table 6.3). However, it has been evident for some time that tumor grade, as quantified by mitotic activity, carries significant prognostic weight for neuroendocrine neoplasms. The World Health Organization (WHO) refined their classification system in 2010 to accommodate this variable (Table 6.4). Although histologic grade does stratify prognostic outcomes, a number of series have shown that variables such as tumor size, nodal metastases, and resection margin are prognostically informative variables for patients with resected pancreatic neuroendocrine neoplasms. As a result, optimal staging of this disease is likely to undergo further evaluation and modification in the future.

TABLE 6.2	Summary of Recent Retrospective Analyses of Patients Undergoing Surgical Resection of Pancreatic Neuroendocrine Neoplasms			
Authors	**Year**	**Number of Patients**	**Median Follow-up (Months)**	**5-Year Survival**
Kazankian, et al.	2006	70	50	89%
Schurr, et al.	2007	45	55	64%
Ferrone, et al.	2007	183	44	87%
Bilimoria, et al.	2008	3,855	51	59%
Hill, et al.	2009	1,815	26	~70%
Ballian, et al.	2009	43	68	91%

TABLE 6.3 AJCC Classification System of Pancreatic Neuroendocrine Neoplasms

Primary tumor (T)

		Stage	T	N	M
Tx	Primary tumor cannot be assessed	0	Tis	N0	M0
T0	No evidence of primary tumor	IA	T1	N0	M0
Tis	Carcinoma in situ	IB	T2	N0	M0
T1	Tumor limited to pancreas, ≤2 cm in greatest dimension	IIA	T3	N0	M0
T2	Tumor limited to pancreas, >2 cm in greatest dimension	IIB	T1	N1	M0
T3	Tumor extends beyond pancreas but without involvement of the celiac axis or the superior mesenteric artery		T2	N1	M0
			T3	N1	M0
T4	Tumor involves the celiac axis or the superior mesenteric artery (unresectable primary tumor)	III	T4	any N	M0
		IV	any T	any N	M1

Regional lymph nodes (N)

Nx	Regional lymph nodes cannot be assessed
N0	No regional lymph node metastases
N1	Regional lymph node metastases

Distant metastasis (M)

M0	No distant metastasis
M1	Distant metastasis

	WHO Classification of Pancreatic Neuroendocrine Neoplasms		
Differentiation	**Grade**	**Mitotic Figures**	**Ki-67 Staining Positivity**
Well differentiated	Low grade (G1)	<2 per 10 HPF[a]	<3%
	Intermediate grade (G2)	2 – 20 per 10 HPF[a]	3% – 20%
Poorly differentiated	High grade (G3)	>20 per 10 HPF[a]	>20%

[a]high-power fields

Suggested Readings

Ballian N, Loeffler AG, Rajamanickam V, et al. A simplified prognostic scoring system for resected pancreatic neuroendocrine neoplasms. *HPB (Oxford)* 2009;11:422–428.

Bilimoria KY, Bentrem DJ, Merkow RP, et al. Application of the pancreatic adenocarcinoma staging system to pancreatic neuroendocrine tumors. *J Am Coll Surg* 2007;205:558–563.

Ferrone CR, Tang LH, Tomlinson J, et al. Determining prognosis in patients with pancreatic endocrine neoplasms: can the WHO classification system be simplified? *J Clin Oncol* 2007;25:5609–5615.

Hill JS, McPhee JT, McDade TP, et al. Pancreatic neuroendocrine tumors: the impact of surgical resection on survival. *Cancer* 2009;115:741–751.

Kazanjian KK, Reber HA, Hines OJ. Resection of pancreatic neuroendocrine tumor: results of 70 cases. *Arch Surg* 2006;141:765–770.

Martin RC, Kooby DA, Weber SM, et al. Analysis of 6,747 pancreatic neuroendocrine tumors for a proposed staging system. *J Gastrointest Surg* 2011;15:175–183.

Norton JA, Fraker DL, Alexander HR, et al. Surgery increases survival in patients with gastrinoma. *Ann Surg* 2006;244:410–419.

Raymond E, Dahan L, Raoul JL, et al. Sunitinib malate for the treatment of pancreatic neuroendocrine tumors. *N Engl J Med* 2011;364:501–513.

Schurr PG, Strate T, Rese K, et al. Aggressive surgery improves long-term survival in neuroendocrine pancreatic tumors. *Ann Surg* 2007;245:273–281.

Yao JC, Shah MH, Ito I, et al. Everolimus for advanced pancreatic neuroendocrine tumors. *N Engl J Med* 2011;364:514–523.

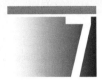

Technical Aspects of Pancreatic Surgery

Charles H. C. Pilgrim, Douglas B.
Evans, and Kathleen K. Christians

PREOPERATIVE CONSIDERATIONS

Pancreatic resection, in particular, pancreaticoduodenectomy, is a technical and perioperative tour de force in abdominal surgery and should be performed only in carefully selected patients. As with any major abdominal procedure, preoperative evaluation for pancreatic surgery should include a detailed history and physical examination (including functional status), laboratory studies, and optimization of medical comorbidities. Tumor markers (serum carbohydrate antigen [Ca19-9], carcinoembryonic antigen [CEA]) have prognostic value, and CA19-9 is being used to identify those patients at very high risk for harboring subclinical, radiographically occult, distant metastases. High-resolution abdominal computed tomography (CT) imaging is the mainstay of clinical staging. Contrast-enhanced multidetector pancreas protocol CT provides important information regarding tumor–vessel relationships. In particular, direct assessment of the relationship to the major vascular structures (superior mesenteric artery [SMA], superior mesenteric vein [SMV], SMV–portal vein confluence [SMV–PV], celiac axis, and common hepatic artery [CHA]) is readily determined in a reproducible manner. In addition, arterial and venous anomalies that affect the technical aspects of the operation should be noted and potential sites of metastatic disease identified. Resectability status must be established on the basis of high-quality imaging prior to treatment as it forms the basis for which stage-specific therapy is delivered both as part of a clinical trial and as off-protocol therapy. Resectability criteria utilized by the Medical College of Wisconsin pancreatic cancer team are found in Table 7.1.

PANCREATICODUODENECTOMY

Pancreaticoduodenectomy involves resection of the pancreatic head, duodenum, gallbladder, and bile duct with or without removal of the gastric antrum. Our recommended technique includes a brief staging laparoscopy to exclude liver and peritoneal metastases followed by a midline upper abdominal incision.

The surgical resection is divided into the following steps:

1. Isolation of the infrapancreatic SMV and separation of the colon and its mesentery from the duodenum and pancreatic head: The lesser sac is entered by mobilizing the greater omentum up off of the transverse colon. The loose attachments of the posterior gastric wall to the anterior surface of the pancreas are divided. The hepatic flexure of the colon is freed from its retroperitoneal attachments, exposing the pancreatic head and duodenum. The visceral peritoneum along the inferior border of the pancreas is incised starting from the left of the middle colic vessels toward the patient's right and inferiorly to expose the junction of

TABLE 7.1 Medical College of Wisconsin CT-based Clinical Staging of Pancreatic Cancer

	Tumor–Artery Relationship	Tumor–Vein Relationship	Extrapancreatic Disease
Resectable	No radiographic evidence of arterial abutment (celiac, SMA, or hepatic artery)	Tumor-induced narrowing <50% of SMV, PV, or SMV–PV	Nil
Borderline	Tumor abutment (<180 degrees) of the SMA or celiac artery Tumor abutment or short-segment encasement (>180 degrees) of the hepatic artery	Tumor-induced narrowing of >50% of SMV, PV, or SMV–PV confluence Short-segment occlusion of SMV, PV, SMV–PV with suitable PV (above), and SMV (below) to allow for safe vascular reconstruction	CT scan findings suspicious, but not diagnostic of metastatic disease (e.g., small indeterminate liver lesions that are too small to characterize)
Locally advanced	Tumor encasement (>180 degrees) of the SMA or celiac artery	Occlusion of SMV, PV, or SMV–PV without suitable vessels above and below the tumor to allow for reconstruction (no distal or proximal target for vascular reconstruction)	No evidence of peritoneal, hepatic, or extra-abdominal metastases
Metastatic	N/A	N/A	Evidence of peritoneal or distant metastases

SMA, superior mesenteric artery; SMV, superior mesenteric vein; PV, portal vein; SMV–PV, superior mesenteric–portal vein confluence the middle colic vein and SMV. The retroperitoneal attachments of the small bowel and right colon mesentery are taken down to a much greater extent in patients with uncinate tumors extending into the small bowel mesentery. When necessary, the small bowel mesentery can be mobilized by incising the visceral peritoneum all the way up to the ligament of Treitz (Cattell-Braasch maneuver).

2. The Kocher maneuver is begun at the third part of the duodenum by identifying the inferior vena cava. All tissue medial to the right gonadal vein and anterior to the inferior vena cava is elevated along with the pancreatic head and duodenum. This dissection is continued to the left lateral edge of the aorta, with exposure of the anterior surface of the left renal vein. A complete Kocher maneuver is necessary for the subsequent dissection of the pancreatic head from the SMA (step 6). Particularly important is the division of the leaf of peritoneum that extends from the retroperitoneum to the root of mesentery; incision of this portion of peritoneum is perhaps the most important part of the Kocher maneuver.

3. The portal dissection is commenced by exposing the CHA proximal and distal to the right gastric artery and the gastroduodenal artery (GDA). Both the right gastric and the GDA are then ligated and divided. Division of the GDA allows mobilization of the hepatic (common-proper) artery off the underlying PV. Cholecystectomy is then performed, and the common hepatic duct is transected at or above its junction with the cystic duct. Following transection of the bile duct, bile cultures are sent and indwelling endobiliary stents are removed. A bulldog clamp is placed on the transected hepatic duct to prevent bile from soiling the right upper quadrant until biliary reconstruction is completed. Note, the PV should always be exposed and the location of the right hepatic artery noted prior to dividing the common hepatic duct.

The PV should be identified but not extensively mobilized until step 6, at which time the stomach and pancreas have been divided. Care must be taken to avoid injury to the superior pancreaticoduodenal vein draining the pancreatic head at the superolateral aspect of the PV, or significant bleeding may occur when one does not yet have adequate exposure and vascular control.

4. The terminal branches of the left gastric artery are ligated and divided along the lesser curvature of the stomach prior to gastric transection. The stomach is then transected with a linear gastrointestinal (GIA) stapler at the level of the third or fourth transverse vein on the lesser curvature and at the confluence of the gastroepiploic veins on the greater curvature to complete a standard antrectomy (Fig. 7.1). The omentum is then divided at the level of the greater curvature transection. In the pylorus-preserving variant, the duodenum is divided just distal to the pylorus.

5. The loose attachments of the ligament of Treitz are taken down with care to avoid injury to the inferior mesenteric vein (IMV) situated immediately to the patient's left running caudal to cranial. The jejunum is then transected with a linear GIA stapler approximately 8 to 10 cm distal to the ligament of Treitz and its mesentery sequentially ligated and divided with an energy device such as the LigaSure. This dissection is continued proximally to involve the fourth and third portions of the duodenum. The duodenal mesentery is divided to approximately the level of the aorta, allowing the devascularized segment of duodenum and jejunum to be reflected beneath the mesenteric vessels into the right upper quadrant.

6. This step is oncologically the most important and difficult part of the operation. Traction sutures are placed on the superior and inferior borders of the pancreas, and the pancreas is then transected with

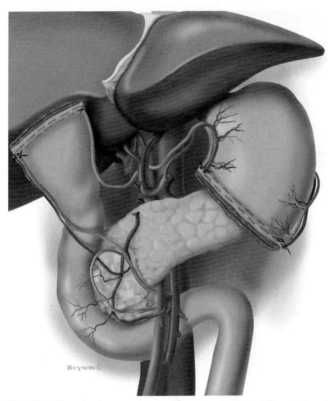

FIGURE 7.1 Illustration demonstrating completion of step 3 and step 4. The porta hepatis has been dissected, with ligation of the gastroduodenal and right gastric arteries. The gallbladder has been removed and the common hepatic duct transected (step 3). The antrum of the stomach has been divided at the level of the third or fourth transverse vein on the lesser curvature (step 4).

electrocautery at the level of the PV. There is usually a small artery that runs along the inferior border of the pancreas that is secured with the traction sutures. If there is evidence of tumor adherence to the PV or SMV, the pancreas is divided more upstream (to the tail) in the preparation for segmental venous resection. The specimen is separated from the SMV by ligation and division of the small venous tributaries to the uncinate process and pancreatic head (Fig. 7.2). Complete removal of the uncinate process from the SMV is required for full mobilization of the SMV–PV confluence and subsequent identification of the SMA. Failure to fully mobilize the SMV–PV confluence risks injury to the SMA and may result in a positive SMA margin. In addition, without complete mobilization of the SMV, it is difficult to expose the SMA. The inferior pancreaticoduodenal arteries (IPDAs) arising from the SMA must be identified and directly ligated. Mass ligation of the IPDAs with mesenteric soft tissue is a common cause of postoperative hemorrhage as the vessels may retract with the usual changes in blood pressure after extubation.

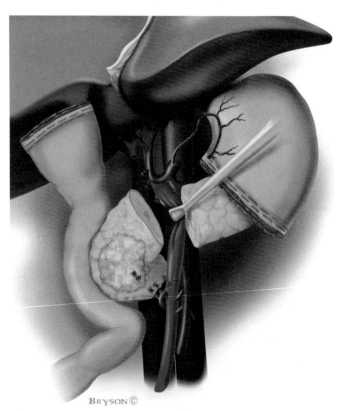

BRYSON©

FIGURE 7.2 Illustration of step 6. The pancreatic head and uncinate process are being separated from the SMV–PV confluence. The pancreas has already been transected at the level of the PV. Small venous tributaries from the PV and SMV are ligated and divided including delicate branches from the uncinate to the first jejunal branch of the SMV.

Proper mobilization of the SMV involves identification of its first jejunal branch. This branch originates from the right posterolateral aspect of the SMV (at the level of the uncinate process), travels posterior to the SMA, and enters the medial (proximal) aspect of the jejunal mesentery. The jejunal branch may course anterior to the SMA in up to 20% of cases, a situation that makes this dissection somewhat simpler. If tumor involvement of the SMV (at the level of the jejunal branch) prevents dissection of the uncinate process from the SMV, the jejunal branch should be divided proximal to the site of tumor encasement and again at its junction with the main trunk of the SMV. Once the uncinate is separated from the distal SMV, medial retraction of the SMV–PV confluence allows exposure of the SMA. The specimen is then separated from the right lateral wall of the SMA, which is dissected to its origin at the aorta; the plane of dissection should be directly on the adventitia of this vessel (Fig. 7.3).

The pancreatic and common hepatic duct transection margins are submitted for frozen-section evaluation. Positive resection margins demonstrating invasive carcinoma on the biliary or pancreatic duct mandate

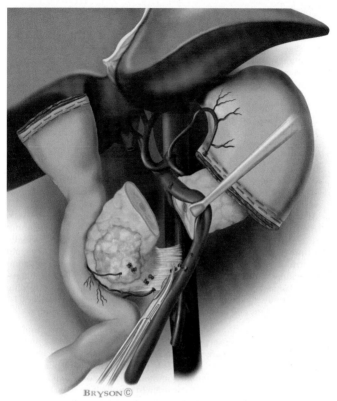

BRYSON©

FIGURE 7.3 Illustration demonstrating sharp dissection of the SMA margin, the most critical component of step 6. Medial retraction of the SMV–PV confluence facilitates dissection of the soft tissues adjacent to the lateral wall of the proximal SMA. The IPDA (or arteries) is identified at its origin from the SMA, ligated, and divided.

further resection until clear margins are achieved. Specimens should be oriented for the pathologist. The SMA margin must be identified and inked for the pathologist, as it cannot be accurately assessed in a retrospective fashion.

Pancreatic, Biliary, and Gastrointestinal Reconstruction

Reconstruction after pancreaticoduodenectomy begins with the pancreatic anastomosis.

1. The pancreatic remnant is mobilized from the retroperitoneum and distal splenic vein for a distance of 2 to 2.5 cm to allow accurate suture placement for the pancreaticojejunal anastomosis. The transected jejunum is brought retrocolic through a generous incision in the transverse mesocolon to the left (rather than the right) of the middle colic vessels. This minimizes tension on the anastomosis and provides a more direct route for the small bowel mesentery to approximate the pancreatic remnant than is afforded using a right-sided mesenteric window. A two-layer, end-to-side, duct-to-mucosa pancreaticojejunostomy is performed.

Occasionally, we use a one-layer anastomosis if the pancreas is small, is firm, and contains a dilated duct. Additionally, a small silastic stent may be used if the pancreatic duct is small. If the duct is too small to allow passage of the stent, an invaginating technique dunking the pancreatic remnant into the jejunal limb may rarely be required. The anastomosis between the pancreatic duct and the small bowel mucosa is completed with 5-0 monofilament absorbable sutures. Each stitch incorporates a generous bite of the pancreatic duct and a full-thickness bite of the jejunum. The posterior knots are tied on the inside and the lateral and anterior knots on the outside. When a stent is used, this is placed into the pancreatic duct and small bowel for a distance of approximately 2 to 3 cm prior to tying the anterior sutures.

2. A single-layer biliary anastomosis is performed using interrupted 4-0 or 5-0 absorbable monofilament sutures at a distance from the pancreaticojejunal anastomosis chosen to eliminate any tension. An interrupted technique is utilized to avoid purse stringing of the anastomosis. A stent is rarely ever used, even when the bile duct is of normal caliber.

3. An antecolic, end-to-side gastrojejunostomy is constructed in two layers. A posterior row of 3-0 silk sutures is followed by a full-thickness inner layer of running absorbable monofilament sutures; an anterior row of silk sutures completes the anastomosis. The distance between the biliary and gastric anastomoses should be at least 45 to 50 cm, allowing the jejunum to assume its antecolic position for the gastrojejunostomy without tension and also minimizing the risk of reflux cholangitis. A 10-Fr feeding jejunostomy tube may be placed approximately 30 cm distal to the gastrojejunostomy and used for feeding in the postoperative period.

Prior to closure, the abdomen is carefully irrigated with water, and the small bowel is run to ensure proper alignment. The use of drains remains controversial although many surgeons still drain both the hepaticojejunostomy and the pancreaticojejunostomy. In patients undergoing neoadjuvant therapy that includes radiation, the authors prefer to only drain the right upper quadrant with a single silastic drain to capture lymphatic fluid in the first 2 to 3 days after surgery. The falciform ligament, which was mobilized at the start of the laparotomy, is now placed between the hepatic artery and the afferent jejunal limb to cover the GDA stump. This maneuver minimizes the risk of pseudoaneurysm formation at this site in the event of a pancreatic anastomotic leak. A tongue of omentum may be used for the same purpose.

Pylorus Preservation

Pylorus preservation may be considered in patients with small periampullary neoplasms but should not be performed in patients with large pancreatic head tumors or in the setting of grossly positive pyloric or peripyloric lymph nodes. The essential differences in technique (compared to standard pancreaticoduodenectomy) involve steps 3 and 4 described above. The duodenum is divided approximately 2 to 3 cm beyond the pylorus with a linear GIA stapler and the gastroepiploic arcade divided at that level. The staple line is removed prior to creation of the duodenojejunostomy leaving approximately 2 cm of the duodenum distal to the pylorus; we usually send the duodenal margin for frozen section evaluation to exclude an unsuspected positive margin from appearing as a surprise on the final pathology report. The pylorus is gently dilated with a Kelly clamp or index finger (or both). The anastomosis is then performed in an end-to-side fashion using a single- (author's preference) or double-layer technique with monofilament absorbable sutures. Placement of a feeding jejunostomy in the setting of pylorus preservation may be considered due to the potentially increased incidence of delayed gastric emptying.

Venous Resection

Venous resection should only be performed in carefully selected patients with tumor adherence to the SMV or SMV–PV confluence without evidence of tumor encasement (>180 degrees) of the SMA or celiac axis. Steps 1 through 5 are completed as described above. Tumor adherence to the lateral wall of the SMV–PV confluence prevents dissection of the SMV and PV off the pancreatic head and uncinate process, thereby inhibiting medial retraction of the SMV–PV confluence (and lateral retraction of the specimen). Division of the splenic vein is performed when tumor abutment (on the lateral wall opposite the splenic vein) or encasement is at the level of the splenic vein junction. Division of the splenic vein allows complete exposure of the SMA medial to the SMV and allows the retroperitoneal dissection to be completed by sharp division of the soft tissues anterior to the aorta and to the right of the exposed SMA. The specimen is then attached only by the SMV–PV confluence. Vascular clamps are placed 2 to 3 cm proximal and distal to the involved venous segment, and the vein is transected, allowing tumor removal (Fig. 7.4). A 2- to 3-cm segment of SMV–PV confluence can safely be resected without the need for interposition grafting as increased SMV and PV length is provided when the splenic vein is divided. Venous resection is always performed with inflow occlusion of the SMA and systemic heparinization. It is important to mark the anterior surface of the SMV and PV prior to venous resection to prevent an inadvertent anastomotic twist.

Upper gastrointestinal hemorrhage due to sinistral portal hypertension following splenic vein ligation can occur if the IMV enters the SMV rather than the splenic vein—in which case there is inadequate venous outflow from the stomach and spleen due to splenic vein ligation. In contrast, when the IMV enters the splenic vein, the IMV provides a route for collateral venous flow from the ligated splenic vein in a retrograde fashion to the systemic venous circulation. When the splenic vein must be divided and the IMV enters the SMV, we create a distal splenorenal shunt to allow decompression of the stomach and spleen into the systemic venous circulation.

Ideally, the splenic vein–PV junction should be preserved. However, this is only possible when tumor invasion of the SMV or PV does not involve the splenic venous confluence. Splenic vein preservation significantly limits mobilization of the PV and prevents primary anastomosis after segmental SMV resection unless the resection is limited to less than 2 cm. Therefore, most patients who need SMV resection with splenic vein preservation require an interposition graft. Our preferred conduit is the internal jugular vein (IJV). Venous resection and reconstruction can be performed either before the specimen has been separated from the right lateral wall of the SMA or after complete mesenteric dissection. We first described the latter "artery-first" approach in the manuscript by Leach et al., and this is our preferred approach. Postoperatively, patients with vascular resection/reconstruction are prescribed aspirin and subcutaneous heparin starting in the recovery room assuming coagulation parameters are acceptable (INR < 1.5).

DISTAL PANCREATECTOMY

This operation can be performed laparoscopically, open, or with a hybrid technique. A distal pancreatectomy can be completed from medial to lateral (transect pancreas at PV–SMV–splenic vein confluence and dissection completed from the patient's right to left) or from lateral to medial (mobilizing the distal pancreas and spleen off of the retroperitoneal attachments and vasculature first, with pancreatic transection and dissection of the root of small bowel mesentery as the final step). Regardless of which technique is used, we always ligate the splenic artery before dividing the splenic vein.

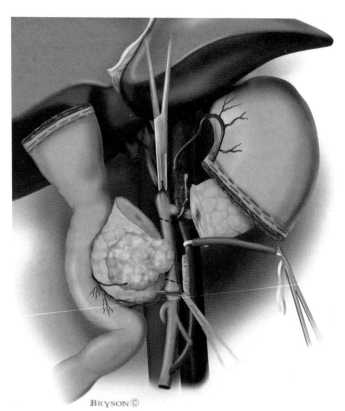

BRYSON ©

FIGURE 7.4 Illustration demonstrating resection of the SMV–PV confluence with splenic vein preservation. Vascular clamps have been placed on the SMV below and the PV above the involved venous segment, and a baby bulldog is utilized to occlude the splenic vein. A Rummel tourniquet is placed on the SMA in preparation for excision of the SMV en bloc with the specimen. The intact splenic vein tethers the PV, making a primary anastomosis impossible in most cases. As such, the reconstruction will require a segmental vein graft (we prefer a conduit of IJV that we prepare prior to the application of vascular clamps). In order to reduce the possibility of performing the anastomosis with a twist in the conduit, the IJV is marked while still in situ to ensure correct orientation.

Frequently, when dealing with a large tumor in the proximal body of the pancreas, we may divide the pancreas before dividing the splenic artery— and sometimes even before ligating the splenic artery. By dividing the pancreas, exposure to the celiac artery and proximal splenic artery is significantly improved.

Lateral to Medial Approach

The greater omentum is separated from the transverse colon, and the splenic flexure is mobilized caudally. The peritoneum lateral to the spleen is then incised in a cephalad direction up to the gastroesophageal junction (GEJ) and the spleen and distal pancreas mobilized out of the left upper quadrant, as the spleen and pancreas are dissected free of their retroperitoneal attachments to the kidney and adrenal gland. The short gastric vessels are ligated and divided, allowing medial and cephalad retraction of the stomach. Before division of the splenic vein, the splenic artery should be ligated, even if it is not divided. The IMV may be divided if it enters the splenic vein, or alternatively, the splenic vein can be divided just proximal (to the left) of the IMV–splenic vein junction. The mesenteric root is divided from the left lateral border of the SMV to the left lateral border of the aorta, staying anterior to the SMA. Exposure of the SMA inferior to the neck of the pancreas allows the dissection to proceed directly anterior to this vessel under direct vision. If the splenic artery was not ligated earlier in the operation (author's preference), this is now completed. Again, the artery is divided before ligation and division of the splenic vein. The pancreas is then transected (before ligation of the splenic artery if increased exposure is needed), a step that can be performed in a variety of manners. The most common techniques include stapler transection or division with electrocautery followed by suture ligation/closure. Regardless of technique, the most important step is identification and suture ligation of the pancreatic duct (we prefer 5-0 monofilament suture). The staple line may also be reinforced with 5-0 monofilament sutures on pledgets. When the pancreas is divided further medially than the level of the pancreatic neck, the point of pancreatic transection is virtually always too thick for a stapling device.

After delivery of the specimen, we routinely bring the mobilized falciform ligament through the lesser omentum to cover the stump of the splenic artery and the pancreatic transection site—analogous to the use of the falciform ligament following pancreaticoduodenectomy discussed previously.

Medial to Lateral Approach

After entering the lesser sac through the gastrocolic ligament, the inferior border of the pancreas is identified, and the peritoneum is incised. The dissection is carried medially until the SMV is identified as it passes beneath the pancreas. A tunnel along the anterior surface of the SMV–PV confluence can then be created, and the superior border of the pancreas is freed from the hepatic artery and PV. During laparoscopy, passing a sling underneath the pancreas and elevating the gland can aid in the further exposure of the pancreatic body and tail as the dissection proceeds laterally. Once sufficient space has been created for the passage of a stapling device, the pancreas is transected. It is then reflected to the left, facilitating its complete dissection from its retroperitoneal attachments.

Splenic Preservation

Distal pancreatectomy may also be performed with preservation of the spleen. Two techniques are available in this context, namely, preservation of the spleen via retrograde flow through the short gastric vessels (Warshaw technique) or by preserving the entire length of the splenic artery and vein. The Warshaw technique involves entering the lesser sac through the gastrocolic omentum but halting the dissection prior to encountering the left gastroepiploic and short gastric vessels. The avascular plane behind the pancreas is then mobilized starting at the inferior border of the gland near its tail, anterior to the splenic vessels. Dissection continues until the superior border is freed from the retroperitoneum. The tail of the pancreas can then be gently reflected to the patient's right, away from the splenic hilum, exposing the vessels for stapler fixation. After division, the dissection of the pancreas (and splenic vessels) proceeds to the right as far as is required to clear the indicated pathology. The pancreatic substance is then divided with a stapler (including the splenic vessels en masse), allowing delivery of the specimen.

Preservation of the splenic vessels is only applicable for certain tumor histologies (i.e., mucinous cystic neoplasms that lack malignant characteristics or symptomatic serous cystadenomas), as dissection in this plane violates oncologic principles of en bloc resection of regional lymphatic tissue. This procedure involves meticulous dissection of the multiple small vessels away from the pancreatic parenchyma that arise from the splenic artery or drain to the splenic vein. This is usually performed from medial to lateral to avoid the labyrinth of tiny vessels often present at the splenic hilum.

Laparoscopic Approach

Any of the approaches described above for distal pancreatectomy may be performed laparoscopically. A Hasson cannula placed supraumbilically allows visualization with a 30-degree laparoscope. A 5-mm working port is placed in the right upper quadrant approximately in the mid-clavicular line, and a second port of 12 mm (to allow passage of an Endo GIA stapler) is placed to the left of the midline at approximately the same level. Another 5-mm port for retraction is often placed further laterally on the left side for the surgical assistant. An umbilical tape or vessel loop passed underneath the pancreas aides in retraction and dissection of the specimen. The resection is then completed as described above with pancreatic transection completed using a stapler with seam guard (Gore).

Hybrid Approach

A laparoscopic-assisted hybrid technique combines the benefits of minimally invasive surgery with the security of precise and direct ligation of the pancreatic duct and splenic artery. The patient is positioned in the right lateral decubitus position (left side up). A Hasson cannula is placed at the umbilicus, pneumoperitoneum is achieved, and a standard four-port laparoscopy is undertaken. The splenic flexure of the colon is mobilized and the greater omentum dissected from the distal transverse colon. The peritoneum lateral to the spleen is incised proceeding cephalad until reaching the GEJ from the patient's left side. The dissection then continues lateral to medial mobilizing the spleen and tail of the pancreas toward the midline. The left crus of the diaphragm marks the medial most extent of the laparoscopic dissection. The short gastric arteries are divided. The patient is then returned to the supine position and a limited upper midline incision created, and the operation proceeds as for the medial to lateral approach. The splenic artery is identified at the superior border of the pancreas and ligated (either before or after pancreatic transection). The splenic vein–SMV junction is identified at the inferior border of the pancreatic body and, after dissection for a short distance, divided with an Endo GIA stapling device either flush with the SMV–PV confluence or just proximal to the IMV–splenic vein junction. Mobilization of the inferior aspect of the pancreas is now completed and the specimen freed from the retroperitoneum. After selection of an appropriate point of transection, the pancreas is divided as described above.

TOTAL PANCREATECTOMY

Total pancreatectomy is accomplished by following steps 1 and 3 of our six-step pancreaticoduodenectomy. After identification of the infrapancreatic SMV and completion of the portal dissection, the proximal splenic artery is exposed and ligated. Resection as described for distal pancreatectomy is then completed. While dissection of the SMA occurs from both the patient's left and right side, it is important, when possible, to leave some of the autonomic nerves on the adventitia of the SMA to preserve small bowel innervation and prevent rapid gastrointestinal transit. Division of the splenic vein is often delayed until the completion of steps 4 (gastric or duodenal transection) and 5 (ligament of Treitz, proximal jejunum, and duodenum). Then, in preparation for completion of the retroperitoneal dissection, the spleen and distal pancreas are again reflected medially, exposing the origin of the splenic vein–SMV junction; the splenic vein is then ligated and divided. Step 6 of pancreaticoduodenectomy is then completed in the standard manner and the specimen delivered intact. With the entire pancreas removed, reconstruction is a simpler procedure, involving only biliary and gastric anastomoses.

CENTRAL PANCREATECTOMY

In rare patients with relatively small tumors of the pancreatic neck of favorable histology (i.e., benign-appearing mucinous cystic neoplasms, branch duct IPMNs, solid pseudopapillary neoplasms), segmental resection of the pancreatic neck and proximal body with preservation of the splenic artery and vein may be utilized to preserve islet cell function. The proximal pancreas and pancreatic duct are oversewn as described above for distal pancreatectomy. Reconstruction includes Roux-en-Y pancreaticojejunostomy to the remaining segment of the distal pancreas. The small bowel is divided 35 to 45 cm distal to the ligament of Treitz. The distal limb is brought through the transverse colon mesentery (retrocolic) and sewn to the distal pancreas as a two-layer, end-to-side, duct-to-mucosa pancreaticojejunostomy as described for pancreaticoduodenectomy. Additionally, the oversewn distal end of the pancreatic head is reinforced by buttressing the serosa of Roux limb, distal to the pancreaticojejunostomy, to the pancreatic transection site. The proximal pancreaticobiliary limb is connected downstream to restore intestinal continuity as a side-to-side jejunojejunostomy.

SUMMARY

A preoperative evaluation that includes detailed patient assessment for comorbid conditions, functional status, and tumor marker trends and assessment of resectability by objective CT criteria minimizes rates of nontherapeutic laparotomy in patients with pancreatic cancer. The operative techniques detailed in this chapter are utilized to minimize intraoperative and perioperative complications. Pancreaticoduodenectomy and total pancreatectomy alone or in combination with vascular resection are technically demanding and should not be undertaken without thorough understanding of the nuances of upper abdominal anatomy. Best outcomes are obtained in high-volume centers by multidisciplinary teams that include experienced pancreatic surgeons, anesthesiologists, and nurses attuned to the intricacies of operative technique. Utilization of postoperative care pathways promotes early recognition of complications. As improved systemic therapies increase survival duration for patients with localized pancreatic cancer, the management of local-regional disease with surgery will become even more complex and the role for extended resection to include vascular resection and reconstruction considered with increased frequency. Patient selection and detailed preoperative planning are simply invaluable to insure the desired results.

Suggested Readings

Balachandran A, Darden DL, et al. Arterial variants in pancreatic adenocarcinoma. *Abdom Imaging* 2008;33(2):214–221.

Christians KK, Lal A, et al. Portal vein resection. *Surg Clin North Am* 2010;90(2):309–322.

Christians KK, Tsai S, Tolat PP, et al. Critical steps for pancreaticoduodenectomy in the setting of pancreatic adenocarcinoma. *J Surg Oncol* 2013;107(1):33–38.

Evans DB, Farnell MB, et al. Surgical treatment of resectable and borderline resectable pancreas cancer: expert consensus statement. *Ann Surg Oncol* 2009;16(7):1736–1744.

Katz MH, Hwang R, et al. Tumor-node-metastasis staging of pancreatic adenocarcinoma. *CA Cancer J Clin* 2008;58(2):111–125.

Katz MH, Fleming JB, et al. Anatomy of the superior mesenteric vein with special reference to the surgical management of first-order branch involvement at pancreaticoduodenectomy. *Ann Surg* 2008;248(6):1098–1102.

Katz MH, Pisters PW, et al. Borderline resectable pancreatic cancer: the importance of this emerging stage of disease. *J Am Coll Surg* 2008;206(5):833–846; discussion 846–838.

Katz MH, Varadhachary GR, et al. Serum CA 19-9 as a marker of resectability and survival in patients with potentially resectable pancreatic cancer treated with neoadjuvant chemoradiation. *Ann Surg Oncol* 2010;17(7):1794–1801.

Leach SD, Davidson BS, Ames FC, et al. Alternative method for exposure of the retroperitoneal mesenteric vasculature during total pancreatectomy. *J Surg Oncol* 1996;61(2):163–165.

Minimally Invasive Pancreatic Surgery

Michael L. Kendrick

INTRODUCTION

Minimally invasive pancreatectomy is rapidly gaining favor in centers specializing in pancreatic surgery. A growing body of evidence suggests several outcome advantages over open approaches; these findings continue to engender enthusiasm for laparoscopy. Laparoscopic distal pancreatectomy (LDP) is the most widely adopted procedure, as it requires basic laparoscopic skills of dissection and no reconstruction. Procedures with more complex resection or reconstruction have seen more gradual acceptance. The predominant challenge preventing the wide application of minimally invasive surgery (MIS) approaches in pancreatic surgery continues to be the lack of adequate surgeon training. Few centers have sufficient experience with more advanced procedures such as pancreaticoduodenectomy and total pancreatectomy; thus, large comparative trials of laparoscopy versus open approach are lacking for these procedures. However, the increasing evidence in support of MIS approaches for all pancreatic operations continues to emerge as larger series are reported, and more centers develop minimally invasive programs.

INDICATIONS AND CONTRAINDICATIONS

The indications for MIS pancreatectomy mirror those for open approaches and include all benign and malignant conditions requiring pancreatic resection. Expanding the indications for pancreatic resection solely based on the ability to perform it with minimally invasive approaches is not recommended. Absolute contraindications for MIS pancreatectomy are also similar to open approaches and include patients with prohibitive comorbidities or poor functional status. The majority of reported contraindications are therefore relative, and experience of the surgeon is the key determinate (Table 8.1).

TECHNIQUE

Laparoscopic Distal Pancreatectomy
Setup, Access, and Initial Exposure
The patient is positioned supine with 15 degrees of reverse Trendelenburg. Whereas some advocate a right lateral decubitus position or place a bump under the left flank, we prefer a supine position that facilitates a right-to-left dissection. A total of four trocars are placed as depicted in Figure 8.1. A periumbilical incision is made, the trocar placed under direct vision, and a pneumoperitoneum established. The remaining three trocars are placed under laparoscopic visualization. The gastrocolic ligament is divided peripheral to the epiploic vessels using the harmonic scalpel, and the lesser sac is entered. The short gastric vessels are preserved, and the splenic flexure of the colon is mobilized inferiorly. Visual inspection of the anterior

TABLE 8.1	Contraindications for Laparoscopic Pancreatic Resection

Absolute	Relative
Prohibitive medical comorbidities	Locally advanced malignancy
Poor functional status	Proximity to major vasculature
	Severe obesity
	Prior major abdominal operations

aspect of the pancreas is performed, and the lesion is identified either through palpation or through the use of laparoscopic ultrasonography. The stomach is sutured anteriorly to the retrocostal peritoneum to facilitate exposure.

Pancreatic Mobilization

The transverse mesocolon is dissected off the inferior border of the pancreas, and the pancreas is dissected out of the retroperitoneum in the anticipated area of transection. Early focus of dissection at the site of anticipated transection and splenic vessels allows excellent access and exposure for a safe dissection. In the event of bleeding during splenic vessel preservation, the vessels can be quickly ligated, reducing blood loss. The splenic vein is dissected off the posterior aspect of the pancreas. The splenic artery is identified and dissected either through an anterior approach at the superior border of the pancreas or via a posterior-inferior approach after elevating

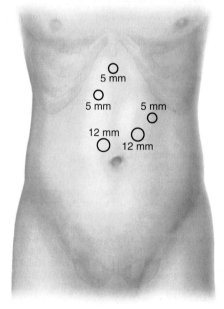

FIGURE 8.1 Trocar positioning for LDP.

the pancreas out of the retroperitoneum. The latter approach is most commonly used when the parenchymal transection is anticipated to occur within the pancreatic body rather than the tail.

Pancreatic Resection

With the pancreas elevated off of the splenic vessels, the pancreatic parenchyma is then divided with either a linear stapler with biologic reinforcement or the harmonic scalpel. If spleen preservation is planned, the assistant retracts the pancreas anteriorly and laterally to expose the dissection plane between the pancreas and splenic vessels. Most tributary vessels can be divided with the harmonic scalpel. Larger vessels (≥ 2 mm) are ligated with suture or are clipped and divided. When planning splenectomy, the splenic vessels are ligated and divided near the pancreatic transection site prior to a right-to-left dissection with division of the short gastric vessels and splenic peritoneal attachments.

Specimen Retrieval

The specimen is placed in an endobag and removed via the periumbilical incision that is extended just long enough to accommodate the specimen. The specimen is inspected on the back table, and a separate pancreatic margin is harvested. We routinely use frozen section histology for evaluation of the primary lesion and the margin prior to termination of the procedure. The extraction site is closed with interrupted suture, leaving the cephalad two sutures untied. The trocar is reintroduced and the carbon dioxide (CO_2) pneumoperitoneum reestablished.

Pancreatic Stump Management and Closure

When the transection is not performed with the stapler, our preferred method of pancreatic stump treatment is with saline-coupled radiofrequency energy source (Salient Surgical Technologies, Portsmouth, NH). The pancreatic resection bed and exposed splenic vessels are then reinspected, and hemostasis is ensured. Prophylactic operative drains are not routinely used in the author's practice. The trocars are removed, and sites are closed with a 4-0 subcuticular monofilament absorbable suture.

Laparoscopic Pancreaticoduodenectomy

Setup, Access, and Initial Exposure

The patient is positioned supine in 15 degrees of reverse Trendelenburg. Initial access is gained through a left subcostal site using a 12-mm transparent, cone-tip trocar. A CO_2 pneumoperitoneum to 15 mm Hg is established, and all visible peritoneal and visceral surfaces are inspected. Five additional 12-mm trocars are placed (Fig. 8.2).

The gastrocolic ligament is divided with the harmonic scalpel (Ethicon Endosurgery, Cincinnati, OH), widely exposing the lesser sac. The gastroepiploic vessels are clipped and divided with the harmonic scalpel. The duodenocolic ligament is resected en bloc with the specimen to facilitate regional lymphadenectomy. A fan retractor is placed under the gastric antrum to provide exposure of the pancreatic head and neck.

Pancreatic Neck Dissection

The pancreatic neck is approached with the surgeon positioned on the left side of the patient. The common hepatic artery lymph nodes are removed, and the common and proper hepatic arteries are identified to verify tumor clearance. The portal vein is exposed at the cephalad border of the pancreatic neck and the superior mesenteric vein at the caudal border. The

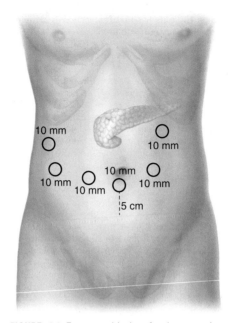

FIGURE 8.2 Trocar positioning for laparoscopic pancreaticoduodenectomy.

gastroduodenal artery is dissected, ligated, clipped, and divided. A plane between the posterior aspect of the pancreatic neck and the portal vein/superior mesenteric vein is developed. An articulating grasper is passed posteriorly and an umbilical tape is placed around the pancreatic neck and secured.

Duodenal Mobilization
The first portion of the duodenum is cleared, and the right gastric artery is ligated and divided. The duodenum is divided 2 cm distal to the pylorus using a linear stapler. The transverse colon is reflected cephalad, and the area of the ligament of Treitz is dissected mobilizing the third and fourth portions of the duodenum off of the aorta and inferior vena cava. The jejunum is divided 15 cm distal to the ligament of Treitz with the linear stapler, and the jejunal mesentery is then divided with the harmonic scalpel back to the uncinate process. The hepatic flexure of the colon is mobilized inferiorly, and the ascending and transverse colon are retracted inferiorly with a fan retractor. The surgeon moves to the patient's right side, and the Kocherization of the duodenum is extended cephalad to the hepatic hilum.

Hepatic Hilar Dissection
A cholecystectomy is performed, leaving the cystic duct intact. The hilum of the liver is dissected, and the common hepatic duct is identified, ligated distally, and divided. All hilar lymphatic tissue is dissected inferiorly with the specimen. The lateral aspect of the portal vein is cleared caudally until

the superior pancreaticoduodenal vein is identified, ligated, and divided. The jejunal stump is brought into the supramesocolic compartment, and the anterolateral aspect of the superior mesenteric vein is dissected proximally to the inferior border of the pancreas.

Pancreatic Head Resection

The pancreatic neck is divided with the harmonic scalpel, with the exception of the pancreatic duct, which is divided sharply with scissors. Using the umbilical tape for retraction, the pancreatic head and uncinate process are dissected off the portal vein, superior mesenteric vein, and superior mesenteric artery (SMA). The inferior pancreaticoduodenal artery and vein are ligated or clipped and divided with harmonic scalpel. Dissection of the uncinate is performed adjacent to the adventitia of the SMA to assure an appropriate oncologic margin.

Specimen Removal

The specimen is placed into an endobag and removed via the infraumbilical trocar site, which is typically extended to a total length of 3 to 5 cm to accommodate the specimen. Specimen inspection is performed on the back table; separate pancreatic neck and bile duct margin are harvested and sent for frozen section analysis. The portal vein groove and SMA margins are inked. The extraction site is closed with interrupted suture and a CO_2 pneumoperitoneum reestablished.

Anastomotic Reconstruction

The jejunum is brought through the duodenal resection bed (retromesenteric tunnel). An end-to-side pancreaticojejunostomy, duct-to-mucosa anastomosis, is constructed with an inner layer of interrupted 5-0 Vicryl suture and an outer layer of interrupted 3-0 PDS suture.

Approximately 10 cm distal to the pancreaticojejunostomy, the hepaticojejunostomy is performed. The surgeon stands on the patient's right with instruments and camera in the right-most trocars. This setup allows sewing toward the surgeon as would be done in an open approach. The end-to-side hepaticojejunostomy is constructed with a single layer of interrupted (duct size ≤6 mm) or running (duct size >6 mm) 5-0 Vicryl suture.

An antecolic end-to-side duodenojejunostomy is constructed approximately 40 cm distal to the hepaticojejunostomy, using two layers of running 3-0 Vicryl suture.

A single, 5-mm round, closed-suction drain is brought through the right abdominal wall and positioned posterior to the hepaticojejunostomy and anterior to the pancreaticojejunostomy. The trocars are removed under direct vision and the skin incisions closed with a subcuticular 4-0 monofilament absorbable suture.

POSTOPERATIVE MANAGEMENT

Postoperative care after MIS pancreatectomy is similar for both distal pancreatectomy and pancreaticoduodenectomy. The orogastric tube is removed at the end of the procedure. Patients are started on clear liquids on the first postoperative day, and diet is advanced over the next 48 hours. Pain is controlled with intravenous ketorolac scheduled every 6 hours and with patient-controlled intravenous administration of morphine. The drain is removed on postoperative day 4 if drain amylase is low and no other signs of pancreatic fistula are present. Hospital discharge is allowed on or after the 5th postoperative day if the patient is tolerating a soft diet and is without evidence of complication.

OUTCOMES

Distal Pancreatectomy

Several large series of minimally invasive distal pancreatectomy have demonstrated the feasibility, safety, and favorable outcomes of this approach. Adequately powered, randomized controlled trials of LDP versus open distal pancreatectomy (ODP) have not been performed, and the assessment of the outcomes of these two approaches is predominantly limited to retrospective comparative trials. Recently, a large meta-analysis of 18 studies including 1,814 patients suggested that minimally invasive distal pancreatectomy is associated with less blood loss, reduced overall and wound-specific complication rates, and shorter length of hospital stay. Importantly, no differences in operative time, margin status, pancreatic fistula rates, or mortality were seen between the two groups.

To further elucidate whether risk factors for operative morbidity differ between LDP and ODP, Cho and colleagues performed an analysis of data from nine separate academic centers comparing LDP and ODP. Of 693 patients undergoing distal pancreatectomy (LDP = 254, ODP = 439), multivariate analysis demonstrated that BMI $\leq$ 27, nonadenocarcinoma, and pancreatic specimen length $\leq$8.5 cm had higher rates of fistula after ODP than after LDP. This study identified no preoperatively variables associated with the increased risk of pancreatic fistula after LDP compared to ODP. Additionally, no patient cohorts were identified that had higher rates of postoperative complication for LDP than for ODP.

Laparoscopic Pancreaticoduodenectomy

Gagner and Pomp published the first report of laparoscopic pancreaticoduodenectomy in 1994 and subsequently published a series of 10 patients in 1997. The conversion rate for this series was 40% and the operative time was long (8.5 hours). The authors concluded that there were no perceivable advantages of the MIS approach. Over a decade passed before the first substantial series of total laparoscopic pancreaticoduodenectomy (TLPD) was published by Palanivelu and colleagues. Of 42 patients undergoing TLPD, the indication was malignancy in 95%. With a mean operative time of 370 minutes, estimated blood loss of 65 mL, and pancreatic fistula rate of 7%, this report not only established the feasibility but also clearly set a challenge to investigate this technique further. To date, only six published series have reported more than 50 patients undergoing TLPD and are shown in Table 8.2. While the outcomes appear comparable to those reported for open approaches, appropriate and intentional selection bias in these early experiences limits validation of equivalency or potential advantages. Asbun and colleagues recently reported a retrospective, comparative analysis of laparoscopic and open pancreaticoduodenectomy. Patients undergoing the laparoscopic approach had significantly less estimated blood loss, fewer transfusions, and shorter length of hospital stay. No differences in overall or pancreas-specific complications were seen; however, operative time was longer for the laparoscopic group. Our institution has now performed laparoscopic pancreaticoduodenectomy in over 300 patients, and a comparative analysis is forthcoming. We continue to observe the typical advantages of MIS approaches with TLPD as reported earlier. Further investigation should be in evaluating the potential impact of laparoscopic approaches on the quality-of-life, oncologic, and long-term outcomes.

Robotic-Assisted Laparoscopic Pancreatic Resection

Robotic assistance has been described as a useful adjunct to pure laparoscopic approaches and is currently gaining interest. Several series have published outcomes of robotic-assisted pancreatic resection. Zureikat and

TABLE 8.2	Selected Series of Laparoscopic Pancreaticoduodenectomy[a]								
Publication	Year	No. of Patients	Procedure	Op Time (Min)	EBL (mL)	PF (%)	DGE (%)	LOS (Days)	Mortality (%)
Palanivelu	2009	75	TLPD	357	74	7	–	8	1.3
Kendrick	2010	62	TLPD	368	240	18	15	7	1.6
Giulianotti	2010	60	RALPD	421	394	21	5	22	3
Kim	2012	100	TLPD	487	–	6	2	20	1
Asbun	2012	53	TLPD	541	195	10	11	8	6
Zureikat	2013	132	RALPD	527	300	7	–	10	1.5
Total[b]		482		453	263	14	9	13	2

[a]Includes only series with ≥50 patients and data sufficient for analysis.

[b]Weighted averages.

TLPD, total laparoscopic pancreaticoduodenectomy; RALPD, robotic-assisted laparoscopic pancreaticoduodenectomy; EBL, estimated blood loss; PF, pancreatic fistula; DGE, delayed gastric emptying; LOS, length of hospital stay.

colleagues reported a large single institutional series of robotic pancreatectomy. Of 250 consecutive robotic pancreatic resections, the most common operations included are pancreaticoduodenectomy (n = 132), distal pancreatectomy (n = 83), central pancreatectomy (n = 13), enucleation (n = 10), and total pancreatectomy. In these selected patients, the safety and feasibility were established with comparable morbidity and mortality rates compared to those reported for open approaches.

In a comparative study of LDP versus robotic-assisted LDP, Kang and colleagues reported greater success with spleen preservation with the use of robotic assistance (56% vs. 5%, P = 0.027). Significant differences in the study group included a younger age and disease indication. Operative time (349 vs. 258 minutes, P = 0.016) was longer, and cost (USD 8,300 vs. 3,862) was significantly higher for the robotic group compared to the laparoscopic group. The small sample size and patient selection may account for these findings. Patients in the robotic-assisted group were also younger and less likely to have intraductal papillary mucinous neoplasm, where pericystic inflammation is frequently noted.

Reported advantages and disadvantages of the robotic platform are listed in Table 8.3. Pertinent advantages may include the relative ease of training and potential avoidance of prerequisite advanced laparoscopic skills. The purported advantages of a three-dimensional view, added maneuverability, and fine motor movement, while enticing, are immeasurable with regard to their independent effect on outcomes over pure laparoscopic approaches. Significant disadvantages of the current robotic systems are the lack of haptic feedback and the cost of the equipment and its maintenance.

With the feasibility and favorable outcomes of pure laparoscopic approaches having already been established, additional comparative trials of robotic compared to open approaches are of questionable value. The pertinent questions are whether the addition of robotic assistance improves outcomes over pure laparoscopic approaches and does the increase cost justify its use? The current literature lacks any adequately powered, appropriately designed trial to address these important questions. Further, the answers are unlikely to be forthcoming for the most complex procedures such as pancreaticoduodenectomy due to the fact that few centers will be able to perform both approaches in sufficient numbers to allow a meaningful comparison.

At present, the main advantage of robotic assistance appears to be centered toward the surgeon rather than the patient. Clearly, surgeons without sufficient laparoscopic skills will be more able to perform complex laparoscopic procedures using robotic assistance. A more widespread application of MIS approaches will provide advantages for patients. Another potential advantage requiring further investigation is the ergonomics of surgeon positioning, which may reduce surgeon fatigue and chronic injuries compared to pure laparoscopic approaches.

TABLE 8.3	Advantages and Disadvantages of Robotic-Assisted Approaches

Advantages	Disadvantages
"Intuitive"—replicates open skills	Lack of haptic feedback
Increased range of motion	Expense (purchase, maintenance)
Fine motor movement	Set-up time
Three-dimensional view	Surgeon remote from the patient
Surgeon ergonomics	Loss of bedside "peripheral" view

Laparoscopic Approaches to Pancreatic Malignancy

A valid concern among many skeptics of minimally invasive approaches to pancreatic resection is the ability of these approaches to maintain oncologic principles. Given the relative recent application of MIS approaches in pancreatic malignancy, long-term oncologic outcomes are not available. Surrogates to assess the quality of the oncologic resection include margin status, number of lymph nodes resected, and short-term recurrence and survival.

In a multicenter, retrospective, matched cohort analysis of patients undergoing laparoscopic versus ODP for adenocarcinoma, Kooby and colleagues identified no difference in oncologic outcomes based on approach. Specifically, margin-negative status (74% vs. 66%, $P = 0.61$), number of lymph nodes harvested (14 vs. 12, $P = 0.41$), and median survival (16 vs. 16 months, $P = 0.71$) were similar.

We have recently evaluated the outcomes of open and laparoscopic pancreaticoduodenectomy at our institution from 2008 through 2013. To avoid the confounding factors of invasiveness, margin-negative rates, and survival among various types of malignancy, we evaluated only patients with pancreatic ductal adenocarcinoma. Of 322 patients undergoing pancreaticoduodenectomy specifically for pancreatic adenocarcinoma, 108 underwent TLPD and 214 underwent OPD. Operative time (379 vs. 387 minutes) and need for major venous resection (13% vs. 22%) were not different. The estimated blood loss and length of hospital stay were less for LPD compared to OPD (492 vs. 867 mL, $P = <0.001$, and 6 vs. 9 days, $P = <0.001$, respectively). With regard to oncologic outcomes, tumor size, margin-negative resection, and number of lymph nodes harvested were not different. A significantly smaller proportion of patients in the TLPD group had a delay greater than 8 weeks from operation to chemotherapy. Despite similar rates of margin-negative resection, local disease as the initial site of recurrence was less common in the TLPD group (15% vs. 27%). While there was no difference in overall survival, TLPD patients had a longer progression-free survival.

Major vascular resection during pancreaticoduodenectomy for pancreatic head adenocarcinoma has been described as feasible and safe in open approaches. Primary objectives of major venous resection are to increase the number of patients eligible for a potentially curative procedure and to increase the rate of R0 resections. Until very recently, the need for vascular resection had been a contraindication for laparoscopic approaches. Our institution reported an early experience suggesting the feasibility and safety of laparoscopic major venous resection at the time of pancreaticoduodenectomy. More recently, a comparative analysis of laparoscopic and open pancreaticoduodenectomy with major venous resection demonstrated less blood loss with comparable graft patency and complication rates for the laparoscopic approach.

CONCLUSION

Minimally invasive approaches for pancreatic resection are feasible and safe. Whereas level I evidence is lacking, existing comparative trials suggest noninferiority and possible advantages for laparoscopic compared to open approaches for both benign and malignant disease. Consistently reported advantages include reduced blood loss and shorter length of hospital stay for most procedures. A more widespread acquisition of advanced laparoscopic skills or access to robotic platforms will continue to advance the use of minimally invasive approaches for pancreatic surgery. Oncologic and quality of life outcomes are needed to assess value in addition to the typical advantages reported for MIS approaches. Careful scrutiny should continue to assure appropriate outcomes and early identification of unexpected complications and to substantiate the perceived advantages of minimally invasive approaches for pancreatic resection.

Suggested Readings

Asbun HJ, Stauffer JA. Laparoscopic vs. open pancreaticoduodenectomy: overall outcomes and severity of complications using the Accordion Severity Grading System. *J Am Coll Surg* 2012;215:810.

Kendrick ML. Laparoscopic and robotic resection for pancreatic cancer. *Cancer J* 2012;18:571.

Kendrick ML, Sclabus GM. Major venous resection during total laparoscopic pancreaticoduodenectomy. *HPB (Oxford)* 2011;13:454.

Kooby DA, Hawkins WG, Schmidt CM, et al. A multicenter analysis of distal pancreatectomy for adenocarcinoma: is laparoscopic resection appropriate. *J Am Coll Surg* 2010;210:779.

Venkat R, Edil BH, Schulick RD, et al. Laparoscopic distal pancreatectomy is associated with less overall morbidity compared to the open technique: a systematic review and meta-analysis. *Ann Surg* 2012;255:1048.

Zureikat AH, Moser AJ, Boone BA, et al. 250 robotic pancreatic resections: safety and feasibility. *Ann Surg* 2013;258:554.

Complications of Pancreatic Surgery

Timothy R. Donahue and Howard A. Reber

INTRODUCTION

At high-volume centers, the operative mortality after pancreaticoduodenectomy (PD) is less than 3%. However, morbidity remains high with an overall rate of postoperative complications ranging from 30% to 65%. These complications can lead to prolonged hospital stays, increased readmission rates, and greater hospital costs. Moreover, in patients who undergo an operation for pancreatic cancer, adjuvant chemotherapy is delayed. Thus, it is important to minimize the complication rate and, when a complication occurs, to treat it promptly and effectively. The complications of pancreatic surgery include pancreatic fistula, delayed gastric emptying (DGE), hemorrhage, biliary fistula, and pancreatic exocrine and endocrine insufficiency. In this section, we will review the diagnosis and treatment of each of these complications.

PANCREATIC FISTULA

Definition and Incidence

A pancreatic fistula is an abnormal communication between the pancreas and adjacent or distant organs or spaces (internal fistula) or the skin (external fistula). Fistulas comprise amylase-rich exocrine pancreatic secretions, and external fistulas are the most common cause of prolonged morbidity and mortality associated with pancreatic surgery. After PD, a fistula forms due to impaired healing of the pancreatic anastomosis or, after distal pancreatectomy, incomplete healing of the cut edge of the pancreas. Fistulas can also form after middle (segmental) pancreatectomy or enucleations of tumors, particularly in the latter case if the main pancreatic duct is injured. Fistulas are arbitrarily described as low output if the volume is less than 200 mL/d and high output if it is greater than 200 mL/d.

Because of variability in how pancreatic fistula has been defined, there is a wide range of the rate of pancreatic fistula formation reported in the literature. To standardize these discrepancies, the International Study Group on Pancreatic Fistula (ISGPF) published a consensus definition in 2005. Postoperative pancreatic fistula was defined as drain output of any measurable volume after postoperative day 3 with an amylase content of at least three times the upper limit of normal in the serum. The ISGPF also developed a grading system (A, B, or C) based on the clinical impact and additional complications caused by the fistula (Table 9.1). Grade A fistulas pose little or no burden on the patient, while grade C fistulas are associated with significant morbidity and occasional mortality.

Numerous risk factors contribute to fistula development. The most widely accepted risks include a soft pancreatic texture that does not hold sutures well for the pancreatic anastomosis in PD or sutures or staples for remnant closure in distal pancreatectomy, a small pancreatic duct (<3 mm

| TABLE 9.1 | Main Parameters for Postoperative Pancreatic Fistula Grading |

Grade	A	B	C
Clinical conditions	Well	Often well	Ill appearing/bad
Specific treatment[a]	No	Yes/no	Yes
US/CT (if obtained)	Negative	Negative/positive	Positive
Persistent drainage (after 3 wk)[b]	No	Usually yes	Yes
Reoperation	No	No	Yes
Death related to POPF	No	No	Possibly yes
Signs of infections	No	Yes	Yes
Sepsis	No	No	Yes
Readmission	No	Yes/no	Yes/no

[a]Partial (peripheral) or total parenteral nutrition, antibiotics, enteral nutrition, somatostatin analog, and/or minimally invasive drainage.
[b]With or without a drain in situ.
US, ultrasonography; CT, computed tomography scan; POPF, postoperative pancreatic fistula.
Taken from Bassi C, Dervenis C, Butturini G, et al. Postoperative pancreatic fistula: an international study group (ISGPF) definition. *Surgery* 2005;138(1):8–13.

diameter), poor nutritional status (albumin <3 g/dL), and high intraoperative blood loss (>1 L). Pancreatic surgeons have also examined different surgical techniques to avoid fistula formation. For PD, the technique used (e.g., duct to mucosa vs. invagination; routine placement of a pancreatic duct stent) or location (pancreaticojejunostomy (PJ) vs. gastrojejunostomy) of the pancreatic anastomosis has been examined. The results of numerous randomized trials and meta-analyses are mixed, with one favoring one technique or location over the other, or no difference observed. We routinely perform a partial invagination technique without the use of stents and have observed an overall fistula rate of less than 15% and a rate of about 7% after PD for pancreatic cancer.

For distal pancreatectomy, the incidence of pancreatic fistula ranges from 15% to 25%. Some studies suggest that the fistula rate is decreased with the use of stapled closure. More recently, there is some evidence that reinforced stapled closure, using a Seamguard, may further decrease the rate of fistula development. We routinely use stapled closure and Seamguard where possible but have found that even the 4.8-mm staples cannot completely seal a thick pancreas. In that case, the pancreas is transected with cautery, and a sutured closure of the cut surface is performed with a running and locking 3-0 Prolene suture and an additional suture (4-0 or 5-0 Prolene) to close the pancreatic duct. The incidence of pancreatic fistula is highest in patients undergoing middle (segmental) pancreatectomy ranging from 20% to 60%. This high incidence is due to the presence of both a closed pancreas surface toward the head of the pancreas and a pancreaticojejunal anastomosis of the distal segment.

Treatment

Pancreatic fistulas are associated with increased patient morbidity, hospital stay and costs, and even occasional death due to sepsis or hemorrhage. Therefore, prompt diagnosis and treatment are essential. Four goals of treatment will be reviewed. These include (a) good drainage, (b) treatment of infection, (c) maintenance of good nutritional status, and (d) correction of electrolyte imbalances.

The most important treatment goal of pancreatic fistula management focuses on complete drainage of extraluminal pancreatic exocrine juices. We routinely place a closed-suction Silastic drain (10 flat or 19 round Jackson-Pratt) anterior to the PJ anastomosis. It is drawn behind the stomach and the left lobe of the liver, which usually maintains its proper position on top of the PJ suture line. It is cut long enough so that its tip lies next to the hepaticojejunostomy anastomosis; thus, it will drain a leak from either site effectively. If the drain output does not appear turbid or contain bile, the drain is routinely removed on postoperative day 5 to 7, when the patient is eating a regular diet. A high-volume output of serous fluid does not influence this decision, but if the character of the fluid is suspicious, the amylase level is checked. If a pancreatic fistula is present, the drain is left in place. If the patient's white blood cell count is elevated, or if they are febrile, broad-spectrum antibiotics are started and a CT scan performed to look for any undrained fluid collections, which should be drained by the interventional radiologist with CT scan or ultrasound guidance (Fig. 9.1). The fluid is sent for culture and amylase concentration, and the antibiotics are then tailored to the specific organisms. Once all signs of infection resolve, the patient is discharged with the surgical drain (and any additional percutaneous drains) in place. Before discharge, around postoperative day 10, the drains are taken off of suction and allowed to drain into a plastic bag. The patient is seen within the next week in the clinic. The drains are removed if their output has been under 10 mL/d for a period of at least 2 to 3 consecutive days. If the fistula persists several weeks after discharge, we obtain a fistulagram and at that time replace the original drain with a red rubber catheter (Fig. 9.2). Occasionally, the tip of the original drain has migrated inside the lumen of the bowel. If this is the case, the replacement tube is positioned more superficially. This will hasten closure of the fistula, and the drain can be removed. If a low-output fistula (<50 mL/d) persists several weeks after drain exchange, rather than immediately removing the drain, it is backed out by 3 to 4 cm each week, so the fistula track can heal behind the drain. Using this strategy, we have never had to reoperate on a patient for a postoperative fistula after a PD.

The use of somatostatin for the prevention or treatment of postoperative pancreatic fistulas has been examined. Overall, it does not decrease fistula development, hasten its closure, or alter its morbidity. Somatostatin does decrease the fistula volume, which can help with management of electrolyte deficiencies, nutritional status, and skin breakdown in high-output fistulas. Short-acting somatostatin is administered as 100 μg subcutaneously three times per day; the long-acting variety, which is effective for 1 month, is preferred.

If a fistula persists for 2 to 3 months in patients who undergo distal pancreatectomy, despite drain exchange as described above, endoscopic retrograde cholangiopancreatography (ERCP) and a pancreatic duct stent are indicated. The ERCP can confirm the site of the leak and identify any downstream ductal strictures that may contribute to the persistence of the fistula. Even without a stricture, a stent in the main pancreatic duct that traverses the duodenal papilla decreases the pressure in the duct, which likely hastens fistula closure. To avoid stent-related complications (migration, erosion, infection, stricture formation, etc.), the stent must be removed within 2 months at most.

If, despite all of these measures, the pancreatic fistula does not close after at least 6 months, then surgical internal drainage may be indicated. A fistulojejunostomy is created with a Roux-en-Y jejunal limb sewn to the fistulous tract as close to the pancreas as possible.

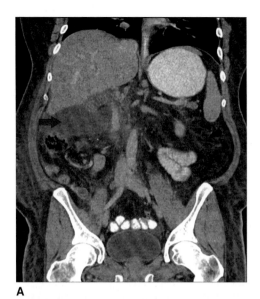

A

B

FIGURE 9.1 Postoperative pancreatic fistula managed with a percutaneous drain. **A.** CT scan (coronal views) taken on postoperative day 6 after a pylorus-preserving Whipple resection for a duodenal cancer reveals a posterior leak from the pancreaticojejunostomy (*arrow* highlights intra-abdominal fluid collection). **B.** Repeat CT scan obtained 5 days after a percutaneous drainage catheter was placed reveals complete resolution of the collection and the tip of the radiology drain (*arrow*).

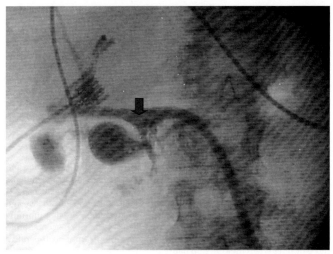

FIGURE 9.2 "Tubogram" reveals presence of pancreatic fistula. A tubogram obtained through a 16-Fr red rubber catheter 3 weeks after a pylorus-preserving pancreatoduodenectomy reveals contrast filling the jejunum at the level of the pancreaticojejunostomy (*arrow*), confirming the presence of a pancreatic fistula.

For nutritional support, patients with pancreatic fistulas should not be kept NPO but allowed to eat a regular diet. Studies have shown that enteric intake is associated with a higher rate of fistula closure. Serum albumin levels should be kept at greater than 3 to 3.5 g/dL. Occasionally, supplemental calories with TPN are required as an adjunct to oral intake to reach that nutritional goal. This is the case particularly in patients with nausea and ileus, which can accompany fistulas and may diminish patients' appetites. Loss of pancreatic exocrine secretions may also be associated with electrolyte imbalances, as the fluid is rich in bicarbonate and other essential electrolytes. Serum electrolyte levels should be routinely monitored in patients in the hospital and after discharge.

DELAYED GASTRIC EMPTYING

Definition and Incidence
DGE is a common complication after PD. It is defined as high nasogastric (NG) tube output in the postoperative setting requiring that the tube be left in place for 10 or more postoperative days, emesis after NG tube removal necessitating replacement of the tube, or failure to progress to a regular diet without the use of prokinetics. DGE is not usually a serious event, but it does prolong hospital stay, temporarily worsens quality of life, and can occasionally lead to additional invasive procedures.

It is difficult to identify the incidence of DGE after PD, as the definition in the literature is quite variable. Randomized trials cite a rate from 0% to 57%, with an overall mean incidence of 15%. The International Study Group on Pancreatic Surgery (ISGPS) published a complex consensus definition in 2007, to standardize its meaning and enable the comparison of new approaches aiming to reduce the rate of DGE.

The etiology of DGE is uncertain. Potential causes include decreased plasma motilin concentrations due to duodenal resection, extended lymph node dissection along the hepatic artery with disruption of vagal and sympathetic innervation to the antropyloric region, relative devascularization or denervation of the pylorus after pylorus-preserving PD (PPPD), anastomotic disruption at the pancreaticojejunostomy, and transient pancreatitis.

The issue of whether DGE is more common after PPPD than standard PD has been debated. The results of studies are mixed, with rates of DGE higher for PPPD in some studies and in PD in others. It is now generally accepted that both operations are equivalent. The routine administration of postoperative prokinetics to reduce the rate of DGE (e.g., erythromycin or metoclopramide) has also not shown benefit. There is evidence that an antecolic duodenojejunostomy (vs. retrocolic) after a PPPD lowers the rate of DGE.

Treatment

Our management of patients with DGE aims to minimize patient burden and has led to universal cure of the condition with only a small minority of patients requiring an additional intervention after surgery. We routinely place an NG tube at the time of surgery, after the patient is under general anesthesia, and leave it to intermittent suction overnight. It is removed on the first morning after surgery unless the output is extremely high (>1 L), which occurs rarely. Patients with DGE usually do not experience symptoms until postoperative day 5 or later when they develop nausea, abdominal distension, or vomiting. An NG tube is reinserted in patients with moderate or severe abdominal distension, vomiting, or an enlarged stomach evident on CT scan. It is placed to intermittent suction and the amount of output recorded. Patients with DGE usually have a high daily volume (>1.5 L) of gastric or bilious output. A CT scan of the abdomen and pelvis with oral and intravenous contrast is obtained to determine the degree of gastric distension and to identify the presence of an early postoperative bowel obstruction or undrained intra-abdominal fluid collections. DGE may be associated with a pancreatic fistula, peripancreatic fluid collections, or an intra-abdominal abscess. The decision to obtain a CT scan is not dependent on the presence of an elevated white blood cell count or fever but rather on the patient's symptoms as previously described. If fluid collections are present on the CT scan, and an infection is suspected, ultrasound- or CT-guided percutaneous drainage is performed. DGE associated with undrained and infected fluid collections usually resolves once the fluid has been drained. If the diagnosis of DGE is still unclear after the CT scan, an upper gastrointestinal (UGI) contrast series is obtained. This confirms delayed emptying of contrast from the stomach.

Once the diagnosis of DGE is suspected, patients are kept NPO. The NG tube decompresses the stomach, which probably hastens its functional recovery. It is left in place at least for 2 to 3 days until the output is minimal and the patient can handle his or her own gastric and salivary secretions. Occasionally, a trial of the NG tube to gravity may be useful.

A promotility agent, usually intravenous metoclopramide, is started immediately after DGE is diagnosed and a bowel obstruction has been excluded. Because metoclopramide is associated with numerous side effects, particularly tardive dyskinesia in elderly patients, all patients should be closely observed during its administration. If it is needed, erythromycin is an alternate promotility agent that binds motilin receptors and may be effective as well. Patients can be transitioned from intravenous metoclopramide or erythromycin to an oral form once their NG tube has been removed.

A peripherally inserted central catheter (PICC) line is placed early after diagnosis, particularly in those patients in whom DGE is predicted to last more than a few days. In these patients, TPN is begun and rapidly compressed to infuse over a 12-hour period. Home health nursing is arranged to assist in home TPN care. Patients are discharged on TPN and a promotility agent and allowed to slowly advance their diet at home. They are seen in the outpatient clinic on a weekly basis until the DGE resolves. Using this strategy, we have found that almost all cases completely resolve within several weeks.

In rare instances, patients have a more prolonged course of abdominal distention, nausea, or even intermittent vomiting that can require numerous hospital readmissions. At each admission, NG tube decompression is repeated. Occasionally, a percutaneous endoscopic gastrostomy tube has been placed to minimize the symptoms and allow for gastric decompression at home. In our experience, reoperation to deal with DGE has not been required.

POSTOPERATIVE HEMORRHAGE

Definition and Incidence

The International Study Group on Pancreatic Surgery (ISGPS) released a consensus definition on postpancreatectomy hemorrhage in 2007, which classifies it according to severity and the time of onset after surgery. The different severity classifications include types A, B, and C with the latter two involving major hemorrhage with a hemoglobin drop of greater than 3 g/dL. "Early postoperative hemorrhage" occurs within the first 24 hours of surgery; "late hemorrhage" occurs after 24 hours. Studies using these definitions cite an incidence of postoperative hemorrhage at 3%.

Prior to the improvement of endoscopic and interventional radiographic angiography techniques, post–pancreatic surgery hemorrhage (PPH) was associated with an overall mortality rate of 50%. Mortality was even higher in those patients presenting 72 or more hours after surgery. The greatest risk of late PPH occurs in patients who develop postoperative pancreatic fistulas from a nonhealing pancreaticojejunostomy anastomosis. Often, these patients also develop vascular abnormalities (e.g., pseudoaneurysms) that further worsen the outcome. The observation that mortality rates have decreased with the development of improved nonoperative techniques has led to the overall goal of avoiding repeat surgery in patients with late hemorrhage. This treatment strategy is in contrast to that for patients with early postoperative hemorrhage, who should generally undergo prompt operative reexploration.

Treatment

Postoperative hemorrhage should be suspected in patients whose hemoglobin decreases by more than 3 g/dL over the first postoperative day or those who develop systemic evidence of hypovolemia and bleeding. Once suspected, resuscitative treatment should be initiated rapidly and urgent steps taken to determine the source of the bleeding, which is either extra- or intraluminal (i.e., within or outside of the intestinal tract). Almost all bleeding within the first 24 to 48 hours is from an extraluminal source and is often due to a technical error during the operation. Nevertheless, the coagulation profile is checked to ensure that there is no evidence of synthetic liver dysfunction, manifested by a high prothrombin time (PT). If the coagulation parameters are abnormal, fresh frozen plasma is promptly administered to correct the deficit. Patients who have had prolonged biliary obstruction and high preoperative bilirubin may also have elevated PT levels due to vitamin K malabsorption and deficiency. They should be given intravenous vitamin K if their PT levels are elevated. If the platelet count is less than 50,000 per dL, platelets should be transfused. However, the surgeon should have a low threshold for return to the operating room for exploration, when most patients will be found to have a correctable source of bleeding. Figure 9.3 illustrates the potential bleeding sources.

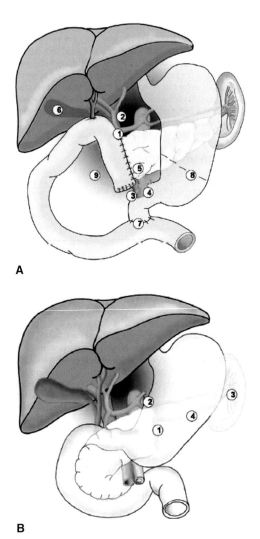

FIGURE 9.3 Common sites of bleeding after **(A)** pancreaticoduodenectomy or **(B)** distal pancreatectomy. (From Wente MN, Veit JA, Bassi C, et al. Postpancreatectomy hemorrhage (PPH): an International Study Group of Pancreatic Surgery (ISGPS) definition. *Surgery* 2007;142(1):20–5. PMID: 17629996.)

Late PPH (>24 hours after surgery) can occur over a long time span that extends to weeks or even months postoperatively. Therefore, it is important for the surgeon to be aware of this possibility and to educate the patients as to the signs and symptoms, since most patients are at home when it occurs. Unlike early PPH, which is almost always extraluminal, late PPH often is intraluminal, although bleeding of either type can occur. Patients with intraluminal hemorrhage present like those with UGI bleeding; they experience hematemesis or melena. The most likely sources are the three surgical anastomoses, and the duodenojejunostomy is the most frequent. An NG tube is inserted to verify that blood is in the stomach. If it is present, a UGI endoscopy is performed for both diagnostic and therapeutic purposes. If the bleeding source is identified, cautery is applied or a clip is placed. Patients must still be closely monitored for the ensuing 48 hours. If the source is not identified, or if the suspected site of bleeding is an extraluminal site, the next step is to employ selective angiography both to identify the bleeding site and to stop the bleeding via various interventional angiographic techniques. Selective angiograms of the celiac axis and superior mesenteric arteries are performed (Fig. 9.4). As illustrated in Figure 9.3, the most common sources of bleeding are the gastroduodenal artery and transverse pancreatic arcades adjacent to the pancreaticojejunostomy anastomosis.

In rare instances, late PPH cannot be controlled via endoscopic or angiographic techniques. If this is the case, the patient should be operated upon urgently. If the source of bleeding is the pancreaticojejunostomy and there is an associated anastomotic dehiscence, the anastomosis may also need to be addressed. This can be done with placement of drainage catheters, reinforcement of the anastomosis with additional sutures, or additional pancreatic resection. However, it should be stressed that surgery for late bleeding is required infrequently today, when the patient is being managed in a "center of excellence" where a skilled multidisciplinary group is available. Reoperative surgery in this setting is still associated with an extremely high mortality rate.

BILIARY FISTULA

Bile leaks from the choledochal/hepaticojejunal anastomosis occur in 1% to 2% of patients undergoing PD and are heralded by the appearance of bile in the drain fluid. If this occurs, the drain should be left in place until the leak stops. If bile is still present when the patient is ready for discharge, they can go home with the drain in place. It can be removed in the office when there is no longer any bile present. If there is no evidence of a bile leak, the biliary drain is removed the day after the patient begins oral intake. Because the PJ anastomosis is close to the bile duct anastomosis, pancreatic fistula fluid can also be tinged with bile. Because a fistula from either site is managed in a similar way, it may not be necessary to determine its origin with certainty. If this is required, a contrast injection through the drain tube can resolve the question. Management of a high-volume (>200 mL/d) bile leak is more complex, often requiring percutaneous transhepatic biliary stent placement.

EXOCRINE AND ENDOCRINE INSUFFICIENCY

The incidence of symptomatic exocrine insufficiency after pancreatic surgery depends on the amount of parenchyma resected, the function of the pancreas that remains, and the adequacy of mixing of the food with pancreatic enzymes and bile. The first two indices can be estimated with some degree of confidence and the last cannot. Thus, we council our patients that if at least 20% of a normal pancreas remains, it should be enough to provide adequate digestive (and endocrine) activity. This is a reliable prediction for patients who will undergo a distal pancreatectomy, including removal of the entire body and tail of gland, but it is less so for patients who will undergo a pancreatoduodenectomy. To some degree, this is because many patients with pancreatic tumors that have obstructed the main pancreatic duct may have obstructive chronic pancreatitis in the remnant pancreas, leading to decreased exocrine function. But it is mostly due to the uncertainty about how well ingested food will mix with the pancreatic secretions and

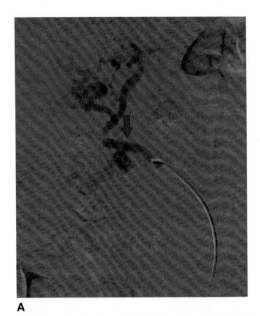

A

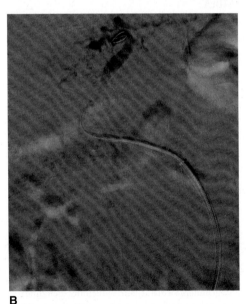

B

FIGURE 9.4 Gastroduodenal artery pseudoaneurysm treated angiographically. **A.** A superior mesenteric artery angiogram reveals a gastroduodenal artery pseudoaneurysm from a completely replaced hepatic artery (*arrow*). **B.** A 5 × 50 Viabahn stent placed across the pseudoaneurysm with complete occlusion of the bleeding site maintaining perfusion to the common hepatic artery distal to the pseudoaneurysm.

bile in the small intestine. This is true for both a standard PD as well as the pylorus-preserving variety; studies show that after either operation, gastric emptying may be normal or faster or slower than normal. So the amount of pancreatic enzymes secreted by the remnant pancreas may be adequate, but if those enzymes do not mix well with the food, they cannot be effective.

It is likely that the majority of patients have some degree of malabsorption and steatorrhea (i.e., >7% excretion of ingested fat) after any major pancreatic resection. We do not treat them unless there are symptoms of weight loss or inability to gain weight, diarrhea, oily stools, and/or abdominal bloating. Treatment consists of supplemental enzymes with at least 30,000 IU of lipase taken with each meal; half that amount should be taken with snacks. Only rarely does fat intake need to be limited. All of our PD patients also are given proton pump inhibitors permanently to minimize the likelihood of marginal ulceration. It is important to make certain that these are given as well to those patients who have had other types of pancreatic resection and who require pancreatic enzymes, especially if a non-enteric preparation is used. This is because gastric acid can denature the ingested enzymes, which makes them ineffective. If patients continue to be symptomatic, they are referred to a gastroenterologist with experience in the treatment of pancreatic exocrine insufficiency.

The incidence of endocrine insufficiency (type I diabetes mellitus, DM) depends mostly on the amount of pancreatic parenchyma removed. Its incidence generally parallels the occurrence of pancreatic exocrine insufficiency for each specific pancreatic operation. The maintenance of gastroduodenal continuity also may be an important factor for the development of DM because it maintains neurohumoral connections between the stomach, the duodenum, and the pancreas. Thus, the development of diabetes appears to be less likely after duodenum-preserving pancreatic resections done for chronic pancreatitis (Beger, Frey), compared to a pylorus-preserving PD.

Patients with preexisting DM can experience worsening of their disease with pancreatic resections. Early in the postoperative period after any type of major surgery including pancreatic resection, blood sugars are generally elevated. Later, if diabetes is suspected after patients resume a diet, we request an endocrinology and dietary consult, and subsequent management of DM is supported by those individuals and, eventually, by the patient's internist. Patients should also be made aware of the signs/symptoms of hypoglycemia, since with the resection of alpha islet cell mass and less available glucagon, the DM may be more brittle than usual.

Suggested Readings

Bassi C, Dervenis C, Butturini G, et al. Postoperative pancreatic fistula: an international study group (ISGPF) definition. *Surgery* 2005;138(1):8–13. PMID: 16003309.

Correa-Gallego C, Brennan MF, D'Angelica MI, et al. Contemporary experience with postpancreatectomy hemorrhage: results of 1,122 patients resected between 2006 and 2011. *J Am Coll Surg* 2012;215(5):616–621. PMID: 22921325.

Kazanjian KK, Hines OJ, Eibl G, et al. Management of pancreatic fistulas after pancreaticoduodenectomy: results in 437 consecutive patients. *Arch Surg* 2005;140(9):849–854; discussion 854–856. PMID: 16172293.

Wente MN, Bassi C, Dervenis C, et al. Delayed gastric emptying (DGE) after pancreatic surgery: a suggested definition by the International Study Group of Pancreatic Surgery (ISGPS). *Surgery* 2007;142(5):761–768. PMID: 17981197.

Wente MN, Veit JA, Bassi C, et al. Postpancreatectomy hemorrhage (PPH): an International Study Group of Pancreatic Surgery (ISGPS) definition. *Surgery* 2007; 142(1):20–25. PMID: 17629996.

Yekebas EF, Wolfram L, Cataldegirmen G, et al. Postpancreatectomy hemorrhage: diagnosis and treatment: an analysis in 1669 consecutive pancreatic resections. *Ann Surg* 2007;246(2):269–280. PMID: 17667506.

SECTION II

Liver

10 | Liver Anatomy, Physiology, and Preoperative Evaluation

Ching-Wei D. Tzeng and Jean-Nicolas Vauthey

INTRODUCTION

Surgical resection remains the first-line treatment of appropriately selected patients with primary and metastatic liver cancer. Until the last two decades, hepatectomies were considered operations of prohibitive risk with frequent hemorrhagic events and high rates of complications and death. Even as surgeons have pushed the limits with resectability criteria, the overall mortality rate has fallen significantly from 10–20% to around 2.5% nationally. This mortality decrease is the result of more advanced surgical techniques, better patient selection and risk stratification, optimization of the future liver remnant (FLR) (including the use of portal vein embolization [PVE] and limiting preoperative chemotherapy), multidisciplinary treatment strategies, and better diagnostic and therapeutic capabilities to rescue patients after complications. This chapter focuses on the preoperative considerations a surgeon must evaluate before performing a hepatic resection.

ANATOMY

In 1888, Rex described the anatomy of the portal vein and the main plane dividing the left and right liver along the middle hepatic vein. His detailed illustrations based on embryology set the stage for modern segmental anatomy (Fig. 10.1). In 1954, Couinaud divided the liver into four sectors based on the right, middle, and left fissures, which follow the vertical planes of the three hepatic veins (Fig. 10.2). They include the right posterior (segments VI + VII), right anterior (segments V + VIII), left medial (segments III and IV), and left lateral (segment II) sectors. The transverse scissura follows the plane of the portal vein, which then divides the sectors into each segment.

The International Hepatopancreatobiliary Association (IHPBA) consensus Brisbane (2000) classification for liver surgery terminology is now widely adopted, with the liver divided into sections rather than sectors. The main difference is that segments II and III now belong together as the left lateral section with segment IV remaining as the medial segment without segment III (Fig. 10.3). In an effort to standardize terminology among surgeons and surgical literature, the terms right/left lobectomy, bilobar, and trisegmentectomy are now mostly replaced with the terms right/left hepatectomy, bilateral, trisectionectomy, sectionectomy, and segmentectomy. Detailed knowledge of the segmental and vascular anatomy is critical to preoperatively planning the amount of liver parenchyma that will need to be resected and how much FLR will remain after resection. Precise terminology is critical for communication among surgeons, radiologists, and the multidisciplinary team.

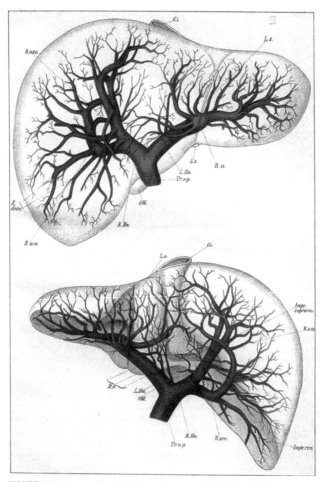

FIGURE 10.1 Intrahepatic portal vein anatomy as depicted by Rex in 1888.

PHYSIOLOGY

For safe resection, the liver parenchyma must have sufficient size, adequate synthetic function, unimpaired biliary drainage and perfusion, and sufficient regenerative capacity. A global assessment of parenchymal quality is important to determine the functional ability of the liver to tolerate resection and to guide the surgeon in choosing a safe maximum volume that can be resected. This can involve the patient's history, physical exam, biochemical tests, and radiologic imaging.

For patients with cirrhosis, the Child-Pugh score classifies the severity of chronic liver disease. This score incorporates albumin, ascites, bilirubin encephalopathy, and international normalized ratio (INR) and, by using a scoring system, stratifies three classes of mortality risk (Table 10.1). Usually, only Child-Pugh A patients are considered operable because the

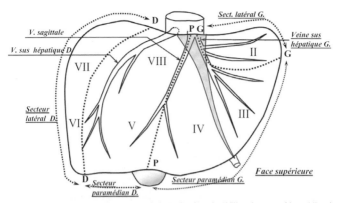

FIGURE 10.2 Liver segments numbered clockwise from I to VIII and sectors (dotted lines) along the planes of the three hepatic veins as described by Couinaud. (Adapted from Couinaud C. Lobes et segments hepatiques: notes sur l'architecture anatomiques et chirurgicale du foie. *Presse Med* 1954;6(2):709–712.)

pathophysiologic consequences of cirrhosis are minimal, and thus they are described as "compensated." Some surgeons will operate on Child-Pugh B patients but with a known increased perioperative risk. The operative mortality of Child-Pugh C patients can approach 50% even for "minor" general surgery operations such as umbilical hernia repair and cholecystectomy. Child-Pugh C patients cannot tolerate any liver resection. The best treatment for hepatocellular carcinoma (HCC) in patients with Child-Pugh B and C cirrhosis is liver transplantation if they qualify.

An alternative system for grading cirrhosis is the Model for End-Stage Liver Disease (MELD), which consists of bilirubin, creatinine, INR, and liver disease etiology, in a formula originally created to predict 3-month mortality after a transjugular intrahepatic portosystemic shunt (TIPS) procedure and validated for predicting mortality in hospitalized and ambulatory patients awaiting liver transplant. As an alternative to Child-Pugh score, MELD score can be used to predict perioperative and long-term mortality after resection of HCC. While patients with high MELD scores (≥9) are inoperable for surgical procedures other than transplant, those with MELD scores less than 9 can be considered for hepatectomy.

While these rules of thumb are easy to follow if a diagnosis of cirrhosis already exists, the real clinical problem occurs when chronic liver disease is unrecognized until surgical exploration. Thus, patients should be carefully screened preoperatively for cirrhosis and portal hypertension based on history (jaundice, hepatitis, upper gastrointestinal [GI] bleeding, encephalopathy), physical examination (skin varices or superficial venous collaterals, ascites, mental examination), serum laboratory tests (bilirubinemia, thrombocytopenia, anemia from bleeding), and imaging (ascites, splenomegaly, scalloping of the liver, left lateral section and caudate hypertrophy, intra-abdominal varices, and venous collaterals). In general, patients with a bilirubin greater than 2 mg/dL are not considered for resection. In patients who present with obstructive jaundice, resection is only considered after resolution of the jaundice using preoperative endoscopic or percutaneous biliary drainage.

Because there is a sliding scale of FLR volume minimums and liver quality, liver biopsy can be used to diagnose preexisting liver damage and

Extended right hepatectomy
or Right trisectionectomy

Right hepatectomy
or Right hemihepactectomy

Bisegmentectomy II + III
or Left lateral sectionectomy

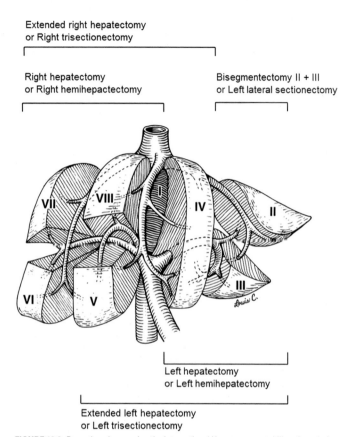

Left hepatectomy
or Left hemihepatectomy

Extended left hepatectomy
or Left trisectionectomy

FIGURE 10.3 Resection planes using the International Hepatopancreatobiliary Association (IHPBA) Consensus Brisbane (2000) classification for liver surgery. (Adapted from Abdalla EK, Denys A, et al. Total and segmental liver volume variations: implications for liver surgery. *Surgery* 2004;135(4):404–410.)

TABLE 10.1	Child-Pugh score for cirrhosis			
	1 point	**2 points**	**3 points**	**Class**
Albumin (g/dL)	>3.5	2.8–3.5	<2.8	A: 5–6 points
Ascites	None	Yes, controlled	Yes, refractory	B: 7–9 points
				C: 10–15 points
Bilirubin (mg/dL)	<2	2–3	>3	
Encephalopathy	None	Grade I–II (controlled)	Grade III–IV (refractory)	
INR	<1.7	1.71–2.20	>2.20	

INR, international normalized ratio.
From Child CG, *The liver and portal hypertension*. Philadelphia, PA: Saunders, 1964.

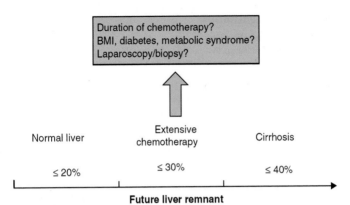

Duration of chemotherapy?
BMI, diabetes, metabolic syndrome?
Laparoscopy/biopsy?

Normal liver   Extensive   Cirrhosis
                    chemotherapy

≤ 20%   ≤ 30%   ≤ 40%

Future liver remnant

FIGURE 10.4 Diagram of the future liver remnant required for hepatectomy depending on the parenchymal quality and any preexisting liver injury. (BMI, body mass index).

evaluate whether this damage is acute, subacute, or chronic in nature (Fig. 10.4). Preoperatively, this can be easily done percutaneously. Or, if diagnostic laparoscopy is being performed for staging or for another minor procedure, a wedge biopsy can be done simultaneously. However, as simple as a biopsy may seem, two major problems must be recognized. First, the distribution of parenchymal diseases, such as fibrosis, steatosis, and chemotherapy-associated liver injury (CALI) such as sinusoidal obstruction syndrome (SOS) and steatohepatitis (SH), is heterogeneous, and thus a small liver biopsy can be associated with false-negative results. Secondly, these histopathologic diagnoses do not accurately predict postresection liver function, FLR regenerative capacity, and protection from postoperative hepatic insufficiency (PHI). Thus, while a positive liver biopsy may be helpful, caution should still be exercised if the biopsy is "normal" but the liver looks clinically damaged. Some parenchymal changes such as fatty liver can be grossly evaluated with cross-sectional imaging by comparing the tissue perfusion and attenuation to that of the spleen and abdominal fat. Many cirrhotic changes from portal hypertension are also readily apparent on imaging as aforementioned. Current work is being done to more precisely correlate computed tomography (CT) and magnetic resonance imaging (MRI) findings with pathologic parenchymal changes.

Indocyanine green retention rate at 15 minutes (ICG R15) is used as a global measure of liver function. In this test, faster clearance (lower retention percentage at 15 minutes) implies better liver function and drainage. Used extensively in East Asia but less so in North and South America and Europe, a decision tree known as the Makuuchi criteria is used to evaluate livers with possible chronic disease before minor hepatectomy (usually for HCC). The qualitative cutoff values of ICG R15 may be less helpful in stratifying livers for major hepatectomy when compared to regeneration criteria such as those provided by PVE (see below). ICG R15 cutoffs for wedge resection and segmentectomy are 30% to 39% and 20% to 29%, respectively. Left hepatectomy or sectionectomy requires 10% to 19% retention or less. Finally, right or extended hepatectomy is considered only if ICG R15 is less than 10%. An important initial consideration in applying these criteria is that patients with ascites and/or elevated bilirubin (> 2 mg/dL) do not qualify for any type of resection irrespective of the ICG cutoffs.

PREOPERATIVE EVALUATION

Risk Factors for Complications

Complications specific to liver surgery include bleeding (both intraoperative and early postoperative), bile leak, and postoperative hepatic insufficiency (PHI or liver failure) with PHI-related mortality. The current authors previously defined PHI as a peak total bilirubin greater than 7 mg/dL, which has a sensitivity and specificity of greater than 93% and an odds ratio of 10.8 for predicting 90-day mortality. Acute PHI often leads to an irreparable slide toward liver failure–related mortality that continues well past 30 days. In regard to measuring surgical outcomes, one-third of posthepatectomy deaths occur between 30 and 90 days, so typical short-term metrics fail to fully capture late liver-related mortalities.

Predictors of major complications can be divided into three categories—medical comorbidities, laboratory abnormalities, and perioperative risk factors (including extent of hepatectomy). These parameters include low albumin, smoking, American Society of Anesthesiologists (ASA) class, elevated alkaline phosphatase, elevated partial thromboplastin time (PTT), extent of hepatectomy, prolonged operative time, and intraoperative or postoperative transfusions. The last three factors are associated with each other, and thus, surgeons should be cautious with patient selection when pairing major simultaneous operations with major hepatectomies. While not every risk factor is reversible, many are potentially modifiable in the preoperative period through optimization of medical issues and planning operations of lesser magnitude when oncologically practical.

Initial Assessment

The initial preoperative assessment of a patient requiring a liver resection takes into account three major factors—patient operability (performance status and comorbidities), liver quality (global function), and tumor extent (balance of oncologic resectability and FLR). An irreversible or unmodifiable issue with the patient or the liver precludes liver resection. The risks of liver resection and PHI are relatively unique, because the liver is the only abdominal visceral organ without which a patient cannot survive. Thus, unless a transplant is planned, enough functional parenchyma must be left behind, or the patient will inevitably die from liver failure.

Patient Operability

The term "operability" describes patient, not tumor, factors. Patients can be operable, inoperable, or borderline operable if they have potentially reversible comorbidities. Operability is dependent on a patient's functional capacity (performance status) and underlying medical comorbidities. If both are good, then the patient is operable. If either is irreversibly poor, then the patient is inoperable. If functional or medical issues are potentially reversible, then the patient is considered borderline operable. The fact that grading performance status is part of the National Comprehensive Cancer Network (NCCN) preoperative assessment for hepatocellular carcinoma (HCC) highlights the importance of assessing patient operability. With aggressive prehabilitation, nutritional counseling, and/or medical optimization, a borderline operable patient may become an operable surgical candidate and has the potential to enjoy the same survival benefit from resection as a patient who was initially operable. If a patient is undergoing preoperative chemotherapy, this time period offers an opportunity to address the aforementioned issues. Even if preoperative therapy is not considered or not indicated, taking appropriate time to optimize patient physiology before surgery will not only decrease surgical complications but will also improve the clinical rescue rate of patients after major complications and decrease the postcomplication mortality rate.

Assessment and Optimization of Future Liver Remnant

The FLR is the predicted volume of remaining liver after resection. Sufficient size, synthetic function, biliary drainage, perfusion, and regenerative capacity are essential to avoid both early and late PHI. Evaluating the FLR's volume is currently the most reliable approach to predict outcomes for patients who are candidates for major resection. Several methods for such evaluation have been described. At the University of Texas MD Anderson Cancer Center (MDACC), the estimated total liver volume (TLV) is calculated using a formula that relies on the linear correlation between the TLV and body surface area (BSA): TLV (in cm^3) = $-794.41 + 1,267.28 \times BSA$ (m^2). The "standardized" FLR is then calculated as the ratio of the predicted FLR volume to the standardized TLV.

In a series of 301 patients without hepatic injury or chronic liver disease undergoing extended right hepatectomy, a standardized FLR of less than 20% was a risk factor for PHI and 90-day postoperative mortality. Generally, the required minimum standardized FLR is greater than 20% for normal livers, greater than 30% for livers with limited parenchymal injury (e.g., extended duration chemotherapy), and greater than 40% for permanently damaged livers (e.g., cirrhosis, Fig. 10.4). Because chemotherapy is used in the majority of cases of colorectal liver metastases (CLM) and often several months of chemotherapy have already been given before the patient sees a liver surgeon, it is imperative that a liver surgeon understands the side effects of oxaliplatin and irinotecan, which, along with 5-fluorouracil, have been the backbone of chemotherapy regimens for CLM since the early 2000s (Table 10.2).

With increased CT volumetry availability, "eyeballing" a CT scan to estimate FLR is highly discouraged. Even with no liver damage, up to 75% of patients at initial presentation are anatomically too small for an extended right hepatectomy based on the volume of segments II + III. Preoperative PVE allows a functional stress test to observe the regenerative capacity of the FLR before, rather than after, a hepatectomy. During a brief 5 weeks between PVE and hepatectomy, surgeons can evaluate the degree of hypertrophy (DH; needs to be > 5%) and the kinetic growth rate (KGR = DH divided by time in weeks). Patients with a KGR less than 2% may be spared hepatectomies of excessive extent that would leave inadequate FLR. Not all PVEs result in adequate hypertrophy, and one putative criticism of PVE is inadequate hypertrophy preoperatively. However, with PVE

TABLE 10.2	Chemotherapy-Associated Liver Injury Characteristics	
Agent	**Liver Changes**	**Clinical Sequelae**
Oxaliplatin	• Sinusoidal dilation • Sinusoidal obstructive syndrome (SOS) • Microvascular damage	• Increased perioperative transfusions with >6 mo of preoperative chemotherapy
Irinotecan	• Steatosis • Steatohepatitis	• Increased complications • Increased overall 90-d mortality (15%) and liver failure–related mortality (6%)

of the right portal vein and segment IV with the combined use of spherical microspheres and coils, an FLR increase of 69% has been documented in the hands of experienced interventional radiologists.

Tumor Extent and Resectability

Besides patient operability, whether a liver tumor can be resected is dependent upon two other major factors—technical resectability and oncologic feasibility. Technical resectability is the ability to surgically remove all liver tumors with R0 (negative microscopic) margins while leaving adequate FLR. Adequate FLR must have regenerative capacity and consist of at least two functional contiguous liver segments with biliary drainage and vascular inflow/outflow. Again, tumor resectability should be differentiated from patient operability, which is the patient's physiologic and medical ability to undergo and recover from major abdominal surgery.

Oncologically, resectability is determined by the tumor biology of the cancer type and the individual patient. For example, while extrahepatic disease is a contraindication for resection in primary liver cancer, patients with limited extrahepatic disease in controllable sites (e.g., small lung metastases or regional lymph nodes) can still benefit from hepatectomy for CLM. However, because these patients are biologically at higher risk of recurrence, they need perioperative chemotherapy. Even patients with limited progression of preexisting CLM while on preoperative chemotherapy, but whose lesions remain anatomically resectable, should undergo resection. However, patients who develop new lesions or interval extrahepatic disease while on preoperative chemotherapy should not undergo surgery until the systemic disease is controlled.

Preoperative Planning with Radiographic Imaging

Four major imaging options are used for liver tumors—ultrasound (US), CT, MRI, and positron emission tomography/CT (PET/CT). US is inexpensive and reliable, but has been replaced by cross-sectional imaging due to limited image reproduction, operator variability, and decreased ability to detect small lesions. However, intraoperative US (IOUS) remains a critically important surgical tool, because it can find additional tumors not seen on preoperative cross-sectional imaging in up to 10% of patients, even with use of improved high-resolution CT and MRI. The greatest value of IOUS is in guiding the resection in relation to hepatic vascular anatomy and directing parenchymal transection to balance optimal tumor margins with maximal FLR preservation.

The current standard for preoperative planning is high-resolution, contrast-enhanced multidetector CT of the chest, abdomen, and pelvis. For enhanced liver characterization, MRI abdomen and pelvis with chest CT is an alternative. CT is generally more useful than MRI for comprehensive imaging for staging, including chest and other abdominal structures. In general, CLM are hypovascular and more prominent in the portovenous phase as hypodense lesions. On the other hand, HCC are hypervascular on the arterial phase with washout on delayed images. Although suboptimal for general abdominal and chest surveillance, MRI is useful for diagnosis and staging of liver tumor burden. Using multiple and newer contrast agents and dynamic phases, high-resolution (3-tesla) MRI offers increased lesion characterization over CT, especially for subcentimeter indeterminate lesions. If preoperative chemotherapy is administered, whichever modality was chosen pretreatment should be repeated after preoperative treatment and before liver resection for accurate FLR assessment.

There has been a recent dramatic increase in the use of PET/CT to identify areas of increased metabolic activity, which are often presumed to be metastases in patients with cancer. Unfortunately, PET can also be nonspecific, and the matched noncontrast CT adds little information for equivocal areas, prompting additional workup. At MDACC, PET/CT is reserved for the detection of occult extrahepatic disease in patients with a high index of suspicion for metastatic disease and equivocal cross-sectional imaging (e.g., elevated carcinoembryonic antigen [CEA] with normal CT) when detection would change the planned treatment strategy.

Percutaneous needle biopsies of suspected liver tumors are unnecessary when imaging identifies new lesions with characteristic imaging features for metastases or primary liver cancer. Needle biopsy may be appropriate when a benign lesion is suspected and cannot be delineated noninvasively with MRI and again importantly, only if the treatment plan would change based on the result.

Radiographic evaluation of treatment response has prognostic value and frequently determines resectability. Although traditionally measured by Response Evaluation Criteria in Solid Tumors (RECIST) and modified RECIST criteria, change in tumor diameter may not provide the best prognostic information. Besides using disease-free interval and tumor factors from published clinical risk scores, biologic selection can be accomplished by stratifying patients by the morphologic response on CT after preoperative treatment for CLM. The morphologic response did not correlate with size-based RECIST measurements, and it was better than RECIST at predicting major pathologic response. When tumors change from heterogeneous consistency and irregular borders to homogenous density, clearly demarcated borders, and no enhancement, this pattern strongly correlates with pathologic response, margin control, and survival (Fig. 10.5). Suboptimal morphologic response is an independent predictor of worse overall survival and thus may offer the surgeon and the patient important prognostic information when counseling about the potential risks versus benefits of hepatectomy. Figure 10.5 details the optimal 1 morphologic response seen in a patient who underwent preoperative chemotherapy for a very large liver metastasis, which encased the right and middle hepatic veins. With such good morphologic response, undergoing the risk of an extended right hepatectomy made oncologic sense in that he was the type of patient who might benefit the most from resection. After PVE, he underwent a margin-negative extended right hepatectomy and is alive more than 5 years later.

PREOPERATIVE THERAPY AND DOWNSIZING

When patients present with anatomically unresectable CLM, the clinician should consider the ability to downsize their lesions to resectability criteria. Effective chemotherapy may achieve this goal in 10% to 20% of initially unresectable patients, and patients who make it to resection share survival rates far better than those associated with palliative chemotherapy with outcomes approaching that of patients with initially resectable CLM. To convert patients from unresectable to resectable, maximal tumor response is required (unlike the goal for preoperative chemotherapy for resectable lesions), frequently involving the addition of targeted agents. With these agents, the conversion rate from unresectability to resectability can be as high as 13% to 23%.

After downsizing with chemotherapy and targeted therapy, the surgical goal should be an R0 resection of all known sites of CLM, including known original sites of any lesions that disappeared with complete radiographic response. A recent "problem" due to improving efficacy of systemic chemotherapy, patients are sometimes presenting to the liver surgeon with

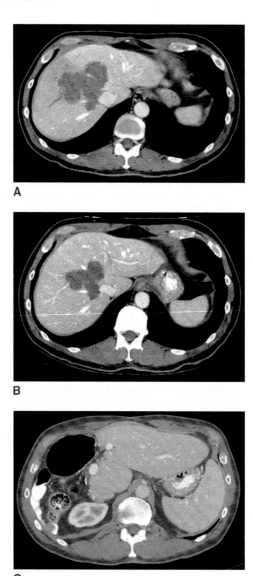

A

B

C

FIGURE 10.5 Optimal response to preoperative chemotherapy. Despite having a positive portal lymph node, this patient was alive with no evidence of disease at 5 years. He has an optimal morphologic (loss of enhancement and well-defined lesion) response during preoperative chemotherapy (from **A** to **B**). His postoperative scan revealed excellent hypertrophy after extended right hepatectomy following preoperative portal vein embolization (**C**).

complete radiographic response in small tumors. However, this does not mean there is complete pathologic response. Approximately 60% of "disappeared metastases" will recur if left unresected. One preoperative consideration when treating multiple metastases of different sizes is the need for fiducial marker placement by interventional radiology for tiny lesions so that if they disappear, the surgeon will know the original site to resect.

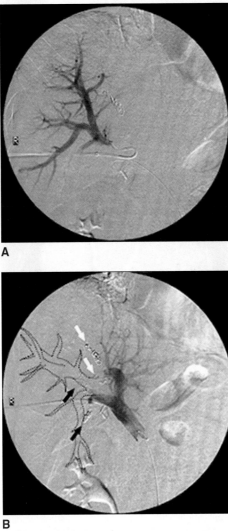

A

B

FIGURE 10.6 Preoperative portal vein embolization (PVE). Figure **(A)** shows preembolization flow to right portal vein branches. Figure **(B)** shows stasis of portal vein flow after embolization of the right portal vein and segment IV portal vein branches with microspheres and coils.

(*Continued*)

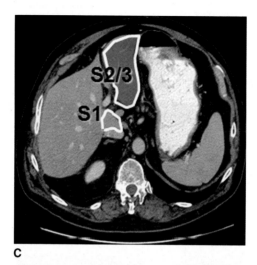

C

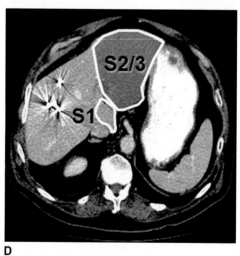

D

FIGURE 10.6 (Continued) Figures **(C)** and **(D)** show the resultant hypertrophy from pre- to postembolization.

Timing of Surgery and Treatment Sequencing Strategy

A key modifiable risk factor for posthepatectomy complications is the duration of preoperative chemotherapy, most often used for CLM. Extended-duration (4 months) chemotherapy only increases the risk of CALI and associated postoperative complications without improving the pathologic response. Thus, every patient with CLM who might be a candidate for surgery (including patients with "initially unresectable" CLM who have bilateral disease, small livers, or resectable extrahepatic disease) should be evaluated at diagnosis by a multidisciplinary team that includes a liver surgeon. The goal of chemotherapy for resectable lesions is not and should not be complete disappearance of the CLM. Further chemotherapy can be given after recovery from hepatectomy.

A second method of decreasing morbidity is treatment sequencing for synchronous CLM with intact primary colorectal cancer. The liver-first, or reverse, approach allows the cleaner operation to be done before resection of the primary tumor while removing the patient's metastatic disease. Used for patients with nonobstructing primary tumors, this is usually chosen for patients requiring preoperative chemotherapy and larger hepatic resections for CLM, which are the real life-limiting process (rather than the primary lesion) for the patient. Concerns about the morbidity of major colorectal operations, even proctectomies, staged after major hepatectomies should not preclude reverse approach sequencing.

Frequently, patients with extensive bilateral liver disease require two-stage hepatectomy. The first stage involves clearing the left liver of small-volume disease. The time in between stages is used for interval percutaneous PVE to grow the FLR (Fig. 10.6). If there will be a significant break in therapy, one or two rounds of chemotherapy can be given without any negative consequence on FLR hypertrophy. The second stage is often an extended right hepatectomy to clear the remaining tumor burden. While this staged sequencing is more time and resource consuming compared to single-stage extended hepatectomy with contralateral ablation or wedge resections, it provides a greater margin of safety for avoidance of PHI-related mortality. Figure 10.6 demonstrates the right portal venography before and after PVE with CT images before and after PVE-induced hypertrophy. With perioperative chemotherapy, two-stage hepatectomy ± PVE can result in prolonged 5-year overall survival of 51% (Fig. 10.7).

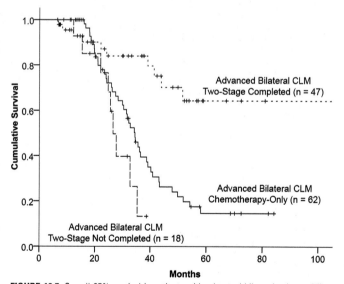

FIGURE 10.7 Overall 65% survival in patients with advanced bilateral colorectal liver metastases (median 6 metastases per patient) treated with chemotherapy and two-stage hepatectomy. This survival was achieved in a subset of patients with advanced metastatic disease by selecting patient candidate for surgery based a combination of response to chemotherapy and adequate regeneration from portal vein embolization. (Reproduced from Brouquet A, Abdalla EK, et al. High survival rate after two-stage resection of advanced colorectal liver metastases: response-based selection and complete resection define outcome. *J Clin Oncol* 2011;29(8):1083–1090.)

CONCLUSIONS

Over the past two decades, hepatectomy has evolved into a safe and effective therapy for a wide range of benign and malignant diseases. Postoperative complications may be related to patient factors, anatomic factors associated with resection extent, or technical factors that result in major intraoperative bleeding. Some patient-related factors (e.g., age, Child-Pugh class, and body mass index) cannot be modified preoperatively. Others can be reversed with prehabilitation and aggressive medical optimization to increase the rescue rate of expected complications. The FLR volume and the degree of hypertrophy after preoperative PVE are important predictors of outcome and can help select appropriate patients for major hepatectomies. Bleeding can be minimized with preoperative anatomic evaluation, image-guided resection, low central venous pressure fluid management, and judicious use of modern surgical instruments. Proper preoperative evaluation and surgical planning before hepatectomy can minimize surgical complications, PHI, and mortality.

Suggested Readings

Abdalla EK, Denys A, et al. Total and segmental liver volume variations: implications for liver surgery. *Surgery* 2004;135(4):404–410.

Adam R, Delvart V, et al. Rescue surgery for unresectable colorectal liver metastases downstaged by chemotherapy: a model to predict long-term survival. *Ann Surg* 2004;240(4):644–657.

Aloia T, Sebagh M, et al. Liver histology and surgical outcomes after preoperative chemotherapy with fluorouracil plus oxaliplatin in colorectal cancer liver metastases. *J Clin Oncol* 2006;24(31):4983–4990.

Aloia TA, Fahy BN, et al. Predicting poor outcome following hepatectomy: analysis of 2313 hepatectomies in the NSQIP database. *HPB (Oxford)* 2009;11(6):510–515.

Brouquet A, Abdalla EK, et al. High survival rate after two-stage resection of advanced colorectal liver metastases: response-based selection and complete resection define outcome. *J Clin Oncol* 2011;29(8):1083–1090.

Brouquet A, Mortenson MM, et al. Surgical strategies for synchronous colorectal liver metastases in 156 consecutive patients: classic, combined or reverse strategy? *J Am Coll Surg* 2010;210(6):934–941.

Child CG. *The liver and portal hypertension*. Philadelphia, PA: Saunders, 1964.

Chun YS, Vauthey JN, et al. Association of computed tomography morphologic criteria with pathologic response and survival in patients treated with bevacizumab for colorectal liver metastases. *JAMA* 2009;302(21):2338–2344.

Couinaud C. Lobes et segments hepatiques: notes sur l'architecture anatomiques et chirurgicale du foie. *Presse Med* 1954;62:709–712.

Giacchetti S, Itzhaki M, et al. Long-term survival of patients with unresectable colorectal cancer liver metastases following infusional chemotherapy with 5-fluorouracil, leucovorin, oxaliplatin and surgery. *Ann Oncol* 1999;10(6):663–669.

Kishi Y, Abdalla EK, et al. Three hundred and one consecutive extended right hepatectomies: evaluation of outcome based on systematic liver volumetry. *Ann Surg* 2009;250(4):540–548.

Kishi Y, Zorzi D, et al. Extended preoperative chemotherapy does not improve pathologic response and increases postoperative liver insufficiency after hepatic resection for colorectal liver metastases. *Ann Surg Oncol* 2010;17(11):2870–2876.

Kodama Y, Ng CS, et al. Comparison of CT methods for determining the fat content of the liver. *AJR Am J Roentgenol* 2007;188(5):1307–1312.

Kopetz S, Chang GJ, et al. Improved survival in metastatic colorectal cancer is associated with adoption of hepatic resection and improved chemotherapy. *J Clin Oncol* 2009;27(22):3677–3683.

Madoff DC, Abdalla EK, et al. Transhepatic ipsilateral right portal vein embolization extended to segment IV: improving hypertrophy and resection outcomes with spherical particles and coils. *J Vasc Interv Radiol* 2005;16(2 Pt 1):215–225.

Makuuchi M, Kosuge T, et al. Surgery for small liver cancers. *Semin Surg Oncol* 1993;9(4):298–304.

Mentha G, Majno PE, et al. Neoadjuvant chemotherapy and resection of advanced synchronous liver metastases before treatment of the colorectal primary. *Br J Surg* 2006;93(7):872–878.

Mullen JT, Ribero D, et al. Hepatic insufficiency and mortality in 1,059 noncirrhotic patients undergoing major hepatectomy. *J Am Coll Surg* 2007;204(5):854–862; discussion 862–854.

Rex H. Beitrage zur morphologie der saugerleber. *Morph Jahrb* 1888;14:517–616.

Ribero D, Abdalla EK, et al. Portal vein embolization before major hepatectomy and its effects on regeneration, resectability and outcome. *Br J Surg* 2007;94(11):1386–1394.

Rubbia-Brandt L, Audard V, et al. Severe hepatic sinusoidal obstruction associated with oxaliplatin-based chemotherapy in patients with metastatic colorectal cancer. *Ann Oncol* 2004;15(3):460–466.

Shindoh J, Loyer EM, et al. Optimal morphologic response to preoperative chemotherapy: an alternate outcome end point before resection of hepatic colorectal metastases. *J Clin Oncol* 2012;30(36):4566–4572.

Shindoh J, Truty MJ, et al. Kinetic growth rate after portal vein embolization predicts posthepatectomy outcomes: toward zero liver-related mortality in patients with colorectal liver metastases and small future liver remnant. *J Am Coll Surg* 2013;216(2):201–209.

Teh SH, Christein J, et al. Hepatic resection of hepatocellular carcinoma in patients with cirrhosis: Model of End-Stage Liver Disease (MELD) score predicts perioperative mortality. *J Gastrointest Surg* 2005;9(9):1207–1215.

Vauthey JN, Chaoui A, et al. Standardized measurement of the future liver remnant prior to extended liver resection: methodology and clinical associations. *Surgery* 2000;127(5):512–519.

Vauthey JN, Pawlik TM, et al. Chemotherapy regimen predicts steatohepatitis and an increase in 90-day mortality after surgery for hepatic colorectal metastases. *J Clin Oncol* 2006;24(13):2065–2072.

Vauthey JN, Zimmitti G, et al. From Couinaud to molecular biology: the seven virtues of hepato-pancreato-biliary surgery. *HPB (Oxford)* 2012;14(8):493–499.

Zorzi D, Laurent A, et al. Chemotherapy-associated hepatotoxicity and surgery for colorectal liver metastases. *Br J Surg* 2007;94(3):274–286.

Cirrhosis and Portal Hypertension

Rachelle N. Damle and Shimul A. Shah

ETIOLOGY

Cirrhosis is a chronic liver disease that results in hepatic failure. Etiologies of cirrhosis range from alcohol abuse to immune disorders to toxin exposure. Regardless of its various causes, cirrhosis is caused by the destruction of hepatic parenchyma with replacement by fibrosis and regenerative nodules. Usually, the damage is done by multiple insults of various etiologies that occur repeatedly over time. In addition to hepatic failure, cirrhosis can lead to hepatocellular carcinoma (HCC). The complications of cirrhosis are devastating and potentially life threatening. Unfortunately, once cirrhosis occurs, the only cure is liver transplantation (LT).

Pathophysiology

Figure 11.1 details the evolution of cirrhosis. Hepatocytes are damaged by an insult or disease, leading to destruction of hepatic parenchyma. Initially, the liver's ability for regeneration can lead to restoration of normal architecture; however, this capacity is finite. The exact mechanism leading to impaired regeneration is poorly understood and remains a key question in current clinical investigation. Impaired regeneration results in disruption of architecture, disturbance to blood supply, poor nutrient supply to hepatocytes, and eventual inhibition of hepatocyte proliferation. Attempts at healing this damage lead to fibrosis and eventual regenerative nodule formation.

Stellate cells play an important role in the development of cirrhosis. They are found at the interface between the basolateral membranes of hepatocytes and sinusoidal endothelial cells, in the space of Disse. Their normal function is paracrine in nature, regulating hepatocyte and endothelial cells as well as the storage of vitamin A. When hepatocytes are injured, cytokine release results in hypertrophy and proliferation of stellate cells. Eventually, the space of Disse becomes thickened with collagen deposits, and the normal architecture of the fenestrated sinusoidal endothelium is distorted. This leads to vascular distortion and portal hypertension.

Under normal circumstances, portal vein pressure ranges from 5 to 8 mm Hg. Any pressure greater than 8 mm Hg or a hepatic portal venous gradient (HPVG) greater 5 mm Hg is defined as portal hypertension. Practically, this measurement is taken via hepatic vein wedge pressure, similar to a measurement of pulmonary arterial pressure using a Swan-Ganz catheter. The normal venous drainage of the gastrointestinal tract is through the portal vein, into the liver, out of the hepatic veins, into the inferior vena cava (IVC), and then back to the heart. The portal vein is formed by the splenic vein and superior mesenteric vein (SMV). Usually, the inferior mesenteric vein (IMV) joins the splenic vein prior to its junction with the SMV; however, this anatomy varies widely. With obstruction of flow at the presinusoidal, sinusoidal, or postsinusoidal level, portal venous pressure

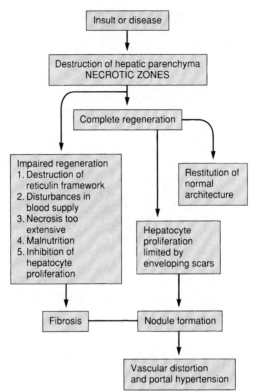

FIGURE 11.1 Evolution of cirrhosis. Fibrosis develops in nonregenerative necrotic areas, producing scars. The pattern of nodularity and scars reflects the type of response to injury (e.g., uniform vs. nonuniform necrosis) and the extent of injury. (From Mulholland MW, Lillemoe KD, Doherty GM, et al. *Greenfield's surgery: scientific principles & practice*, 5th ed. Philadelphia, PA: Lippincott Williams & Wilkins, 2010.)

increases and decompression occurs with flow back to the heart via collaterals. These collaterals are generally thin walled and fragile and, with increased flow, become varicosities. Given their fragility, varicosities rupture easily and can cause life-threatening bleeding. Figure 11.2 depicts the collaterals that can form with portal hypertension.

Causes

Table 11.1 lists the causes of cirrhosis. The most common cause of cirrhosis in the world is viral hepatitis, but alcohol abuse is the most common cause in the United States. Nonalcoholic fatty liver disease (with progression to nonalcoholic steatohepatitis or NASH) is increasing in prevalence in the United States and is linked with hyperlipidemia, non–insulin-dependent diabetes, and obesity. Immune or inflammatory cirrhosis due to cholestasis is caused by primary biliary cirrhosis and primary sclerosing cholangitis. Hemochromatosis, an inborn error in metabolism, leads to cirrhosis secondary to lipid peroxidation of iron deposits in periportal regions of the liver. Wilson disease is an inherited deficiency in hepatocyte transport of

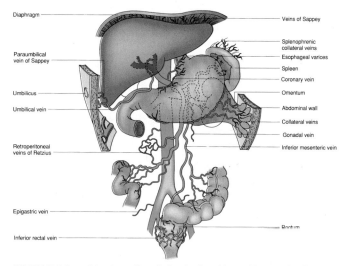

FIGURE 11.2 Potential venous collaterals that develop with portal hypertension. The veins of Sappey drain portal blood through the bare areas of the diaphragm and through paraumbilical vein collaterals to the umbilicus. The veins of Retzius form in the retroperitoneum and shunt portal blood from the bowel and other organs to the vena cava. (From Mulholland MW, Lillemoe KD, Doherty GM, et al. *Greenfield's surgery: scientific principles & practice*, 5th ed. Philadelphia, PA: Lippincott Williams & Wilkins, 2010.)

 Causes of Cirrhosis

Viral

Alcoholic
Nonalcoholic steatohepatitis
Cholestasis
  Extrahepatic
    Stones
    Extrinsic mass
    Strictures
    Primary sclerosing cholangitis
  Intrahepatic
    Primary biliary cirrhosis
    Primary sclerosing cholangitis
    Cystic fibrosis
    Vanishing bile duct syndrome
Genetic disorders
  Hemochromatosis
  Wilson disease
  Cystic fibrosis
  α-Antitrypsin deficiency
  Glycogen storage disease
Venous outflow occlusion
  Budd-Chiari syndrome
Idiopathic

copper into biliary tract, resulting in copper accumulation in the liver, once again causing periportal inflammation and eventual cirrhosis. Obstruction of hepatic venous outflow (Budd-Chiari syndrome) causes sinusoidal congestion and hepatocyte necrosis and, eventually, cirrhosis. Hepatic venous outflow obstruction is associated with "nutmeg" appearance of the liver secondary to multiple small areas of hemorrhage.

DIAGNOSIS

As with any disease, a history and physical examination yield most of the information needed to diagnose a patient with cirrhosis. Clues in the history include acknowledged alcohol abuse, hepatitis, toxin exposure, previous upper gastrointestinal bleeding, hemorrhoids, infections, and increased abdominal girth. Classic physical exam findings in a cirrhotic patient are found in Table 11.2. Fetor hepaticus, bruising, decreased body hair, and purpura are also physical signs associated with cirrhosis.

Diagnostic tests are indicated if the history and physical exam raise suspicion for liver disease. Laboratory evaluation includes hepatic panel, complete blood count, chemistry panel, and coagulation profile. As mentioned in earlier sections of this handbook, functional capacity of the liver is evaluated by coagulation studies, platelet count, and bilirubin. Inability of the liver to produce coagulation factors, thrombopoietin, and bilirubin will lead to abnormal values of these labs. Markers of hepatocyte or cholangiocyte damage are AST, ALT, and alkaline phosphatase. The term liver "function" panel traditionally includes AST, ALT, alkaline phosphatase, bilirubin, and lactate dehydrogenase. It is important to understand this misnomer of "function" as these values do not indicate the liver's functional capacity. *Importantly, abnormal values are not specific for liver dysfunction and may even be normal in the setting of hepatic disease.*

In addition to laboratory values, imaging studies are commonly used to further investigate a suspicion of liver dysfunction. Ultrasonography, computed tomography, and magnetic resonance imaging (MRI) can detect cirrhosis. Generally, these studies will reveal a nodular, atrophic liver and splenomegaly. Ultrasound is nearly 90% sensitive and specific for diagnosing cirrhosis. Cirrhotic livers demonstrate multiple nodular irregularities

TABLE 11.2	Physical Findings in Cirrhosis
Physical Findings	**Incidence (%)**
Palpable liver	96
Jaundice	68
Ascites	66
Spider angiomas	49
Dilated abdominal wall veins	47
Palpable spleen	46
Testicular atrophy	45
Palmar erythema	24
Noninfectious fever	22
Hepatic coma	18
Gynecomastia	15
Dupuytren contractures	5

From Mulholland MW, Lillemoe KD, Doherty GM, et al. *Greenfield's surgery: scientific principles & practice.* 5th ed. Philadelphia, PA: Lippincott Williams & Wilkins, 2010.

Child-Turcotte-Pugh (CTP) Score	Estimated Mortality Rates for Surgical Intervention by CTP Score	Mortality
A		10%–15%
B		30%–40%
C		75%–90%

on the anterior surface of the liver distinct from the abdominal wall. Fibrosis can be seen with disruption in parenchyma, though this is often difficult to detect. Computed tomography and MRI are more expensive modalities and do not yield any more information than ultrasound; however, they may reveal an atrophic liver, evidence of venous thrombosis, and/or splenomegaly.

Invasive diagnostic methods (biopsy) definitively establish the diagnosis of cirrhosis; however, in the presence of strong clinical, laboratory, and radiographic evidence, they are not necessary. Direct visualization of the liver during an abdominal surgical procedure can reveal a nodular, atrophic liver. Percutaneous, laparoscopic, or transjugular biopsy, as well as image-guided fine needle aspiration, can be used. Histology will reveal fatty infiltration, balloon-cell degeneration, Mallory bodies, hepatocyte necrosis, fibrosis, or features of cirrhosis.

Two methods of classifying liver disease severity are the Child-Turcotte-Pugh (CTP) score and the Model for End-Stage Liver Disease (MELD) score. These prognostic models of disease severity are important in operative planning and liver transplant allocation. The CTP score is the best predictive score for most patients with cirrhosis and is used to determine risk of morbidity and mortality for surgical procedures (Table 11.3). Originally, the MELD score was developed to determine survival following transjugular intrahepatic portosystemic shunt (TIPS) procedure. It was then adopted as a prognostic indication of a patient's 90-day survival with optimized medical management. Bilirubin, international normalized ratio, and creatinine are the only values used in calculating the MELD score, so it is a more objective system than CTP score. Because of its objectivity, the MELD score is used as the main determinant of liver transplant allocation in the United States.

CLINICAL MANIFESTATIONS

Renal

Complications of impaired renal function in the setting of cirrhosis are caused by dysregulation of vascular tone. This results in sodium retention, water retention, and ultimately hepatorenal syndrome (HRS) and renal failure. When ascites develops, there is an inability to excrete sodium. Water retention follows sodium retention and is due to the inability of patients with ascites to process free water. Excess water leads to dilutional hyponatremia, which may cause nausea, vomiting, lethargy, and seizures.

HRS is a complex complication of cirrhosis, characterized by renal failure in the absence of intrinsic renal disease. Up to 10% of patients with cirrhosis and ascites develop HRS. Signs of HRS include oliguria, increasing serum creatinine level, rising cardiac output, proteinuria, and decreased arterial pressure. The renin–angiotensin–aldosterone system is overactive, and the renal cortex is markedly vasoconstricted. Prerenal azotemia is difficult to distinguish from HRS, and laboratory values are similar in the two

Diagnostic Criteria for Hepatorenal Syndrome[a]

Major Criteria
1. Low glomerular filtration rate, as indicated by serum creatinine >1.5 mg/dL or 24-hour creatinine clearance 40 mL/min
2. Absence of shock, ongoing bacterial infection, fluid losses, and current treatment with nephrotoxic drugs
3. No sustained improvement in renal function (decrease in serum creatinine to ≤1.5 mg/dL or increase in creatinine clearance to 340 mL/min) following diuretic withdrawal and expansion of plasma volume with 1.5 L of a plasma expander
4. Proteinuria <500 mg/d and no ultrasonographic evidence of obstructive uropathy or parenchymal renal disease

Additional Criteria
1. Urine volume <500 mL/d
2. Urine sodium <10 mEq/L
3. Urine osmolality greater than plasma osmolality
4. Urine red blood cells <50 per high-power field
5. Serum sodium concentration <130 mEq/L

[a]All major criteria must be present for the diagnosis of HRS. Additional criteria are not necessary for the diagnosis but provide supportive evidence.
From Arroyo V, Ginés P, Gerbes A, et al. Definition and diagnostic criteria of refractory ascites and hepatorenal syndrome in cirrhosis. *Hepatology* 1996;23:164, Mulholland MW, Lillemoe KD, Doherty GM, et al. *Greenfield's surgery: scientific principles & practice.* 5th ed. Philadelphia, PA: Lippincott Williams & Wilkins, 2010.

conditions. However, HRS is distinct from acute intrinsic renal failure, with low urine sodium, a high urine/plasma creatinine ratio, high urine osmolality, and normal urine sediment. In an attempt to distinguish HRS from other etiologies, diagnostic criteria for HRS were developed (Table 11.4).

Pulmonary

Although some causes of cirrhosis can also cause pulmonary complications, cirrhosis itself can have effects on the pulmonary system. As ascites develops, lymphatic transdiaphragmatic communication can result in hepatic hydrothorax. The resultant effusion can directly compress pulmonary parenchyma, which impairs gas exchange and may result in hypoxemia. Hepatopulmonary syndrome (HPS) is diagnosed with hepatic dysfunction, oxygen tension less than 70 mm Hg or diffusion gradient greater than 20 mm Hg, and pulmonary vascular dilation in structurally normal lungs. Patients present with shortness of breath when moving from supine to upright position (platypnea) and dyspnea in the absence of primary pulmonary disease. On physical exam, patients may have clubbing and cyanosis of nail beds. Portopulmonary hypertension is defined by a mean pulmonary arterial pressure of greater than 25 mm Hg in the presence of liver disease. This rare entity has a significant risk of mortality and is a relative contraindication to liver transplant. The exact mechanism of HPS is not known; interestingly, portal hypertension is not required for its development.

The goal of treating and preventing pulmonary complications of cirrhosis and portal hypertension centers around fluid management. With the previously discussed fluid derangements, extracellular fluid increases and intravascular volume decreases. Increasing ascitic fluid can impair respiration due to increased intra-abdominal pressure, so therapeutic paracentesis can help relieve this pressure and improve air exchange. Prevention of fluid accumulation is done through sodium restriction. The more complex treatment of HPS and portopulmonary hypertension is beyond the scope of this chapter.

Hepatic Encephalopathy

Hepatic encephalopathy is manifested by mental status alterations. Although a debated topic, the pathophysiology of hepatic encephalopathy is related to ammonia. Interestingly, the serum concentration of ammonia does not correlate with the severity of encephalopathy. Normally, after bacterial digestion of proteins, ammonia is absorbed through the gut and then undergoes degradation in the liver. With impaired hepatic function, ammonia reaches the peripheral circulation, permeates the blood–brain barrier, and causes alterations in mental status. Evidence exists both in favor of and against elevated serum ammonia as the cause of hepatic encephalopathy. Serum ammonia levels are elevated in up to 90% of patients with hepatic encephalopathy, and treatments that reduce ammonia levels improve or resolve this condition. Alternatively, there is poor correlation of ammonia level with severity of encephalopathy; direct administration of ammonia to patients with cirrhosis does not cause encephalopathy, and the same treatments that reduce ammonia levels also reduce other toxin levels. Signs and symptoms of hepatic encephalopathy include early findings of memory loss, mood disturbances, and sleep pattern alteration. As the condition progresses, confusion, lethargy, obtundation, and coma can occur. Asterixis, elevated ammonia levels, and altered mental status are strongly suggestive of hepatic encephalopathy.

Treating hepatic encephalopathy involves dietary modifications and medications that reduce ammonia production and/or neutralize its effects. Initially, any precipitating factors need to be identified including infectious source, electrolyte abnormalities, and medications. These factors should be treated if possible. Secondly, intravenous fluids are administered to expand intravascular volume and dilute the concentration of the toxins. In addition to marked dietary restriction of proteins, nitrogenous compounds should be removed from the gut. This is done via medications that inhibit the metabolism of such compounds in the gut, thereby reducing ammonia levels. The preferred medication is lactulose, which can be administered orally, through a nasogastric tube, or per rectum. Lactulose is administered three to four times daily, with the goal of producing two to three soft bowel movements per day. Dosing ranges from 45 to 90 g/d. Its mechanism has been debated, but is possibly through alteration of bacterial metabolism to increase bacterial uptake of ammonia. Other medications include neomycin and metronidazole, which work to decrease the concentration of ammonia-forming bacteria in the gut.

Ascites

Ascites is present when free fluid within the peritoneal cavity reaches over 150 mL. In addition to cirrhosis and portal hypertension, the differential diagnosis for ascites is broad. Congestive heart failure and renal insufficiency both commonly cause ascites. Other causes of ascites include hypoalbuminemia; bile, chylous, or pancreatic urinary ascites; ovarian disease; peritoneal dissemination of carcinoma; and myxedema. In the setting of cirrhosis, increased sinusoidal pressure results in leaking of protein-rich fluid directly from the liver into the peritoneal cavity. Ascites is of prognostic significance in a patient with portal hypertension. One-year mortality with new-onset ascites in a cirrhotic patient is estimated at 50%, compared to 10% in cirrhotic patients without ascites. This fluid cannot be absorbed secondary to the increased hydrostatic pressure and accumulates in the peritoneal cavity.

Physical exam findings include shifting dullness, bulging flanks, increased abdominal girth, and fluid waves. With enough ascites accumulation, increased intra-abdominal pressure can cause respiratory distress. Increased intra-abdominal pressure in combination with muscle wasting can result in abdominal wall and inguinal hernias, which are difficult to manage.

Management of renal sodium and water retention, dietary sodium restriction, and bed rest are the initial steps in the treatment of ascites. Sodium retention is exacerbated in the upright position secondary to venous pooling and relative hypovolemia; therefore, bed rest is recommended; up to 15% of patients respond with this therapy alone. In addition, dietary salt restriction is implemented; however, compliance with this recommendation is generally poor. If these lifestyle modifications are ineffective, diuretics are the mainstay of treatment. Furosemide and spironolactone are generally prescribed in combination to maximize effectiveness. Intermittent large-volume paracentesis can be performed for patients with large volumes of fluid that are not responding to lifestyle or medication interventions. Up to 30 L of fluid can be removed with infusion of concentrated albumin repletion. Ascites can also be treated with shunts, either peritoneovenous (surgical) or portosystemic (i.e., TIPS), which are discussed later in this chapter. Surgical portovenous shunts that are associated with significant complications are rarely used. Table 11.5 lists treatments of ascites, including doses for antibiotic prophylaxis for spontaneous bacterial peritonitis (SBP) (see below).

TABLE 11.5	Treatment of Ascites

Bed rest
Sodium restriction
  1–2 g/d (45–90 mEq/d)
Fluid restriction
  1–1.5 L/d
Diuretics
  Spironolactone
    50 mg PO q8h
    Maximum of 100 mg q6h
  Furosemide
    40–370 mg/d
Antibiotics
  Cefotaxime
    2 g IV q12h
  Ofloxacin
    400 mg PO q12h
  Prophylaxis
  Norfloxacin
    400 mg/d while hospitalized
  Ciprofloxacin
    750 mg PO weekly
  Norfloxacin
    400 mg/d for 6 mo
  Trimethoprim/sulfamethoxazole
    One double-strength tablet five times a week

Mulholland MW, Lillemoe KD, Doherty GM, et al. *Greenfield's surgery: scientific principles & practice.* 5th ed. Philadelphia, PA: Lippincott Williams & Wilkins, 2010.

Spontaneous Bacterial Peritonitis

Up to 10% of patients with portal hypertension and ascites will develop SBP. The etiology of SBP is unclear, but often patients have had preceding gastrointestinal hemorrhage. Ten to twenty percent of cases are detected by evaluating routine paracentesis fluid, but most patients present with clinical symptoms of abdominal pain, fever, progressive encephalopathy, and impaired renal function. Specific criteria for SBP include a serum–ascites–albumin gradient of ≥ 1.1 g/dL, a polymorphonuclear count of ≥ 250 cells/ mm^3, and a single organism (usually G+) on culture. The presence of more than one organism cultured from peritoneal fluid raises suspicion for secondary bacterial peritonitis and mandates evaluation for sources such as a perforated viscus and appendicitis.

Antibiotic prophylaxis against SBP is given to patients with a low protein count in their ascitic fluid or patients with gastrointestinal hemorrhage, as those patients are at high risk for development of SBP. Patients with hemorrhage are given ofloxacin alone or neomycin, colistin, and nystatin in combination. These medications can reduce the incidence of SBP from up to 20% to about 9% with few side effects. Patients with diagnosed SBP are treated with intravenous cefotaxime or oral ofloxacin.

Esophageal Varices

Esophageal varices are a life-threatening complication of portal hypertension and can be quite difficult to manage. Esophageal varices are the most common site for life-threatening variceal bleeding. Typically, they are located in the distal esophagus, in the submucosal venous plexus. As these vessels dilate, they become more superficial and they erode into the lamina propria. Variceal development is dependent upon the pressure in the portal system. In general, a hepatic vein–portal vein gradient of about 12 mm Hg is present in patients with varices, although not all patients with this gradient or higher will develop varices. Incidence varies widely in the literature, ranging from 8% to 90% of patients with cirrhosis. Nevertheless, once varices develop, the risk of bleeding is 25% to 35%. Predictors of bleeding include a combination of CTP class, variceal size, and specific markings present on endoscopy.

The mainstay of therapy for esophageal varices is medical, the goal being decreased splanchnic blood flow and prevention of first bleeding episode. Beta-blockade is the first-line treatment, with nadolol and propranolol being the agents of choice. The mechanism of nonspecific beta-blockade includes decreasing cardiac output as well as increasing splanchnic vasoconstriction; combined, they result in decreased portal blood flow and decreased hepatic portal venous gradient. Beta-blockers are effective regardless of the etiology of portal hypertension, even in the absence of ascites. They can also reduce mortality from subsequent bleeding episodes in patients with large varices. Organic nitrates are also effective in primary and secondary prevention of bleeding. These medications cause splanchnic vasoconstriction and arterial vasodilation, thereby decreasing collateral resistance. Nitrates also decrease hepatic resistance, likely a result of stellate cell contractility inhibition. Patients with a contraindication to beta-blocker treatment receive nitrates as the first-line therapy. The combination of nitrates with beta-blockers decreases in the incidence of variceal bleeding to a greater degree than either alone.

MANAGEMENT OF ACUTE VARICEAL BLEEDING

Medical Treatment

Acute variceal bleeding requires prompt attention. Basic management includes securing a protected airway, establishing intravenous access with large-bore catheters, close hemodynamic monitoring, thorough laboratory evaluation, intensive care monitoring, and blood product administration as needed. Medications used in the situation of acute bleeding include continuous intravenous administration of vasopressin and/or octreotide. Octreotide infusion is very effective. It is the first-line therapy in acute variceal bleed, as it results in splanchnic vasoconstriction without any unintended consequences. Its mechanism is indirect, by reducing the levels of other gut hormones that normally cause vasodilation. Vasopressin decreases portal venous flow to reduce portal pressure by splanchnic vasoconstriction. Its vasoconstrictive effects on the coronary circulation can lead to cardiac complications, so it is often used in combination with a vasodilator such as nitroglycerin.

Endoscopic Treatment
Endoscopy has been established as a definitive intervention to stop variceal bleeding through interventions such as sclerotherapy or band ligation. Sclerotherapy involves visualization of the varices through a flexible endoscope and injection of sclerosing agent in close proximity to the varices. Sclerotherapy has largely been replaced by band ligation secondary to its complication rate of 10% to 30%, including esophageal perforation due to ulceration caused by the sclerosing agent. Success rates for initial control of esophageal variceal bleed range from 60% to 90%; often more than one session is required to completely stop bleeding. Band ligation is performed by insertion of an endoscope over a sheath, suctioning each individual varix into the lumen of a channel, and placement of a rubber band around the tissue to ligate it. In a few days, the tissue is sloughed off, leaving only a small ulcer. Multiple bands can be placed during each procedure; the exact number is dependent upon the equipment used. Ligation has a success rate of 80% to 100% in the first session. A significant reduction in the incidence of rebleeding, death from bleeding, and overall mortality has been found with band ligation in comparison to sclerotherapy.

Balloon Tamponade
Balloon tamponade represents a third-line treatment for patients who fail medical and endoscopic management for acute variceal bleed. In the 10% to 25% who fail first-line treatment strategies, balloon tamponade has a high success rate. The Sengstaken-Blakemore and Minnesota tubes are most commonly used. The concept is similar for both. The tube has an esophageal balloon and a gastric balloon that sits at the gastroesophageal junction in the cardia of the stomach. After insertion via nasogastric route and radiographic evidence of proper position is demonstrated, the two balloons are inflated, resulting in tamponade of any gastric or esophageal varices. The esophageal balloon is inflated between 15 and 40 mm Hg of pressure and the gastric balloon initially inflated with 30 mL of air and then with a total of 300 to 400 mL. It is imperative to secure the tube in place, using a facemask or helmet to prevent inadvertent removal. About 10% to 20% of patients suffer from significant complications including aspiration, perforation, and necrosis; however, 70% to 80% are treated successfully. These severe complications limit the use of balloon tamponade to 24 hours. Up to half of these patients rebled when the balloons are deflated. Balloon tamponade can be very effective in the initial control of bleeding, but is merely a temporizing measure until a more definitive procedure such as TIPS or transplant can be performed. Figure 11.3 shows the algorithm for management of a patient with variceal bleeding when medical and endoscopic treatment fails.

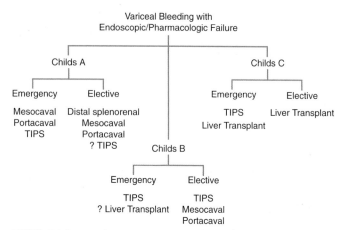

FIGURE 11.3 Suggested treatment options for patients who fail to undergo medical management for variceal bleeding. (From Mulholland MW, Lillemoe KD, Doherty GM, et al. *Greenfield's surgery: scientific principles & practice*, 5th ed. Philadelphia, PA: Lippincott Williams & Wilkins, 2010.)

Transjugular Intrahepatic Portosystemic Shunt

Unsuccessful treatment of esophageal variceal bleeding by medication, endoscopy, or balloon tamponade results in 90% mortality. Therefore, a more definitive procedure is required that can temporize until LT can be performed. Traditionally, surgically created portosystemic shunts were the mainstay of treatment. However, the significant morbidity and mortality associated with these procedures has led to the development of the less invasive and lower-risk TIPS procedure. When medical, endoscopic, and balloon tamponade fail, TIPS is the next line in therapy. This stent effectively shunts blood from the portal vein into the hepatic vein, bypassing the hepatic parenchyma and avoiding the area of increased resistance. The goal hepatic portal venous pressure gradient to stop bleeding is less than 12 mm Hg. However, a gradient of less than 5 mm Hg results in liver ischemia secondary to decreased hepatic flow. Care needs to be taken to achieve an adequate pressure to resolve varices, but maintain hepatic perfusion.

Surgical Shunt Creation

Surgical shunt creation is the most effective method of reducing portal venous pressure and preventing recurrent variceal bleeding. TIPS is preferential, as the surgical creation of a shunt is associated with significant morbidity and mortality. Portosystemic shunts are divided into three types depending on their diversion of flow: nonselective, selective, and partially diverting.

Nonselective shunts involve anastomosis of the portal vein or SMV to the IVC or the portal vein to the proximal renal vein. "Hepatofugal flow" is the reversal of blood flow out of the liver and into the systemic circulation. It is achieved by the large diameter of these anastomoses and allows for decompression of the high-pressure portal venous system into the low-pressure systemic circulation. A portacaval shunt can be done in an end-to-side or side-to-side fashion. Mesocaval shunts are created via a prosthetic or vein interposition graft. To create a central splenorenal shunt, a splenectomy is performed and the proximal splenic vein is anastomosed to the left renal vein. Remember that ascites is caused by leaking of protein-rich fluid from the liver secondary to high pressure at the level of the sinusoids. Therefore, these nonselective shunts, by reduction of portal venous pressure, allow for a decrease in ascites in addition to resolving varices.

The goal of a *selective shunt* is to create two distinct drainage pathways for the portal circulation. By diverting flow from the esophagogastric circulation into the systemic circulation, a low-pressure system is created and maintains a high pressure in the mesenteric system. This is done by creating a distal splenorenal shunt. Unlike the proximal splenorenal shunt, the very distal aspect of the splenic vein is anastomosed to the left renal vein in an end-to-side fashion. This allows decompression of the short gastric veins through the systemic circulation and relieves varices. It is important to note that portal venous pressure is not reduced in this procedure. Therefore, ascites may persist or even worsen after a splenorenal shunt is created. Another selective shunt involves anastomosis of the left gastric vein to the IVC and works in the same way as a distal splenorenal shunt.

Partial shunts use small-diameter interposition polytetrafluoroethylene or Dacron grafts to create mesocaval or portacaval shunts. These shunts allow for a decrease in the hepatic venous–portal pressure gradient to less than 12 mm Hg and maintain hepatopetal flow, thereby reducing the risk of hepatic encephalopathy and accelerated hepatic dysfunction due to lack of trophic hormones from the gut.

Complications and Outcomes with TIPS and Surgical Shunts

The major complication of TIPS is in-shunt stenosis, via either neointimal hyperplasia or thrombosis. At 1 year, approximately 50% of shunts will be occluded, but these results have improved dramatically with newer technology. Intervention is possible with thrombolysis, balloon dilation of the stent, or placement of a second stent. About 15% of patients sustain nonreversible shunt occlusion. Ultrasonography to assess shunt patency should be performed every 3 months. Given the relatively short duration of efficacy of TIPS, it is ideal as a bridge to LT or for those that have severe enough hepatic decompensation that they are unlikely to live long enough to experience TIPS failure. TIPS is not only effective in treatment of uncontrolled variceal bleeding, it also reduces the rate of rebleeding episodes.

Both TIPS and surgically created shunts may be complicated by accelerated hepatic dysfunction and hepatic encephalopathy. With diversion of blood flow from the liver, important trophic hormones present in the portal circulation bypass the liver. Shunts that involve dissection near the porta hepatis result in adhesions that make future LT difficult, another reason that TIPS is preferred over the surgical portosystemic shunts. When it comes to control of variceal hemorrhage, both nonselective and selective shunts are successful in greater than 90% of cases.

LIVER TRANSPLANTATION: MANAGEMENT OF PORTAL HYPERTENSION

The ideal management in selected patients with cirrhosis and at least one clinical manifestation of portal hypertension is LT. There are currently close to three times the number of patients listed compared to available organs in the United States. Due to the shortage of donors and the complexity of the surgery, donor and recipient selection is key to successful treatment. Patients typically undergo an exhaustive pretransplant workup to be considered candidates. Current 1-year survival rate after LT is 85%. Perioperative mortality is roughly 5%. Graft failure commonly results from sepsis. Other common complications include hepatic artery thrombosis (5%), biliary stricture (10%), biliary leak (<5%), and primary nonfunction (1%).

PREOPERATIVE CONSIDERATIONS

Cirrhosis portends a high risk for surgical and anesthetic complications, including death. Careful assessment of the status of a patient's liver disease is warranted prior to any elective procedure. Even with preoperative risk stratification, cirrhosis may not be discovered until the time of surgery. Most studies evaluating surgical risk in cirrhosis exclude Child class C patients, and the majority of included cases are Child class A. This heterogeneity leads to poor generalizability of study results and, often, a misclassification of surgical risk. As with any disease process, emergency surgery is extremely high risk, with a high mortality rate. Estimates of mortality rates for surgery in cirrhotics range from 11% to 25% versus 1.1% in noncirrhotic patients. In general, the postsurgical 30-day mortality rate in Child class A is 10% to 15%, Child class B is 30% to 40%, and Child class C is 75% to 80%. Despite advances in surgical and anesthetic technique, these numbers are largely unchanged over several decades.

The cause of these high mortality rates in cirrhosis is related to four main organ systems: circulatory, pulmonary, immune, and hematologic. Cirrhotics have a hyperdynamic circulation, and decreased hepatic perfusion and anesthetic administration can exacerbate this, causing increased hypotension and hypoxemia. Hypoxia may be exacerbated by previously mentioned pulmonary complications due to ascites, hepatic hydrothorax, portopulmonary hypertension, or HPS. Cirrhotic patients are more susceptible to bacterial infection and subsequent sepsis, as well as wound healing complications. Additionally, thrombocytopenia and coagulopathy lead to bleeding complications. Malnutrition is prevalent among cirrhotic patients and can exacerbate the aforementioned complications. Given the baseline fluid derangements in these patients, fluid management intra- and postoperatively may be quite challenging.

The CTP class is used most widely in the literature to classify severity of liver disease and surgical risk. It is easy to calculate, but it can have interobserver variability, as the category of ascites and encephalopathy is subjective in nature. The MELD score is more objective and gives weights to each variable. It has been proven to be a good predictor of 30-day postoperative mortality, demonstrating a linear relationship to mortality. Both CTP and MELD score may be used in practice when determining surgical risk and guiding clinical management of a cirrhotic patient. Certainly, risk is optimized when a cirrhotic patient is treated at a transplant center with an intensive care unit available.

CONCLUSION

Cirrhosis and subsequent portal hypertension are serious, life-threatening diseases that may go undetected for years and may eventually lead to HCC. Eventually, patients will succumb to the disease without a liver transplant, although there are various ways to optimize medical management as a bridge to transplant. Portal hypertension can result from cirrhosis, hepatic vein obstruction, or portal vein thrombosis, all of which have many potential causes and may not be related to liver dysfunction. Variceal bleeding is a life-threatening complication of portal hypertension and may be the presenting symptom of end-stage liver disease. Detection of the subtle signs and symptoms on history and physical, as well as careful interpretation of laboratory and diagnostic imaging, can lead to early identification of cirrhosis cessation of the inciting factors of liver damage.

EDITORIAL NOTE

The profound clinical importance of hepatic cirrhosis is impossible to understate. For example, contemporary 1-year *mortality* of cirrhotic patients after a first episode of esophageal variceal hemorrhage or new onset of ascites is 50%!

Many surgeons have experienced the disastrous consequences of operating on cirrhotic patients (even those with seemingly well-compensated cirrhosis)—intraoperative and occasionally delayed postoperative bleeding, development of postoperative ascites (often leaking through abdominal incisions) with secondary bacterial peritonitis; hepatic insufficiency; encephalopathy (commonly accompanied by aspiration/pneumonia); and almost astonishingly high mortality, even after simple procedures. Cirrhotic patients have no physiologic reserve and little margin for error. These patients should be approached by an experienced surgical team.

Suggested Readings

Albano E. New concepts in the pathogenesis of alcoholic liver disease. *Expert Rev Gastroenterol Hepatol* 2008;2:749–759.

Al-Gusafi SA, McNabb-Baltar J, Farag A. Clinical manifestations of portal hypertension. *Int J Hepatol* 2012:2012:203794.

Anthony PP, Ishak KG, Nayak NC, et al. The morphology of cirrhosis: definition, nomenclature, and classification. *Bull World Health Organ* 1977;55:521–540.

Chedid A, Mendenhall CL, Gartside P, et al. Prognostic factors in alcoholic liver disease. VA Cooperative Study Group. *Am J Gastroenterol* 1991;86:210–216.

Csikesz NG, Nguyen LN, Tseng JF, et al. Nationwide volume and mortality after elective surgery in cirrhotic patients. *J Am Coll Surg* 2009;208:96–103.

Grattagliano I, Ubaldi E, Bonfrate L. Management of liver cirrhosis between primary care and specialists. *World J Gastroenterol* 2011;17(18):2273–2282.

Kahn S, Tudur SC, Williamson P. Portosystemic shunts versus endoscopic therapy for variceal rebleeding in patients with cirrhosis. *Cochrane Database Syst Rev* 2006(4);CD000553.

Nicoll A. Surgical risk in patients with cirrhosis. *J Gastroenterol Hepatol* 2012;27: 1569–1575.

Shaw JJ, Shah SA. Rising incidence of hepatocellular carcinoma in the USA: what does it mean? *Expert Rev Gastroenterol Hepatol* 2011;5:365–370.

12 Intraoperative Ultrasound of the Liver, Bile Ducts, and Pancreas

Nicholas J. Zyromski

INTRODUCTION

Intraoperative ultrasound (IOUS) plays a critical role in HPB surgery. In general, IOUS has four purposes: (1) acquisition of new information (such as identifying occult metastatic disease), (2) complementing preoperative and intraoperative radiologic imaging (cross-sectional imaging, intraoperative cholangiography), (3) guiding surgical procedures (biopsy, ablation), and (4) confirming operation completion (clearance of stones from the common bile duct, confirming vascular flow following reconstruction).

Structured ultrasound instruction has been developed by the American College of Surgeons, ranging from trauma uses (focused abdominal sonography for trauma—FAST) to endocrine (thyroid/parathyroid), breast, vascular, and other applications. Similarly, leaders in HPB surgery education recognize IOUS as an essential part of HPB training and are currently working to formalize training objectives. The goal of this chapter is to provide a review of ultrasound basics and a practical approach to IOUS of the liver, biliary tree, and pancreas.

BASIC PHYSICS

Sound energy passes through matter at various frequencies. The human ear perceives sound waves ranging in frequency from 20 to 20,000 hertz (Hz, cycles per second). "Ultrasound" by definition includes sound waves above the level of human hearing, that is to say greater than 20,000 Hz. Medical ultrasound applications typically range between 1 and 15 million Hz (mega hertz or MHz).

Sound waves move through tissues at different speeds depending on the tissue density. Some of the sound waves are reflected, while other sound waves will attenuate at different rates depending on tissue density. The relative amount of sound wave reflection and attenuation is a function of the tissue impedance.

Electrical current applied to crystals in the ultrasound probe generates sound waves at specific frequencies (typically a range or "bandwidth" of frequencies, i.e., 4 to 9 MHz). These sound waves pass through tissue and reflect from tissue. The probe "listens" for returning sound waves—in fact, up to 99% of a probe's time is spent "listening" as opposed to sending out sound waves. These returning sound waves are then converted or transduced back to electrical energy from which an image is generated. This signal transduction from electrical voltage to sound wave and back is known as the piezoelectric effect.

BASIC ULTRASOUND MECHANICS—"KNOBOLOGY"

The appearance of an ultrasound console may be quite intimidating. (Fig. 12.1 shows the console of a typical IOUS unit.) The next few paragraphs

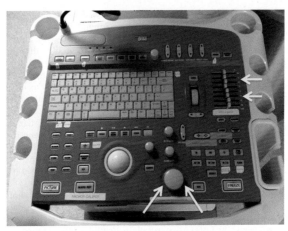

FIGURE 12.1 Console of Aloka ultrasound unit. Gain knob is on **bottom** (*long arrows*); TGC slider pots are on **top right** (*short arrows*).

will break down this big picture to smaller, usable, practical segments. Pattern recognition is important in IOUS.

Echogenicity refers to the ultrasound appearance of tissues and structures. Anechoic structures appear to be without echoes; hypoechoic structures have fewer echoes, and hyperechoic structures have brighter echoes than surrounding structures. (Fig. 12.2 shows the gallbladder lumen

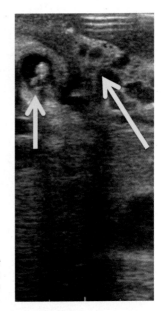

FIGURE 12.2 IOUS of the gallbladder (*short arrow*, note hyperechoic stones) in a patient with portal vein thrombosis and cavernous transformation (darker veins, *long arrow*).

that is anechoic or hypoechoic relative to the adjacent liver parenchyma, as well as hyperechoic stones in the gallbladder lumen.)

Signal transmission: begins with coupling of the transducer and the structure being imaged. Coupling may be generated by direct probe placement on the tissue to be imaged (liver, pancreas, etc.) or via "standoff" through an acoustic window such as the stomach/duodenum. Flooding the operative field with saline and using this fluid as an acoustic window is a useful standoff technique with which to evaluate superficial lesions.

Probe types: Transducer frequencies ranging from 5 to 10 MHz are useful for IOUS. Many IOUS probes are set at 7.5 MHz. The sound penetration of these frequencies is 6 to 10 cm, which is acceptable for most IOUS applications. Most IOUS probes are linear array; the crystals may be arranged in a linear fashion (which generates rectangular images) or curved orientation (also called convex probes). Probes may be of the "finger" or "T" shape. Each probe shape has advantages and limitations. The operator should try as many probes as possible; most will gravitate to one probe type or another (i.e., finger or T). Laparoscopic probes may be rigid or articulate in one or two orientations; the latter are particularly helpful when scanning the posterior liver sections (Fig. 12.3).

Orientation: Two basic planes are recognized in ultrasound—longitudinal and transverse. The operator should orient the probe (particularly the T probe) by pattern recognition—the left lateral section of the liver is a useful landmark with the "point" of the left lateral section aiming to the left upper corner of the screen (Fig. 12.4). The right kidney also serves as a good landmark.

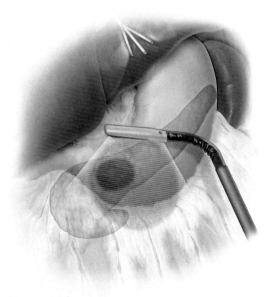

FIGURE 12.3 Articulating laparoscopic transducers provide more range of tissue coverage.

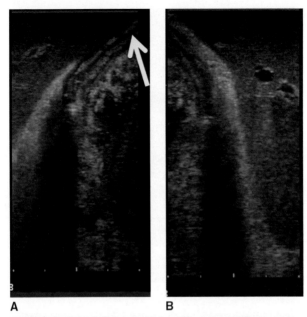

A   **B**

FIGURE 12.4 Orientation relative to left lateral liver section. **A.** Correct orientation, edge of the liver at top right of screen (*arrow*). **B.** Backward orientation.

Depth: can be adjusted in many ultrasound units (Fig. 12.1). Users should remember that image "magnification" typically sacrifices some clarity.

Image refinement: Once orientation and ideal scanning depth have been established, the image is refined by adjusting the gain and time gain compensation (TGC). Adjusting gain amplifies the returning echo signal (makes the image on the screen brighter). The gain should be set initially to make structures known to be anechoic (such as blood vessels) black. Too little gain results in nonvisualization of some structures; too much gain results in image artifact. Sound waves attenuate as they pass through tissue. The TGC controls are used to "fine tune" the depth of focus of IOUS images, using the most sensitive area of the sound wave (the focal region of transition from near field to far field) to interrogate the structure of interest.

Scanning techniques: systematic scanning is undertaken using four basic probe movements—sliding, rotating, rocking, and tilting. The novice ultrasonographer's initial impulse is to slide the probe; however, a remarkable amount of information can be learned simply by rocking and tilting the probe from one discrete position. The operator must be aware of the effect probe pressure exerts on the underlying tissue. Too much pressure may compress vascular structures (Fig. 12.5) or obscure lesions. On the other hand, deliberate compression ("compression scanning") is a useful technique for defining some structures. For example, in the porta hepatis, the portal vein will compress, while the hepatic artery will not compress.

Special techniques: such as standoff, acoustic window use, or intravascular contrast-enhanced ultrasound may be applied to appropriate situations.

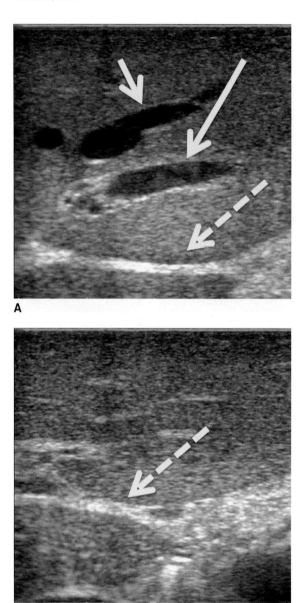

A

B

FIGURE 12.5 Compression. **A.** Liver without compression. Note hepatic vein (*short arrow*), portal vein branch (*long arrow*, note hyperechoic edges from extension of Glisson capsule around the portal triad), and hyperechoic ligamentum venosum (*dashed arrow*). **B.** Probe is in the same position, though with compression. Note ligamentum venosum (*dashed arrow*) as anatomic reference; the vascular structures have been obliterated by the compression.

Mode: most ultrasound images are in gray scale "B" mode (brightness modulation). Doppler mode may be used to evaluate vascular flow. In Doppler mode, spectral analysis is plotted against time. Color flow uses computer transformation of Doppler direction and velocity. By convention, flow toward the transducer is red and flow away from the transducer is blue. Velocity is typically shown in shades—darker shades indicate reduced velocity, and brighter hues representing more rapid velocity.

Annotation and storage: Images may be stored either as static images or as "cine" loop recording real-time scans.

Biopsy/ablation: biopsy or ablation may be directed precisely by ultrasound. It is critical to confirm needle position in two planes. A helpful technique is to apply color flow: moving the biopsy needle or ablation probe under color flow visualization produces color motion marking.

Table 12.1 illustrates basic approach to IOUS scanning.

INTRAOPERATIVE ULTRASOUND OF THE LIVER

Intraoperative liver ultrasound is used to evaluate known lesions, identify new lesions, and guide procedures (resection, ablation, biopsy). This guidance also includes precisely localizing a lesion's location relative to intrahepatic vascular structures, which has obvious therapeutic implications. Despite advances in cross-sectional imaging, IOUS remains the most accurate way to detect liver lesions; as many as 10% of patients will have unanticipated additional liver lesions found at the time of IOUS evaluation. This situation is particularly true for neuroendocrine tumors, many of which have numerous occult intrahepatic metastases.

Intrahepatic metastases have a discrete acoustic character—they may be isoechoic, hyperechoic, or hypoechoic relative to the surrounding liver parenchyma (Fig. 12.6). Multiple metastases in the same patient nearly always have similar echogenicity. Therefore, the best approach to a patient with known hepatic metastases is to first identify a known lesion (i.e., one that is palpable or easily seen on cross-sectional imaging) to determine echogenicity. After identifying the echogenic characteristics of the known lesion, the entire hepatic parenchyma should be scanned systematically, keeping in mind the lesions' character. Isoechoic lesions obviously are the most challenging to detect intraoperatively.

In general, the approach to liver IOUS involves documenting vascular inflow and outflow, followed by systematic evaluation of the parenchyma with particular attention paid to target lesions' relationship to vascular

	Basic Approach to IOUS Scanning[a]

1. Orientation—relative to known patterns such as left lateral liver section
2. Depth adjustment—will sacrifice resolution for magnification
3. Image refinement—gain and TGC
4. Systematic scanning
   a. Movements—sliding, rotating, rocking, tilting
   b. Compression scanning
   c. Special techniques—standoff, acoustic windows
   d. Mode adjustment—duplex, color flow
   e. Biopsy/ablation (if indicated)
5. Annotation and storage
6. Completion scan

[a]IOUS should be performed both prior to and after any dissection.

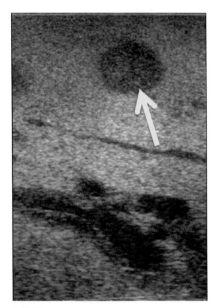

FIGURE 12.6 Metastatic cholangiocarcinoma to the liver (*arrow*). The lesion is hypoechoic to the surrounding hepatic parenchyma.

structures. Mobilization of the liver permits more accurate ultrasonographic examination, though also creates superficial artifact. Therefore, liver IOUS should be performed both before and after mobilizing dissection.

Systematic Approach

Again, IOUS of the liver consists of inflow, outflow, and parenchymal evaluation. Pattern recognition is important: an example is the fact that hepatic veins have more acute angles of articulation than portal veins, which join at more of a right angle. Particularly important to inflow is evaluation of known tumor relationship to vascular structures. An example of this concept is a caudate tumor's relationship to the inferior vena cava and portal vein. Outflow imaging documents hepatic vein drainage to the suprahepatic vena cava as well as documentation of accessory right hepatic vein. Although this anatomy is ideally known from preoperative imaging, the actual spatial relationship to the vena cava is well visualized with the ultrasound. The relationship of central tumors to the intrahepatic vasculature (particularly the middle hepatic vein) is similarly quite important. Intravascular tumor thrombus may be diagnosed by IOUS; this finding may dramatically alter operative approach.

Hepatic parenchymal pathology such as cirrhosis, steatosis, and post-chemotherapy changes significantly affects ultrasound characteristics. The hyperechogenicity of fatty liver or cirrhotic liver limits IOUS resolution. Evaluation of the parenchyma should be performed in a systematic fashion, that is, "lawn mowing" or segmental approach. No one perfect method for parenchymal scanning exists; the operator should become familiar with an approach and apply this approach consistently. As mentioned above, intrahepatic metastases may be hyper-, hypo-, or isoechoic to the underlying parenchyma; identifying the echogenicity of a known lesion early facilitates systematic interrogation of the hepatic parenchyma. Parenchyma should be scanned slowly. The operator should be cautious of superficial lesions that may not be completely captured by ultrasound without using standoff techniques. The operator should also be aware of compression, too much of which may obscure intrahepatic lesions. With increasing experience, the ultrasound operator will become more comfortable adjusting TGC to obtain more precise visualization of deep liver lesions. Perihepatic lymph nodes particularly the portal nodes, celiac nodes, and retropancreatic (aortocaval) nodes should also be evaluated at this point. Finally, postresection, evaluating flow in vascular structures with Doppler/flow mode, is particularly useful after vascular reconstruction or to document portal flow following a Pringle maneuver.

Pearls

- Interoperative ultrasound of the liver may be limited in the setting of hepatic parenchymal pathology such as cirrhosis and steatosis.
- Do not "directly observe" intrahepatic radiofrequency ablation; the heat may damage the sensitive ultrasound crystals as they contact the liver surface.
- For ultrasound-guided needle localization (radiofrequency ablation or biopsy), the angle of needle placement may be challenging, and experience is helpful in determining this approach. Needle placement directly adjacent to the ultrasound probe may not be the best position.
- Validating probe position *in two planes* is mandatory prior to ablation. This maneuver must be performed prior to ablation to avoid artifact. Also, remember that ablation defects are not spherical.
- Simple cysts of the liver are easily characterized; these lesions are anechoic with posterior shadow (Fig. 12.7).

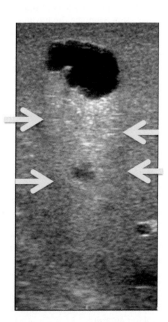

FIGURE 12.7 Classic features of simple liver cyst: anechoic cyst with posterior shadowing (*arrows*).

- Hemangioma of the liver may be confirmed by documenting flow through the lesion (although this diagnosis is almost always secure preoperatively with adequate IV contrast-enhanced cross-sectional imaging).
- The ultrasound character of focal nodular hyperplasia and hepatic adenoma is very similar—these heterogeneous lesions are not possible to distinguish by IOUS.
- The posterior section and segment VII in particular is most challenging to visualize with the laparoscopic ultrasound probe. A two-way articulating probe is quite helpful evaluating these areas. Mobilizing the falciform and coronary ligaments also helps expose the posterior section for IOUS.
- It is important to complete laparoscopic IOUS through multiple port sites.
- Scoring the liver capsule with electrocautery provides a useful artifact that helps define the intrahepatic plane of resection.

INTRAOPERATIVE ULTRASOUND OF THE BILIARY SYSTEM

IOUS of the biliary system is most commonly used to visualize intrahepatic and extrahepatic stones as well as to evaluate the relationship of biliary tumors to intra- and extrahepatic vascular structures. Less commonly, the diagnosis of biliary cystadenoma may be confirmed by visualizing septa and/or rarely a direct communication between cyst and the biliary tree. The later is usually seen more clearly with magnetic resonance cholangiography.

Systematic Approach

It is helpful to use an acoustic window (i.e., viewing through hepatic segment III or IV) to visualize the extrahepatic biliary tree. Similarly, either the stomach or the duodenal bulb provides a good acoustic window to visualize the intrapancreatic common bile duct. Of note, no Kocher maneuver is necessary to image the intrapancreatic bile duct. If Kocher maneuver is planned, ultrasonography should be performed both before and after disrupting these tissue planes. The quality of ultrasound images decreases significantly after dissection.

The course of the biliary tree should be defined. Particular attention should be paid to the aberrant biliary anatomy such as a low-lying right posterior sectoral duct. The relationship of the biliary tree to vascular structures (particularly the right hepatic artery) should be defined. Figure 12.8 shows aberrant right hepatic artery coursing anterior to the common bile duct. The presence of shadowing defects (e.g., intraductal stones) should be sought. Three classic sonographic criteria for stones are (1) presence of hyperechoic focus, (2) posterior shadowing, and (3) mobility (Fig. 12.9). Most stones are mobile with movement of the gallbladder or bile duct—this distinguishes them from polyps or tumors, which are fixed. Gallbladder polyps may not shadow; generally, neoplastic polyps are less echogenic than cholesterol polyps. Infiltrating tumors may show irregular wall thickening; attention should be paid to the interface of the gallbladder wall with the hepatic parenchyma. Tumors of the gallbladder fundus or extrahepatic biliary tree should be evaluated relative to their relationship with adjacent vascular structures—portal veins and hepatic arteries.

Although some skilled operators advocate IOUS as the sole modality to diagnose bile duct stones, it is important to realize that the learning curve for biliary IOUS is relatively steep. Many biliary surgeons feel comfortable confirming ultrasound findings with intraoperative cholangiography.

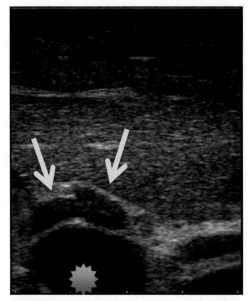

FIGURE 12.8 Transhepatic acoustic window visualizing extrahepatic biliary tree. Aberrant right hepatic artery (*arrows*) passing anterior to dilated common bile duct (*star*).

Pearls

- IOUS is helpful in identifying the course of an aberrant arterial structure (i.e., replaced right hepatic artery, right hepatic artery anterior to the common hepatic duct).
- IOUS of the biliary system may actually be most useful in laparoscopic surgery, where decreased tactile sensation is available.
- IOUS is quite useful to evaluate the intrahepatic and intrapancreatic extension of choledochal cysts.
- With practice, ultrasonography allows identification of the common bile duct and main pancreatic duct junction in the pancreatic head, that is, an abnormal biliopancreatic junction.
- IOUS is useful to localize the papilla for "targeted" (limited) duodenotomy for papillary exploration, such as sphincteroplasty, ampullectomy, transsphincteric exploration.
- IOUS is helpful to identify enlarged and possibly pathologic involved second echelon lymph nodes in patients with cholangiocarcinoma and gallbladder cancer (i.e., celiac, retropancreatic, aortocaval nodes). Many authorities consider involvement of these nodes to be a contraindication to resection.
- In gallbladder cancer, ultrasound is important in evaluating tumor relationship to the portal vein and the hepatic artery.
- In Mirizzi syndrome, ultrasound is quite useful for evaluating the biliary tree in relationship with the surrounding vascular structures and position of the stone.
- Pressure from the ultrasound probe in the porta hepatis will compress the portal vein but not the hepatic artery.
- Intrahepatic bile ducts are typically not visible on ultrasound scanning. Therefore, any intrahepatic biliary dilation visible on IOUS suggests biliary pathology.

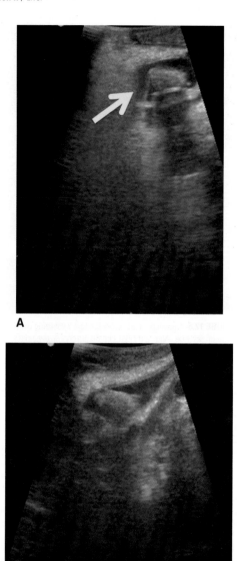

A

B

FIGURE 12.9 Laparoscopic IOUS of common bile duct stone (*arrow*) shown in transverse **(A)** and sagittal **(B)** orientation. The stone is hyperechoic with posterior shadowing.

INTRAOPERATIVE ULTRASOUND OF THE PANCREAS

Ultrasound is a remarkably useful but generally underused modality with which to evaluate pancreatic pathology. Similar to most tools, the more one uses ultrasound for pancreatic evaluation, the more comfortable the operator becomes with the approach and the more they appreciate the broad variety of applications of this modality.

Systematic Approach

Ultrasound of the pancreas should be performed both using an acoustic window such as the stomach or duodenum as well as by placing the probe directly on the pancreatic parenchyma to appreciate improved resolution. Systematic approach to the pancreatic ultrasound involves evaluation of the parenchyma, pancreatic duct, vascular relationships, and the target lesion (i.e., tumor, stone, dominant stricture). The pancreas relationship to adjacent vascular structures such as the splenic vein/superior mesenteric vein confluence (Fig. 12.10) provides useful points of reference (i.e., pattern recognition).

Pancreatic Parenchyma

Normal pancreatic parenchyma is usually homogeneous, with a small, anechoic or hypoechoic duct visible. The typical "salt and pepper" speckled features of the pancreatic parenchyma is due to the hyperechogenic intra-parenchymal fat. Pancreas echogenicity is usually similar to or greater than that of the liver.

Features of chronic pancreatitis have been defined to include parenchymal (hyperechoic foci, hyperechoic strands, hypoechoic lobules, and cysts) and ductal (dilation, dilated side branches, main duct irregularity, hyperechoic duct margins, and stones) criteria (Fig. 12.11). Table 12.2 outlines these criteria.

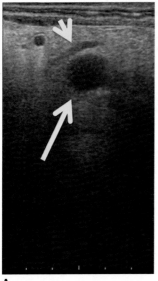 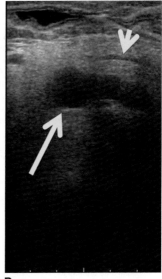

A   **B**

FIGURE 12.10 Transverse orientation at the pancreatic head. Superior mesenteric vein (SMV) (in **A**) and SMV/splenic vein confluence (in **B**) are shown with *long arrow*; pancreatic duct at the genu **(A)** and body **(B)** is shown with *short arrows*.

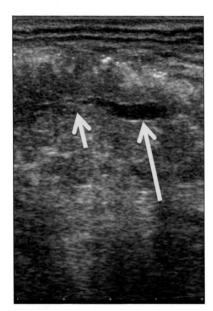

FIGURE 12.11 Chronic pancreatitis showing main pancreatic duct stricture (*short arrow*) with dilation of MPD upstream to the tail (*long arrow*).

Pancreatic Duct

The pancreatic duct should be evaluated for size, tortuosity, known (or unappreciated), strictures, the presence of pancreatic divisum, and/or size of accessory pancreatic duct, which has implications when planning transduodenal sphincteroplasty. A minimally dilated or tortuous pancreatic duct may be very challenging to open longitudinally if one is considering a lateral pancreaticojejunostomy; direct IOUS guidance is quite helpful in this circumstance. Perhaps, the most important relationship of the pancreatic duct is that of the main pancreatic duct to a cyst or neuroendocrine neoplasm if the operator is considering enucleation. Injury to the main pancreatic duct results in a high-volume, morbid pancreatic fistula.

TABLE 12.2	Ultrasound Characteristics of Chronic Pancreatitis

Parenchymal
    Hyperechoic foci
    Hyperechoic strands
    Hypoechoic lobules
    Cyst
Ductal
    Irregular duct contour
    Visible side branches
    Hyperechoic duct margin
    Dilated main duct
    Stones

The intrapancreatic portion of the common bile duct should be evaluated routinely for size, intraluminal lesion, and relationship to pancreatic ducts.

Vascular Relationships

Vascular relationships include relation of the pancreas and target lesion to the surrounding arterial and venous structures: portal, splenic, and superior mesenteric veins, and celiac, hepatic, gastroduodenal, and superior mesenteric arteries. This relationship is unique to individual lesion/tumor position. Often the splenic artery is intraparenchymal in the body and the tail of the pancreas. Therefore, understanding splenic artery anatomy is important when the operator is considering spleen preserving distal pancreatectomy or lateral pancreaticojejunostomy (which should be extended to the tail). Unusual anatomy such as a replaced right or left hepatic artery is important and may be recognized with the IOUS. The presence and/or extent of portal vein/superior mesenteric vein or splenic vein thrombosis can be identified and again may have direct implications on operative planning.

Target

Finally, in the systematic approach to pancreas IOUS is evaluation of the target lesion. Tumors should be evaluated for their relationship to adjacent vasculature (i.e., superior mesenteric/portal veins, superior mesenteric artery,) as well as to adjacent organ structures such as the stomach, adrenal, and colon in the case of pancreas tail tumors. Deliberate characterization of tumor echogenic features will inform the operator's future practice. For example, pancreatic adenocarcinoma is typically hypoechoic; distal cholangiocarcinoma may not obstruct the pancreatic duct (Fig. 12.12);

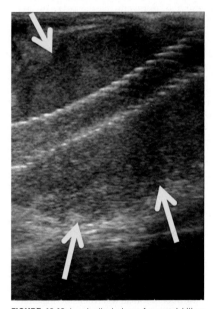

FIGURE 12.12 Longitudinal view of a metal biliary stent passing through well-circumscribed, hypoechoic distal cholangiocarcinoma (*arrows*). The pancreatic duct in this patient was not dilated.

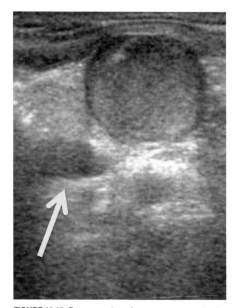

FIGURE 12.13 Transverse view of a pancreas neuroendocrine tumor is hyperechoic and well circumscribed, with hypoechoic edges and faint posterior shadowing. Superior mesenteric vein is shown with *arrow*.

and neuroendocrine neoplasms are typically hyperechoic and well-circumscribed relative to surrounding parenchyma (Fig. 12.13).

Dominant strictures in the pancreatic duct should be identified; in addition, ultrasound provides a sensitive method to interrogate the entire ductal system for other unexpected strictures, which may influence the choice of operation, particularly in chronic pancreatitis patients.

Pancreatic cysts are easily identified and characterized by IOUS (Fig. 12.14). Attention should be directed toward communication with the main pancreatic duct, wall irregularity, or mural nodularity. In addition, the relationship of the cyst to surrounding structures including the main pancreatic duct is important, especially if considering enucleation.

IOUS is the most accurate method with which to characterize peripancreatic inflammatory collections in the setting of necrotizing pancreatitis (Fig. 12.15). The volume of solid necrosis has major implication in treatment planning.

Pearls

- Fine tuning TGC is particularly useful when evaluating the vascular/tumor interface.
- Knowledge of the relationship between cysts or islet cell tumors and the main pancreatic duct is critical when considering enucleation.
- In laparoscopic IOUS evaluation of the pancreas, port placement is important. The pancreas should be scanned from at least two separate ports. The operator should also be aware that probe orientation and the resulting image will change significantly with different fulcrum of laparoscopy.

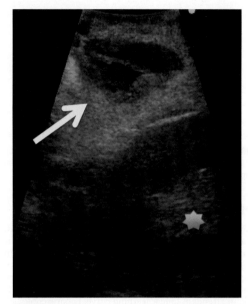

FIGURE 12.14 Transverse orientation, laparoscopic IOUS of pancreatic tail mucinous cystic neoplasm (MCN; *arrow*). Note thick walls and internal septae. Note also relationship to the left kidney (*star*).

- Evaluation of the pancreatic duct is important when considering opening a small pancreatic duct for lateral pancreaticojejunostomy.
- It bears repeating that ultrasound is the most accurate way to identify solid versus fluid peripancreatic necrotic debris in the setting of necrotizing pancreatitis.

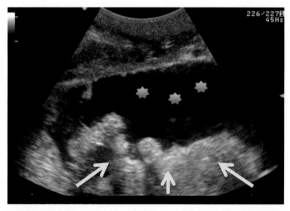

FIGURE 12.15 Transgastric view (transverse orientation) of peripancreatic collection in necrotizing pancreatitis patient. This collection has fluid (*stars*) and solid (*arrows*) components.

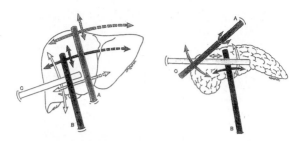

FIGURE 12.16 Laparoscopic ultrasound scanning from several different ports. (From Machi J, Staren E, eds. *Ultrasound for surgeons*, 2nd ed. Philadelphia, PA: Lippincott Williams & Wilkins, 2005.)

INTRAOPERATIVE LAPAROSCOPIC ULTRASOUND

Laparoscopic ultrasound follows the same principles as other IOUS techniques. The major difference is limited probe motion based on probe rigidity and the fulcrum of the probe interface through the abdominal wall (Fig. 12.16). Laparoscopic probes that articulate in one and two directions provide better tissue coverage than rigid probes (Fig. 12.3). Laparoscopic ultrasound is technically and intellectually more demanding than open IOUS, with an attendant longer learning curve. Laparoscopic IOUS should be performed through multiple ports (i.e., umbilical, subxiphoid, lateral). The operator should concentrate on understanding image patterns that may be markedly different from traditional (open) IOUS patterns.

CONCLUSION

In summary, intraoperative ultrasonography is an extremely valuable addition to the HPB surgeon's armamentarium. Performing ultrasound on every case is helpful to understand both normal parenchymal and anatomic relationships as well as becoming familiar with pathology and unusual relationships.

Suggested Readings

Choti MA, Kaloma F, de Oliveira ML, et al. Patient variability in intraoperative ultrasonographic characteristics of colorectal liver metastases. *Arch Surg* 2008;143(1):29–34.

Connor S, Barron E, Wigmore SJ, et al. The utility of laparoscopic assessment in the preoperative staging of suspected hilar cholangiocarcinoma. *J Gastrointest Surg* 2005;9(4):476–480.

Hagopian EJ, Manchi J, eds. *Abdominal ultrasound for surgeons*. New York, NY: Springer, 2014.

13 Energy Devices for Parenchymal Transection in Liver Surgery

Prejesh Philips and Robert C.G. Martin II

BACKGROUND

The first well-documented reports of deliberate resection of liver tumors come from A. Luis in 1886 and Carl von Langenbuch in 1887, both of which were marred by postoperative bleeding. Control of the hepatic bleeding was accomplished with "well-placed sutures and well-timed prayers." William Williams Keen was credited with first liver resection in America and also described the "finger fracture" technique and individual cauterization. In1888, Hugo Rex and, in 1897, James Cantlie from Liverpool rediscovered the work of Glisson from 1654 and described the avascular plane through the gallbladder bed toward the vena cava, now known as the Rex-Cantlie line. This was followed by description of the Pringle maneuver, and finally the seminal work of Claude Couinaud, in 1954, on the segmental architecture of the liver, led to the blossoming of modern-day hepatic surgery. The finger fracture technique was initially described and was followed later by the clamp–crushing technique or Kelly-clysis, which has since become the reference parenchymal transection method. Following these anatomical principles and improvement in anesthesia, surgeons could attain anatomical resection with less blood loss, but the problem of bleeding parenchyma, erratic vasculature, high mortality, and morbidity persisted. At the same time, it has been shown clearly that the use of blood transfusions in liver surgery is associated with worse outcomes. In an attempt to decrease blood loss and improve transection speed and quality, various hemostatic assist energy devices have been designed.

Although great advances have been made in technology, the ideal hemostatic energy device and mechanism is a topic of much debate. The ideal coagulation mechanism would include ease of use, minimal lateral energy damage, the ability to cut as well as coagulate, control of tissue temperature (so that charring is avoided), reliability, noninterference with medical devices, and the versatility to work on a variety of tissues. We will individually examine the commonly used energy sources, review current literature, and compare their strengths, weaknesses, and uses.

ELECTROSURGERY

Thermal and chemical cauteries were the first tools for hemostasis. This technique evolved over time to the use of electrocautery or more accurately electrosurgery, since it involves the use of an alternating current in which the patient is part of the circuit. The principle is generation of electricity from the Electro-generator unit, delivered to a handheld device, which then uses tissue impedance to produce heat. The complementary part of the circuit, return electrode, or grounding pad takes the electrons back to complete circuit.

Monopolar high-frequency electrical energy is the oldest method used to coagulate vessels. The first commercial electrosurgical device is credited to William T. Bovie and used for the first time in 1926 in Boston. It uses a generator to create high-frequency current (200 kHz) in order to prevent nerve conduction and generate local thermal energy while at the same time preventing remote electrical injury. Because of this, a local thermoablative zone is created. There are different modes that monopolar electrocautery can be used. "Cut" causes a high enough voltage (> 400 V peak to peak) to create a vapor pocket and results in an incision. It typically uses a modulated periodic sine waveform. When the system is operating in "coag mode," the voltage output is usually lower than in the cut mode and less power is delivered. Typically, sine wave is turned on and off in a rapid succession. This therefore generates less heat, and a vapor pocket is not generated. The overall effect is a slower heating process that causes tissue to coagulate and smaller vessels are destroyed and sealed, stopping capillary and small arterial bleeding. In simple coagulation/cutting mode machines, the lower-voltage cycle typical of coagulation mode is usually heard as a lower frequency.

Monopolar electrocautery is versatile, almost universal in availability, and cheap, acts quickly, and is relatively safe to use. It can be used in a variety of settings and can effectively help control bleeding from small vessels and capillaries.

Limitation of Electrosurgery

Patients with electrical implants such as cardiac pacemakers require special precautions, especially when using monopolar devices. Conventional monopolar electrosurgery should not be used to control larger vascular structures, around vascular compromised tissue, bowel, and other visceral structures such as the bile duct and ureter. The limitations of monopolar electrocautery include poor efficacy with vessels greater than 3 mm, a wide collateral zone of thermal injury, and lack of an effective feedback mechanism except visual approximation.

Complications of Electrosurgery

Electrosurgery-related complications are relatively uncommon, occurring in 2 to 5/1,000 procedures. Lack of experience and knowledge of the device's mechanism of action is the major contributing factor with approximately 60 procedures being the inflection point for injuries from electrothermal devices in laparoscopy.

The mechanism of electrosurgical injury includes direct injury, lateral thermal spread, direct coupling, capacitive coupling, and insulation failure. Direct coupling results from inadvertent contact of two noninsulated instruments, and the current flows from the primary to the secondary instrument. Severe injury may result from a second conductor if it is in contact with sensitive structures. Capacitive coupling is alternating current flowing through the primary electrosurgical device inducing unintended stray current in any conductor (such as metal trocars of liver retractors) in close proximity with the monopolar instrument.

Hollow viscus injury is uncommon but is often missed and can have fatal consequences. The nature of the thermal injury is such that intraoperatively, the injury may be masked and will manifest usually about 4 to 10 days postoperatively, depending upon the severity of the coagulation necrosis. In the context of liver surgery, electrocautery has caused duodenal injury and late bile duct strictures. These injuries can be avoided by minimizing the use of electrocautery in extrahepatic pedicle control techniques. While assessing the efficacy of the coagulation, attention should be paid to the whitening of tissue surrounding the tip of the electrosurgical instrument and formation of bubbles. Whitening suggests adequate hemostasis and bubbles represent water vapor; thus, the tissue is desiccated, and the bubbles disappear, marking adequacy. Other visceral and vascular injuries from electrocautery have been reported. Severe skin burns caused by a partially detached grounding pad/return electrode can occur, but most modern electrosurgical monopolar devices have a return electrode monitoring system to prevent this problem. Use of lowest-effective power settings, intermittent activation, and direct visual feedback for adequacy are good practices for the prevention of injury. With bipolar electrosurgery, termination at the end of the vapor phase and alternating between desiccation and incision are a good practice.

Our preference is to use the monopolar electrosurgical device to gain access to the abdomen and use it for mobilization of the right hepatic lobe off the triangular ligaments. We also use it to "score" the liver capsule while delineating resection lines. This demarcation defining the line of resection can be seen with high-quality ultrasound imaging and helps to ensure an adequate margin prior to resection. This line of demarcation for resection is even more important when performing laparoscopic resections given the limited visualization and lack of tactile feedback during resection.

Conventional Bipolar Electrosurgery

In bipolar electrosurgery, both the active electrode and return electrode functions are performed at the site of surgery. The two tines of the forceps perform the active and return electrode functions. Only the tissue grasped is included in the electrical circuit. Because the return function is performed by one tine of the forceps, no patient return electrode is needed. Most bipolar units use a low-voltage waveform that achieves hemostasis without excessive charring. For the same reasons, bipolar electrosurgical devices are less effective for cutting tissue since adequate vaporization is difficult to achieve. Effective hemostasis can be achieved by coapting and thermally welding the blood vessels. Conventional bipolar is widely used in neurosurgery and gynecologic surgery.

Bipolar electrosurgery technology is very safe because of limited tissue conduction. Use of lower voltages in a smaller circuit leads to less lateral thermal spread and injury. Bipolar energy is also safer to use when there is a question about the safety of using more powerful monopolar electrosurgical units (i.e., implantable medical electromagnetic devices such as pacemaker, defibrillator, pumps). There are some disadvantages to the use of bipolar: Bipolar cannot spark to tissue, and the low voltages make it less effective on large vessels.

BIPOLAR VESSEL-SEALING DEVICES

Ligasure

Vessels sealing devices stemmed from refinement of bipolar electrosurgery technology. The bipolar vessel-sealing system (LigaSure) applies a precise amount of bipolar energy and pressure to fuse collagen and elastin within the vessel walls. This fusion is done using a feedback-controlled energy delivery through a generator that senses adequate coaptation and coagulation. In addition, the device minimizes lateral thermal spread. The seal with this device can withstand three times the normal systolic pressure and seals vessels up to 7 mm. The sealing is achieved with minimal sticking and charring; thermal spread to adjacent tissues is approximately 2 mm. Vessel sealing has steadily gained acceptance in various surgical disciplines due to its ease of use and ability to seal relatively large vessels. To underscore this point, vessel sealing has been successfully used on the splenic hilum. The disadvantages include the need to fully engage and lock the clamps before delivery of energy can occur and the nonuniform compression it delivers over the length of the prongs. This technology is fast growing with proponents arguing the ease of use, fast sealing, and relative cost–benefit versus other devices. It is also one of the few devices with a cost–benefit analysis in its favor in published literature.

Ligasure has fast been gaining ground in laparoscopic surgery and has been used extensively in colorectal and bariatric procedures. A systematic review of six randomized controlled trials of hemostatic devices in colectomy was favorable for the use of Ligasure over conventional electrosurgery but did not demonstrate clear superiority over other ultrasonic vessel-sealing devices. A Japanese randomized control trial (RCT) demonstrated Ligasure's superiority with respect to blood loss, transection times, and lower number of ties required. They also showed a cost–benefit in using Ligasure over conventional techniques. This was however followed shortly later by another Japanese trial showing no benefit over the crush–clamp technique. Another RCT, which showed superiority of the clamp–crush technique, was conducted under inflow control and that needs to be taken into consideration in the era of minimally invasive surgery where inflow control is the exception rather than the norm.

EnSeal

Enseal is another vessel-sealing system that uses bipolar electrosurgical principles. EnSeal delivers vessel sealing by using a combination of compression and thermocoagulative energy to ensure hemostasis. It is capable of achieving seal strengths up to seven times the normal systolic pressures on vessels up to 7 mm with a typical thermal spread of approximately 1 mm. It differs from Ligasure in its compression mechanism, which applies uniform pressure along the full length of the instrument jaw, achieving compression forces similar to those of a linear stapler of up to 7,800 psi. Compression is combined with controlled energy delivery utilizing Nanopolar thermostats to reach collagen denaturation temperatures in seconds: temperatures maintained at approximately 100°C throughout the power delivery cycle. The device also has a simultaneous cutting mechanism to allow one-step sealing and transection of vessels and soft tissues. The big cost advantage is the ability to use conventional bipolar generators for its use, thereby obviating a large new capital investment for generators. EnSeal also has a large jaw width and produces minimal smoke (or steam). The dynamic dual mechanism mandates active operator effort and cognizance and has a modest learning curve as compared to other lock-fire devices.

This device is about 3 cm in length at the functional portion of the head, which is comprised of jaws. The instrument head is designed to facilitate atraumatic dissection. In a comparative porcine model, Enseal devices were reported to achieve higher burst pressures with a sub-mm lateral thermal spread. Another ex vivo study reported longer sealing times and variable burst pressures with Enseal as compared to Ligasure device. There have been few clinical studies of Enseal in published literature and no randomized controlled trials. Initial studies demonstrated the safety profile of this device. A single-center study on laparoscopic liver resection using the EnSeal versus ultrasonic dissector showed shorter parenchymal transection time. However, head-to-head comparisons with conventional clamp–crush are not available in current literature. Despite this paucity of clinical data, its performance in preclinical studies, ease of use, and ability to simultaneously seal and divide large vessels without significant lateral thermal spread have made Enseal popular among many centers.

Inherent limitations of the device remain the need for the operating surgeon to feel when the tissue is desiccated–sealed with a gradual compression of the device. The device differs from other devices as its mechanism of action is initiated prior to complete closure of the device giving the operating surgeon feedback on the type of tissue that is being transected.

Salient Dissecting Sealer (Formerly TissueLink Monopolar)

The TissueLink floating ball is a saline-cooled, high-density monopolar radiofrequency probe used for dissection and coagulation. Saline irrigation at the tip maintains the surface temperature below 100°C, preventing charring and tissue "sticking," reducing smoke, and decreasing lateral thermal spread. The saline facilitates energy transfer between the device–tissue interface, maintaining contact with the hepatic tissue even when the tip is moving and evenly dispersing thermal energy. The mechanism of sealing is primarily by heat and shrinking, and it provides a clean transection bed and can seal vessels up to 3 mm in size. It will isolate larger vessels, which can then be controlled by other techniques.

TissueLink is useful in transecting cirrhotic livers and in resecting lesions in close proximity to major vessels. Theoretically, the saline cooling prevents lateral thermal spread, thus making it safer around biliary and larger vascular structures. It is however expensive and slow. It has been used in many centers in combination with ultrasonic dissection device. Various nonrandomized studies showed efficacy in cirrhotic and noncirrhotic liver transection with respect to blood loss and postoperative liver dysfunction, albeit with an increase in operative time. It has been used in living donor hepatic transection showing superiority in one study over CUSA and bipolar electrocautery. One randomized study, using water-jet, ultrasonic dissector and aspirator, and salient dissecting sealer, found that the dissecting sealer group used less hemostatic agents but was slower and more expensive than Hydrojet and CUSA. Randomized trials however have showed no significant benefit over the crush–clamp technique. The benefits of this device remain its hemostatic potential and action, while not requiring any type of compression. This can be very helpful when performing nonanatomic resections in cirrhotic patients when the hepatic parenchyma is more fibrotic that the portal inflow or hepatic outflow and thus a crushing technique can lead to more bleeding. The limitations of the device remain its methodical method of action and limited efficiency when used alone.

PlasmaKinetic Tissue Management System

This system delivers pulsed bipolar energy through the instrument to the tissue, allowing intermittent tissue cooling, which limits lateral thermal spread and tissue sticking. The generator detects the optimal settings for the specific instrument, and there are visual and audible tissue impedance indicators. The system has two different modes: the vapor pulse coagulation mode and the PlasmaKinetic tissue-cutting mode. In the vapor pulse mode, high energy is delivered to grasped tissue, creating vapor zones. The current then travels around the high-impedance vapor zones, following the path of least resistance. The vapor zones subsequently collapse, and with each new energy pulse, more and more tissue between the instrument jaws is coagulated, ultimately resulting in uniform coagulation of tissue. It is capable of sealing vessels 5 to 6 mm in diameter and has burst pressure up to three times the systolic blood pressure with half of the lateral thermal spread compared to conventional bipolar devices. In a recent study, PlasmaKinetic was used for hepatic resections in 51 cirrhotic and noncirrhotic livers, with acceptable morbidity and transection speeds. The authors point to the statistical similarity between the outcomes of the cirrhotics and noncirrhotic patients as evidence that it is efficacious in cirrhotic liver. There are various effector instruments including hook, needle, and dissecting and cutting forceps.

ARGON BEAM COAGULATORS

The argon beam coagulator is a noncontact, monopolar electrocoagulation device that transmits radiofrequency electrical energy from a handheld electrode across a jet of argon gas. The argon gas jet clears the field of pooled blood and evenly distributes electrical energy to the target tissue. Argon photocoagulation is used very commonly to control bleeding from the cut parenchymal edge. It allows for rapid and diffuse superficial coagulation at the plane of transection. It is usually used in conjunction with another dissecting technique such as Kelly-clysis and CUSA. It cannot be used to control large vascular and biliary structures, but with its low penetrance contact coagulation, it is extremely effective in surface hemostasis. Its use is almost ubiquitous in transplant and cirrhotic settings. There have been various reports of bowel injury with its use when used by untrained hands or because of a lack of understanding of the method of action of the device. There remains a myth regarding the potential risk of venous gas embolism, which can occur in any open case when the central venous pressure (CVP) is low and/or inadvertent injury to the hepatic outflow structure occurs. We have successfully utilized argon beam coagulation following over 300 laparoscopic cases and have not had a single venous embolism event, and thus, we believe this risk is unproven when good surgical transection technique is utilized.

ABLATIVE TECHNOLOGIES

Radiofrequency-Assisted Parenchymal Transection (RF-PT): Habib 4×

Radiofrequency (RF) devices have been used for more than a decade to thermoablate nonresectable hepatic lesions. The Habib was an extension of this technology. It was one of the first devices to create a bloodless field at the purported site of transection using thermocoagulative properties. It uses RF probes, which can be inserted into the liver surface. This leads to a plane of coagulative necrosis to be developed along the line of parenchymal transection, with subsequent reduction of blood loss and transfusion. This concept of precoagulation deep in the parenchyma of the liver before transection allows nonanatomical resections. It can seal intrahepatic vessels and bile ducts. The radiofrequency energy is typically applied in sequentially overlapping segments to ensure adequate hemostasis. This technique, however, is time consuming and costly. Despite the ability for nonanatomical resection, it does lead to a large area of hepatic eschar and more tissue necrosis than other techniques.

In the RF-PT or radiofrequency-assisted parenchymal transection, the Habib device 4× has been used widely in various centers. Various nonrandomized studies showed benefit especially in reduction of blood loss and postoperative complications. However, there have been increasing reports of liver failure and infectious complications in part due to the wide zone of ablation that the RF device induces. In some randomized studies and two meta-analyses, Habib was shown not to be superior to the crush–clamp technique. Proponents argue that the use of RF-assisted device is especially useful in cirrhotic livers where traditional transection methods can lead to significant more blood loss. This claim has been backed up by at least one randomized study that showed significantly lower blood loss and a trend to decreased complications with the use of RF devices in cirrhotic livers.

It is useful in cirrhotic patients, but the risks of the large ablation zone leading to liver failure in these patients with marginal liver reserve need to be taken into account. Additional challenges with this device for laparoscopic use are the large trocar that is required and the lack of any type of transection feature leading to inefficient of movements during transection.

Microwave

Microwave energy technology has been used as an ablative therapy in patients with nonresectable hepatic lesions. Similar to the RF-PT device, it utilized the precoagulation principle. A microwave tissue coagulator (Alfresa Ind., Osaka, Japan) generates a 2,450-MHz microwave, which is transmitted to a monopolar type of needle electrode, called a microwave scalpel, by way of a coaxial cable. This endoscopic surgical device has a hand piece with needle-shaped monopolar applicators. Microwave emission is started after the liver tissue is punctured with a microwave probe or scalpel. Molecular excitation by microwave causes thermal energy, which results in zone of tissue coagulation around the microwave scalpel. The coagulation region reaches a depth equal to the length of the scalpel. It can be recognized as a superficial yellow-whitish coagulation zone approximately 1 cm in diameter.

Microwave precoagulation has been gaining favor among some surgeons. It has shown to be a safe and effective mode of precoagulation before transection in a nonrandomized study with respect to bile leak, hospital stay, and blood loss as compared to historical controls with other transection devices. It has a smaller ablation zone compared to radiofrequency ablation. This technique however is time consuming and needs precoagulation as a separate step. No randomized controlled trials have compared microwave to other technologies or to the clamp–crush technique. Current technologies have not been optimized for precoagulation and transection with the use of microwave and thus remain limited to open resections.

DISSECTION-ONLY DEVICES

Ultrasonic Dissectors: (CUSA)

The Cavitron Ultrasonic Surgical Aspirator (CUSA) is a dissecting device that uses ultrasonic frequencies to fragment tissue. In combination with the aspiration of the dissected contents (i.e., hepatic parenchyma), CUSA skeletonizes small vessels and bile ducts allowing control by clips, ligatures, or other energy devices. Utilizing a hollow titanium tip that vibrates along its longitudinal axis, fragmentation of susceptible tissue occurs while concurrently lavaging and aspirating material from the surgical site. The CUSA selectively ablates tissues with high water content such as liver parenchyma, glandular tissue, and neoplastic tissue. Among CUSA's benefits, it provides a very well-defined transection plane, which is useful in situations of close proximity between tumors and major vascular structures. Also, it can be used in the cirrhotic as well as noncirrhotic livers and is associated with a low blood loss and low risk of bile leak.

Noninferiority studies comparing CUSA to the clamp–crush technique have shown similar outcomes. One of the first randomized studies comparing the ultrasonic dissector versus the clamp–crush technique showed that the ultrasonic dissector is more frequently associated with tumor exposure at the resection margin and with incomplete appearance of landmark hepatic veins on the cut surface. Subsequent retrospective studies showed superiority with respect to blood loss but with longer operating times compared to conventional surgery. Other studies comparing CUSA with water dissectors (Hydrojet) showed CUSA to have longer transection times but less blood loss. Several RCTs looking at the effectiveness have not shown any improvement in operative times, blood loss, or complication rates with CUSA. Proponents of CUSA highlight the selective vascular isolation and visualization of the CUSA, the clean operative field, and the fact that it has been used clinically for close to two decades. Opponents argue that is takes longer, has similar transection outcome, and is expensive. The incidence of air embolism with ultrasonic dissectors is also a common phenomenon, which is usually asymptomatic but may lead to adverse outcomes.

Water-Jet Dissector (ERBEJET 2, ERBE USA Inc., Marietta, GA)

This technique employs a high-pressure water jet to break apart the liver tissue and selectively isolate small vascular and biliary structures, potentially decreasing blood loss. These vessels and ducts must then be ligated and divided individually according to preference. Its advantage is having a precise delineation of the transection plane, which can be used to expose major vessels effectively, especially in the context of closely adjacent tumors. Water-jet dissection does not use thermal energy and thus spares the surrounding tissue from any thermal damage. Water-jet dissection was noted in one randomized study to be superior to CUSA with regard to transection speed and blood loss, Pringle time, and operative duration. A randomized trial comparing four techniques of clamp–crush (under pedicle control), CUSA, Hydrojet, and dissecting sealer was recently conducted. The clamp–crush method was noted to be superior in transection speed, blood loss, transfusion rate, number of ligatures, and transection time. The ultrasonic and water-jet dissection devices have remained a useful tool for precoagulation dissection and thus do require an additional coagulation device and cosurgeon of adequate experience to assist during the transection steps. This requirement can limit efficiency, but overall remains a very safe and effect method of dissection.

ULTRASONIC CUTTING AND COAGULATING DEVICE

The ultrasonic cutting and coagulating surgical device (Harmonic scalpel, not to be confused with ultrasonic dissector such as CUSA) converts sound energy into mechanical energy at the functional end of the instrument. A piezoelectric crystal in the hand piece generates vibration at the tip of the active blade at 55,500 times per second. This leads to production of heat from rupture of hydrogen bonds, which leads to denaturation of proteins at tissue temperatures of 60°C to 80°C, resulting in coagulum formation without the desiccation, charring, or smoke caused by conventional electrosurgical methods. The main disadvantages of Harmonic scalpel are the limited ability to coagulate vessels larger than 3 to 5 mm, increased cost of disposable instruments, and potential for extensive thermal spread at high energy levels (level 5) for more than 5 seconds. The quality of vessel seal also depends on the amount of tissue tension delivered and the setting used, and in this aspect, it is surgeon dependent.

Use of Harmonic scalpel has become more widespread in the era of laparoscopic surgery, with varied uses from thyroid surgery to upper gastrointestinal (GI) tract procedures. Harmonic scalpel is capable of sealing vessels from 3 to 5 mm and has shown to have less lateral thermal spread than conventional electrosurgery and minimal smoke formation or charring. It is also a versatile instrument, allowing the surgeon to dissect, cut, and coagulate using one instrument. The presence of an active exposed blade can be both an advantage in mobilizing coapted tissue but can also be dangerous if unintentional tissue contact with the active blade occurs. Initial reports used Harmonic scalpel in both open and laparoscopic liver resections, with no biliary leakage reported in a study of 41 patients. In contrast, a nonrandomized study showed an increased rate of postoperative bile leakage, raising some concerns of its safety sealing biliary structures. Another large published series comparing clamp–crushing with ultrasonic plus Harmonic scalpel dissection showed longer operative time, but with a reduced blood loss and a lower rate of biliary fistula. However, the retrospective method of the study and the relatively long period of inclusion may have biased these results against the clamp–crush technique. The merits of Harmonic device in cirrhotic livers, or in preventing bile leaks, remain to be proven. Similarly, the device has not been optimized for prolonged 20- to 30-second continuous use during transection, and thus, care should be taken to avoid collateral heat transfer and to ensure device integrity.

COMPARISON

The techniques of finger fracture technique or the use of Kelly-clysis along with individual ligation with clips or sutures for vascular and biliary structures have long been employed in liver resection. There has since been an increase in the use of precoagulation, or making the transection plane avascular with coagulation devices before transection. Examples of precoagulation devices are microwave and radiofrequency energy devices, which ablate and coagulate along the transection plane leaving a rim of avascular tissue. Broadly speaking, Ligasure, Enseal, and Harmonic devices use the precoagulation principles to effect subsequent parenchymal division. This is in contrast to resistance-modulated devices, which fragment low-resistance tissue (hepatic parenchyma) preserving fibrous (high-resistance) components such as vessels and bile ducts for subsequent ligation by the surgeon. These vascular-sparing structures include the ultrasonic dissector (CUSA) and the Hydrojet devices.

The advent of laparoscopy and its increased use in hepatic surgery led to an increased need for improved transection technology. The use of inflow control in laparoscopic surgery is less common than with conventional techniques due to technical difficulty. Newer transection devices have allowed parenchymal transection without the need for prolonged inflow control in laparoscopic procedures.

Although the Kelly-clysis or clamp–crush technique has long been the cornerstone of parenchymal transection in combination with inflow control, there is a greater risk of blood loss associated with this technique, when performed incorrectly. Despite a plethora of published literature with respect to parenchymal transection devices, no clear consensus of the optimal device exists. One of the major problems encountered in performing trials in this setting is rapid advance of technology. Newer variations of existing technology and refinements in current devices do not present enough time for planning and conduct of appropriately powered trials. Again, when these trials do happen, they are quickly outmoded by a more novel technology. This is due to the constant feedback from the operator of the devices and manufacturers trying to retain a niche market. Also, the operative mortality is about 1% in recent studies with a similar low morbidity of 8%. Therefore, sample size needed for adequately powered randomized controlled trials using surgery-related mortality or specific complications as a primary end point is very high, and most single-center studies are unable to reach those numbers. Multicenter trials are marred by nonuniformity of technique, which can lead to aberrant interpretations. At this current point in time, no specific claims of superiority can be made based on the evidence-based literature of one energy device over another.

Published studies have mixed results and design flaws and are underpowered. In an attempt to resolve this issue, a few meta-analyses have been performed; these have showed no clear benefit of one device over another or in fact even over the conventional clamp–crush technique. In this void of definitive literature or consensus, the individual surgeon's technique, prior training, and familiarity with the device are the key to maintain the current quality standards for hepatic transection and postoperative morbidity and mortality.

In summation, most parenchymal transection devices have certain advantages and niche users. Ligasure has the most published literature, is capable of sealing vessels up to 7 mm, has low lateral thermal imprint and spread, and is easy to use. Similarly, the newer Enseal device has a similar vessel-sealing ability, with lower thermal imprint, uses compression forces in addition, and can cut and coagulate at the same time but needs a trained measured input from the user. Harmonic scalpel is often used in combination with CUSA, Hydrojet, or the clamp–crush technique, but is not suitable for controlling larger biliary or vascular structures. Using of resistance-modulated devices, such as CUSA or Hydrojet, provides clean lines of transection. Proponents argue that in performing hepatectomies in which small margins are anticipated, the Harmonic scalpel could be beneficial in achieving R0 resections. Primary precoagulation technology of RF-PT (Habib) is popular among many centers, with reported bloodless transection field especially for nonanatomical resections but leaves a large area of necrosis in its wake. Microwave devices are newer energy platforms with a smaller zone of necrosis. Some large centers use salient dissecting sealer often in conjugation with another hemostatic device and prefer the clean transection with minimal thermal spread. It would be remiss to discuss parenchymal transection without mentioning hepatectomy with staplers. Stapler-directed parenchymal transection is safe and fast and leads to less blood loss and shorter hospital stay. Initial studies have yet to be confirmed, and the increase in cost may deter some surgeons. The CRUNSH study is a randomized controlled trial to evaluate stapler hepatectomy versus the clamp–crush technique with the primary end point being intraoperative blood loss; this trial has recently been completed.

Most of these devices when used properly are safe and can facilitate parenchymal transections. Therefore, the choice of hemostatic assist technology in liver transection should be based on individual surgeon preference, training, and practice setting. Surgeons should use mentors, industry workshops, animal labs, and current literature to train themselves to the device(s) they use. As a word of caution, some of these powerful energy devices, if used inappropriately, can have severe consequences. For example, in aberrant anatomy, or anatomy distorted by tumors, large vascular or biliary structures could be easily sealed off with disastrous consequences (Table 13.1).

Our Perspective

The published literature in hepatic parenchymal transection is heterogeneous. Some technologies have been shown to be superior in histologic models and animal studies, but randomized controlled trials or similar high-quality clinical data do not exist. At this point, no single energy source has shown to be superior to others, and it behooves the operator to be aware of the risks and benefits of the technology that they are using. Currently, many surgeons are using an "energy device"–clysis technique in which they replace the Kelly clamp with hemostatic device as the crush–clamp device. This was originally used with harmonic focus and was described as focus-clysis but is being used with other devices.

TABLE 13.1   Vessel-Sealing Devices' Comparison

	Ligasure	Enseal	PK-Gyrus	Harmonic
Mechanism	Bipolar	Bipolar	Bipolar	Ultrasonic shear
Vessel size	Up to 7	Up to 7	5	5
Lateral thermal spread	2–3	1	2–6	1
Burst pressure (2–3 mm)	744	1,025	910	789
Burst pressure (4–5 mm)	1,261	927	647	390
Burst pressure (6–7 mm)	645	720	284	532
Seal times (2–3 mm)	2.8	4	2	4
Seal times (4–5 mm)	3	6.8	4	3.9
Seal times (6–7 mm)	3.5	8.25	4.5	5.2
Failure rates	0–13.3	0–5.8	11–40	0–22
Smoke/vapor (ppm)	12.5 ± 3.6	21.6 ± 5	74.1 ± 12	2.9 ± 0.6
Operator-dependent sealing	No	Yes	No	Yes
Tactile feedback during actuation	No	Yes	No	No
Learning curve	Minimal	Moderate	Minimal	Moderate

Our current practice is to use a similar technique in open and laparoscopic as well as in cirrhotic livers. The mobilization of the liver is done with combined use of sharp Bovie dissection and Enseal. Pedicle clamping is the exception rather than the norm, and this helps reduce blood loss in patients who have steatohepatitis or cirrhosis. After performing intraoperative ultrasound and marking the planned line of liver transection, a combined crush and vessel sealing is performed with the Enseal device. Dissection is advanced from the liver surface in 2- to 3-mm layers and 3 cm depth, avoiding making "tunnels" or "holes." The inflow and outflow tract is controlled with a single vascular stapler. Our preference for the Enseal device is due to its high-burst pressures, low lateral thermal spread, ability to engage the coagulation without locking or clamping down the instrument, uniform application of pressure along the length of the jaws, comparative cost efficacy and the ability to use the same device across a spectrum of liver resections including open or laparoscopic cases.

Suggested Readings

Gurusamy KS, et al. Techniques for liver parenchymal transection in liver resection. *Cochrane Database Syst Rev* 2009;(1):CD006880.

Kluger MD, Cherqui D. Minimally invasive techniques in hepatic resection. In: Jarnagin WR, Blumgart WH (eds.), *Blumgart's surgery of the liver, pancreas and biliary tract*, 5th ed. Philadelphia, PA: Elsevier, 2012.

Newcomb WL, et al. Comparison of blood vessel sealing among new electrosurgical and ultrasonic devices. *Surg Endosc* 2009;23(1):90–96.

Pamecha V, et al. Techniques for liver parenchymal transection: a meta-analysis of randomized controlled trials. *HPB(Oxford)* 2009;11(4):275–281.

Rahbari NN, et al. Clamp-crushing versus stapler hepatectomy for transection of the parenchyma in elective hepatic resection (CRUNSH)—a randomized controlled trial (NCT01049607). *BMC Surg* 2011;11:22.

14

Hepatocellular Carcinoma

Mashaal Dhir and Chandrakanth Are

INTRODUCTION

Worldwide, hepatocellular carcinoma (HCC) is the fifth most common cancer and a leading cause of cancer-related mortality. The major risk factors for HCC include presence of cirrhosis and chronic viral hepatitis due to hepatitis C virus (HCV) and hepatitis B virus (HBV). HBV is the predominant risk factor in the developing world, whereas HCV is the major risk factor in the United States. HBV and HCV coinfection as well as human immunodeficiency virus and HCV coinfection may accelerate the development of HCC. Nonalcoholic fatty liver disease or nonalcoholic steatohepatitis (NASH) is commonly seen in obese and diabetic individuals and is currently on the rise worldwide and may become a major cause of HCC in future. HCV and NASH account for majority of cases of HCC in the United States. Alcohol, although not a mutagen itself, can cause HCC through alcohol-induced cirrhosis and can act synergistically with other risk factors, including viral hepatitis. Aflatoxin B1 exposure, autoimmune disorders such as primary biliary cirrhosis and autoimmune hepatitis, and several inherited liver disorders such as hemochromatosis, Wilson disease, alpha1-antitrypsin deficiency, hereditary tyrosinemia, and glycogen storage disorders, although rare, can also predispose to HCC.

HCC is the result of chronic injury to the liver cells leading to repeated cycles of cell damage and proliferation with accruals of several genetic and epigenetic changes. Major molecular alterations in HCC include TP53 mutation (approximately 50%), Wnt–beta-catenin signaling pathway mutations (20% to 40%), activation of the insulin-like growth factor signaling pathway, and PI3/PTEN/AKT signaling pathway activation. The PI3/PTEN/AKT pathway plays a role in cell invasion through activation of MMP-9; therefore, kinases in this pathway could prove to be exciting therapeutic targets.

SURVEILLANCE AND DIAGNOSIS

Several societies including the American Association for the Study of Liver Diseases (AASLD) and the National Comprehensive Cancer Network have published guidelines for screening and surveillance of HCC. The AASLD prefers the use of term surveillance over screening for early detection of HCC as it involves repeated use of screening test at repeated intervals. Surveillance for HCC is indicated in all cirrhotic patients. Surveillance is also recommended for other specific groups such as hepatitis B carriers with positive family history of HCC and those with high HBV DNA levels.

Both radiologic and serologic tests are used for surveillance of HCC in the above-mentioned populations. Ultrasound (US) examinations and alfa-fetoprotein (AFP) levels are the most widely used methods for surveillance. A surveillance interval of 6 months is based on tumor doubling times of approximately 6 months.

Among the serologic methods, AFP is the most commonly used diagnostic test although sensitivity and specificity vary with the size of the nodule and the cutoff values utilized. Sensitivity and specificity range from 55% to 60% and 88% to 90% for a cutoff value of 20 μg/L compared to 17% and 99.4%, respectively, for a cutoff value of 400 μg/L. In addition, AFP may be elevated in patients with intrahepatic cholangiocarcinoma. Therefore, per AASLD, diagnosis should rest on the radiologic and histopathologic criteria, and AFP alone is considered as an inadequate screening test for HCC. US is the most commonly recommended test overall for surveillance with sensitivity (65% to 80%) and specificity (48% to 94%) varying depending on the size of the nodule. Importantly, US is operator dependent, and all focal lesions on US should be verified using four-phase multidetector CT (MDCT) or a dynamic contrast-enhanced MRI as these modalities have higher sensitivity (89%) and specificity (99%) for lesions greater than 1 cm. A contrast-enhanced study is required to demonstrate the typical "washout" of the contrast seen in HCC. HCC has arterial blood supply exclusively, whereas the rest of the liver has both portal venous and arterial supply. In the arterial phase, HCC enhances more than the liver as it has only arterial supply, whereas arterial contrast in nontumorous liver is diluted by the portal venous blood. In the venous phase, HCC enhances less than the liver as it has no venous blood supply and the arterial blood flowing through HCC no longer contains contrast, whereas the nontumorous liver is enhanced by contrast in the venous blood. This phenomenon is known as "washout" and is characteristic of HCC. A four-phase study (unenhanced, arterial, venous, and delayed—MDCT or dynamic MRI) is required to document this radiologic finding. Figure 14.1 summarizes the AASLD-recommended diagnostic algorithm for suspected HCC (Fig. 14.1).

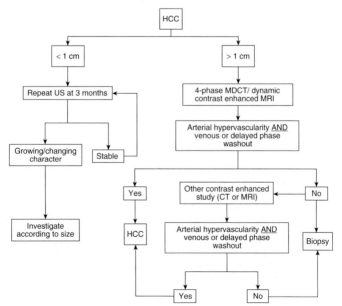

FIGURE 14.1 Algorithm for investigation of small nodules found on screening in patients at risk for HCC. Adapted from AASLD practice guidelines 2010. Bruix et al. 2010, with permission.

STAGING SYSTEMS FOR HCC

HCC arises in the background of a preneoplastic cirrhotic liver, and both HCC and the underlying cirrhosis along with the patient's condition may affect the mortality of the patient. Similarly, the biology of the disease and the risk factors are different in the East and West. HCC is the one of the few tumors that can be treated by both resection and transplantation. Because of these unique challenges, it is difficult to devise a uniform staging system and, consequently, several staging systems for HCC exist. An ideal staging system should take into account the tumor burden, functional state of the liver, and performance status of the patient. The Barcelona Clinic Liver Cancer (BCLC) staging system is currently the most widely utilized staging system worldwide as it includes tumor stage, liver functional status, and physical status of the patients and links the various stages to treatment modalities and estimated life expectancies. Figure 14.2 summarizes the BCLC staging system (Fig. 14.2).

TREATMENT OF HCC

There are several treatment options available to patients diagnosed with HCC. The treatment algorithms are guided by the extent of tumor burden (extrahepatic spread, vascular invasion, number of tumors, tumor diameter), severity of underlying liver dysfunction, size of future liver remnant (FLR), functional status, and comorbidities of the patient.

Transplantation and resection continue to be the major curative-intent therapeutic options available to patients with HCC. Patients with early-stage disease (i.e., HCC falling within the Milan criteria—solitary lesion ≤ 5 cm or ≤ 3 lesions with the largest diameter ≤ 3 cm and absence of macroscopic vascular invasion or extrahepatic disease) and advanced cirrhosis including Child-Pugh class B/C and portal hypertension are thought to be candidates for transplantation, whereas resection remains the treatment of choice for patients without any significant underlying liver disease. Ablative treatment, chemoembolization, and systemic therapies play an important role as well.

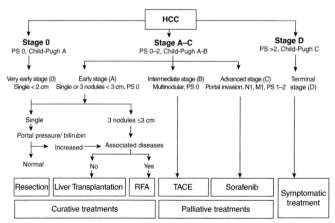

FIGURE 14.2 Barcelona Clinic Liver Cancer (BCLC) staging system. PS, performance status; N, nodal status; M, metastases. Adapted from AASLD practice guidelines 2010. Bruix et al. 2010, with permission.

Liver Resection

Liver resection may be considered the primary treatment modality in some patients with HCC in the absence of cirrhosis. Patients with well-compensated cirrhosis, that is, Child-Pugh A cirrhosis, absence of portal hypertension, and Model for End-Stage Liver Disease (MELD) score of less than 10, may be considered for resection as well. Resection is usually contraindicated in patients with advanced liver disease, that is, Child-Pugh C and majority of patients with Child-Pugh B with portal hypertension.

Liver resection provides specimen for pathologic confirmation of diagnosis and can also help to ascertain other pathologic tumor factors, which may help provide information on the biology of tumor. Unlike orthotopic liver transplant (OLT), liver resection is not usually limited by tumor size/number or macrovascular invasion, and there is no waiting time. Unfortunately, the recurrence rates tend to be higher as resection does not address the premalignant potential of the FLR.

Preoperative Assessment of Liver Function

Careful preoperative assessment of liver function is important since postoperative liver failure in patients undergoing liver resection is associated with high mortality and morbidity. A complete metabolic panel is one of the most basic tests that can be performed to assess the liver function. Candidates who have evidence of active hepatitis as indicated by elevated bilirubin, AST, or ALT may be poor candidates for resection. In the Western world, the Child-Pugh scoring system has been used traditionally to estimate the hepatic functional reserve prior to liver resection. Patients with Child-Pugh class A and those with highly select Child-Pugh B are considered candidates for resection. More recently, the MELD score has been applied to preoperative selection of HCC resection candidates, as well.

Portal hypertension is considered to be present when hepatic venous pressure gradient is greater than 10 mm Hg. Portal hypertension increases the risk of major postoperative complications in the form of variceal bleeding, endotoxemia, and postoperative hepatic decompensation. Therefore, clinical or radiologic criteria to diagnose portal hypertension are a key step in the evaluation of candidates for resection. Platelet count of less than 100,000/μL associated with splenomegaly, ascites requiring drug treatment or intervention, esophagogastric varices on upper endoscopy, and presence of abdominal wall collaterals may point toward significant portal hypertension.

In the East, further functional assessment of the liver is performed preoperatively most commonly using indocyanine green (ICG) clearance. Functionally, ICG is taken up by hepatocytes and excreted in the bile in an adenosine triphosphate-dependent fashion. Therefore, its clearance from the systemic circulation is an indicator of hepatic function. The amount of ICG remaining in the bloodstream of a patient with normal liver function 15 minutes after the injection should be less than 10%. The ICG clearance test is not commonly used in the United States.

Evaluation of Future Liver Remnant Volume

Major or extended hepatectomy may lead to an inadequate FLR that can be associated with significant risk of hepatic insufficiency and subsequent mortality and morbidity. Although the risk of hepatic insufficiency is determined by several factors as highlighted above, the size of FLR continues to be one of the major determinants of postoperative hepatic failure. Precise measurements of hepatic volume are needed before operating on any patient that is likely to be left with an inadequate FLR. The FLR can be calculated using three-dimensional (3D) CT volumetry. FLR has been used as a surrogate to predict postoperative outcomes. In patients with normal liver function, FLR of at least 20% is recommended. For patients with cirrhosis and those treated with systemic chemotherapy, a higher FLR is recommended (40% for cirrhosis, 30% after systemic chemotherapy) due to the underlying liver dysfunction.

Portal Vein Embolization

A small FLR may increase the risk of posthepatectomy liver failure (PHLF). However, this can be avoided by inducing ipsilateral atrophy of the tumor-bearing liver and compensatory hypertrophy of the FLR by selectively occluding the blood flow to the tumor-bearing part of the liver. Hypertrophy of the nonembolized, non–tumor-bearing liver could be secondary to increased portal blood flow through redistribution as well as release of cytokines such as hepatocyte growth factor and transforming growth factor α and β. In general, portal vein embolization (PVE) is offered to patients with (1) normal liver function and an FLR of 25% to 30% and (2) with compromised liver function such as postchemotherapy liver damage, cirrhosis/fibrosis, cholestasis, and FLR of 35% to 40%. In the post-PVE period, the FLR undergoes rapid hypertrophy in the ensuing 3 to 4 weeks. In patients who have diabetes or cirrhosis, the hypertrophy may be delayed, and an additional 3 to 4 weeks may be required to assess the complete response. A small percentage of patients undergoing PVE may develop severe complications in the form of severe cholangitis, large abscesses, sepsis, portal venous, or mesentericoportal venous thrombosis, precluding liver resection. In a different strategy, PVE embolization can be utilized as a "stress test" for the liver. Patients who undergo sufficient hypertrophy may do well with resection, whereas those with insufficient hypertrophy are more likely to experience complications and posthepatectomy liver failure. Similarly, any disease progression seen during the period of PVE may indicate aggressive tumor biology, and resection may not change the course of the disease in these patients.

Outcomes

Most major centers report a perioperative mortality of less than 5% after liver resection for HCC. Cirrhosis and portal hypertension may impair liver regeneration, increase intraoperative blood loss requiring transfusion, and increase the risk of liver failure. PHLF is one of the most serious complications after liver resection and is reported in approximately 5% to 10% of patients. Careful patient selection, limiting resection to patients with well-compensated cirrhosis (Child A) in the absence of portal hypertension, and parenchymal-sparing resections are all strategies to help prevent postoperative liver failure. Additionally, intraoperative blood loss can be limited by reducing the central venous pressure and intermittent portal clamping.

The overall 5-year survival after hepatic resection ranges from 25% to 50% depending on the size and number of HCC nodules, vascular invasion, and level of AFP. Multifocal HCC and major vascular invasion are associated with poor survival. Resection does not address the residual (usually cirrhotic) liver whose function may continue to worsen and in which new tumors may develop. In patients with small solitary HCC and well-preserved liver function, the 5-year survival may exceed 50%.

Orthotopic Liver Transplant

Generally speaking, OLT is the preferred treatment approach for cirrhotic patients falling within the Milan criteria as long-term outcomes are comparable to patients with similar stage of cirrhosis in the absence of malignancy. The Milan criteria include (1) single HCC less than 5 cm in size, (2) three or fewer nodules each less than 3 cm in size, and (3) absence of extrahepatic spread or major vascular invasion. Extrahepatic staging should include CT of the chest and CT/MRI of the abdomen and pelvis. In patients with cirrhosis undergoing transplantation for early stage HCC, the 5- and 10-year survival may vary from 60% to 80% and 50% to 60%, respectively. However, most studies do not take into account the mortality while awaiting liver transplant or dropout from the waitlist as some patients experience disease progression.

At most centers, organ allocation is based on the MELD score. Researchers at the University of San Francisco have proposed expanded size criteria for HCC in transplant candidates (UCSF criteria), that is, single HCC less than 6.5 cm, maximum of three total tumors with none greater than 4.5 cm, and cumulative tumor size less than 8 cm. The overall 1- and 5-year survival rates were 90% and 75%, respectively, for patients meeting the UCSF criteria. Therefore, selected patients with stage 3 disease may be candidates for transplantation.

Downstaging

Many times, HCC is detected at an advanced stage, and such patients are no longer candidates for OLT. The goal of downstaging is to decrease the size and number of tumors in patients who do not meet the criteria for transplantation on initial evaluation. Liver transplantation after successful downstaging should achieve a 5-year survival comparable to HCC patients undergoing transplantation without downstaging.

No clearly defined upper limits for size and number of lesions qualify or preclude a patient downstaging. However, the presence of extrahepatic disease and major vascular invasion are often considered as contraindications for downstaging. Transarterial chemoembolization (TACE) and radiofrequency ablation (RFA) are commonly used downstaging techniques. In patients who are successfully downstaged, a minimum wait period of 3 months is recommended prior to transplantation. Failure of downstaging may be defined as (1) before listing— failure to achieve listing criteria, tumor progression with or without development of major vascular invasion, and extrahepatic spread or tumor size or spread beyond the inclusion criteria—and (2) after listing—tumor progression requiring delisting.

Management of Patients on the Waiting List

Dropouts of HCC patients on the waiting list are common due to cancer progression or other medical reasons. Current consensus guidelines recommend at least three monthly monitoring of listed patients using imaging (dynamic CT, dynamic MRI, or contrast-enhanced US) and AFP measurements to identify those who undergo disease progression. Bridging strategies with locoregional therapies may be used to decrease tumor-related dropout rates and are usually beneficial for patients with a wait time of 6 months or more. The most common bridging strategies include TACE, RFA, a combination of TACE and RFA, ^{90}yttrium radioembolization, or hepatic resection.

LOCOREGIONAL THERAPIES

Locoregional therapies in the treatment of HCC are aimed at inducing selective tumor necrosis. These therapies can be broadly divided into two categories, that is, ablation versus embolization. The extent of tumor necrosis induced by locoregional therapies can be assessed by imaging as well as biochemical criteria. Posttreatment dynamic CT/MRI and AFP can be used to assess the response to locoregional therapies.

Ablation

Liver cancer cells can be destroyed by chemical substances such as ethanol or acetic acid or by modulation of temperature of the cancer cells by radiofrequency, microwaves (MW), laser, or cryoablation.

Percutaneous ethanol injection (PEI) and RFA are the two most commonly used ablative treatments. Any ablative treatment can be performed by laparoscopic, percutaneous, or open technique. In patients who receive PEI, distribution of ethanol may be blocked by intratumoral septa and/or tumor capsule, resulting in heterogenous distribution. As a result of this anatomic compartmentalization, curative capacity of PEI decreases as the size of tumor increases. PEI can achieve complete tumor necrosis in almost all patients with tumors smaller than 2 cm and approximately 70% of patients with tumors smaller than 3 cm.

In contrast, RFA causes destruction of the tumors and surrounding liver parenchyma through high-frequency alternating electrical current, generating temperatures in the range of 70°C to 105°C, which leads to coagulative necrosis. Ablation also generates a margin of ablated nontumoral tissue, which might eliminate any undetected satellite nodules. One of the major limitations of RFA includes inability to ablate lesions located close to major vascular structures, which act as a heat sink.

In patients with small HCC (< 3 cm) and well-preserved liver functions, RFA may be considered the first-line ablative treatment. In contrast, PEI may be reserved for lesions not suitable for RFA such as pericholecystic lesions or those near the hepatic hilum. The efficacy of percutaneous ablative treatments may be assessed by contrast-enhanced CT or MRI at 1 month after therapy. Absence of contrast uptake at 1 month is associated with tumor necrosis, and persistence of contrast uptake indicates treatment failure.

Proximity to large blood vessels can lead to absorption of heat by the rapidly flowing blood (heat-sink phenomenon); this heat sink can lead to reduced efficacy and is a relative contraindication to RFA. There is higher chance of tumor rupture after RFA of lesions located near the liver capsule. Caution is advised for lesions located near the major bile ducts, bowel, gallbladder, diaphragm, heart, and stomach as these structures may be damaged.

Other Ablative Strategies

MW are electromagnetic waves that can produce thermal effects leading to tumor destruction. MW ablation has some advantages over RFA, such as a higher temperature at the target tissue, a shorter duration of therapy, a less pronounced cooling effect of adjacent vessels (less heat-sink effect), an effective treatment of cystic lesions, and lack of need for neutral electrodes, thus avoiding the risk of related skin burning. Irreversible electroporation (IRE) is a recent addition to the armamentarium of ablative strategies. In IRE, small electrical pulses cause disintegration of the cell membranes leading to cell death without producing the thermal effect. Functionally, IRE causes either definite cell death or no death, so the area of damage is very well defined. In theory, and unlike RFA or MW, there is little damage to the surrounding vessels, bile ducts, or bronchioles.

Embolization

Embolization is based on catheter-based infusion of particles targeted at the arterial branch of the hepatic artery feeding the portion of the liver in which the tumor is located. The liver has dual blood supply derived from the portal vein and hepatic artery. Tumors such as HCC are supplied predominantly by the hepatic artery and are hypervascular resulting from increased blood flow to the tumor compared to normal liver tissue. The blood supply to the tumor is carefully isolated, and embolization is performed to the subsegment, segment, or lobe of the liver containing the tumor. Nontarget embolization to the liver may result in serious liver damage. Embolization can be performed using bland particles, chemotherapy or drug-eluting beads (DEB-TACE), or beads tagged with a radionuclide (^{90}Yttrium).

Embolization plays multiple roles in the management of HCC. Major indications include (1) palliative treatment for patients with unresectable/inoperable disease with tumors not amenable to ablation treatment only and minimal or absence of large-volume extrahepatic disease; (2) treatment for postresection intrahepatic recurrence; (3) primary treatment for ruptured HCC; (4) adjuvant treatment to prevent postoperative recurrence; (5) neoadjuvant treatment for large resectable HCC to reduce tumor volume; (6) bridging treatment to inhibit tumor growth in patients awaiting transplant.

Selection Criteria

Preoperative procedure workup includes evaluation of hepatic functional reserve and baseline tumor markers and cross-sectional imaging to assess the size, number, and macroscopic vascular invasion of the hepatic or portal vein. Assessment of the patient's comorbidities, functional status, and evaluation for metastatic disease also play important roles in treatment planning. The endpoint of treatment includes stasis in tumor-feeding arteries and appearance of embolization material in the peritumoral portal vein tributaries. Patients are routinely followed at 2- to 4-week intervals with liver function tests and tumor marker assays. Similar to ablative treatment, tumor necrosis by embolization can be assessed by contrast uptake on dynamic CT/MRI 4 to 8 weeks posttreatment.

OTHER STRATEGIES

External beam radiation therapy (EBRT) allows focal administration of high-dose radiation to HCC tumors in patients with unresectable tumors or inoperable liver disease. Unlike ablation treatment, EBRT is not limited by tumor location.

Systemic therapies including sorafenib are being explored. Sorafenib is an oral multikinase inhibitor that suppresses tumor cell proliferation and angiogenesis and has been evaluated for the treatment of advanced or metastatic HCC.

In conclusion, treatment of HCC is evolving. Resection and transplantation remain major surgical options. Locoregional therapies including ablative treatments and transarterial embolization are increasingly utilized in the management of HCC patients. The role of systemic therapies is evolving. The evolution of these varied treatment strategies combined with a better understanding of the biology of the disease should contribute to further improvements in outcomes for patients with HCC.

Suggested Readings

Belghiti J, Carr BI, Greig PD, et al. Treatment before liver transplantation for HCC. *Ann Surg Oncol* 2008;15(4):993–1000.

Benson AB, III, Abrams TA, Ben-Josef E, et al. NCCN clinical practice guidelines in oncology: hepatobiliary cancers. *J Natl Compr Canc Netw* 2009;7(4):350–391.

Bruix J, Sherman M. Management of hepatocellular carcinoma: an update. *Hepatology* 2011;53(3):1020–1022.

Clavien PA, Lesurtel M, Bossuyt PM, et al. Recommendations for liver transplantation for hepatocellular carcinoma: an international consensus conference report. *Lancet Oncol* 2012;13(1):e11–22.

El-Serag HB. Epidemiology of viral hepatitis and hepatocellular carcinoma. *Gastroenterology* 2012;142(6):1264–1273 e1.

Forner A, Llovet JM, Bruix J. Hepatocellular carcinoma. *Lancet* 2012;379(9822): 1245–1255.

Jarnagin W, Chapman WC, Curley S, et al. Surgical treatment of hepatocellular carcinoma: expert consensus statement. *HPB (Oxford)* 2010;12(5):302–310.

Jemal A, Bray F, Center MM, et al. Global cancer statistics. *CA Cancer J Clin* 2011;61(2):69–90.

Llovet JM, Ricci S, Mazzaferro V, et al. Sorafenib in advanced hepatocellular carcinoma. *N Engl J Med* 2008;359(4):378–390.

Mazzaferro V, Regalia E, Doci R, et al. Liver transplantation for the treatment of small hepatocellular carcinomas in patients with cirrhosis. *N Engl J Med* 1996;334(11):693–699.

Rahbari NN, Garden OJ, Padbury R, et al. Posthepatectomy liver failure: a definition and grading by the International Study Group of Liver Surgery (ISGLS). *Surgery* 2011;149(5):713–724.

Rahbari NN, Mehrabi A, Mollberg NM, et al. Hepatocellular carcinoma: current management and perspectives for the future. *Ann Surg* 2011;253(3):453–469.

Schwarz RE, Abou-Alfa GK, Geschwind JF, et al. Nonoperative therapies for combined modality treatment of hepatocellular cancer: expert consensus statement. *HPB (Oxford)* 2010;12(5):313–320.

Management of Patients with Colorectal Liver Metastases

Danielle A. Bischof and Timothy M. Pawlik

ETIOLOGY

In the United States, approximately 140,000 people are diagnosed with colorectal cancer (CRC), and 50,000 people die of CRC, yearly. CRC currently represents the second leading cause of cancer deaths in the United States. During the course of their disease, half of patients with CRC will develop colorectal liver metastases (CRLM). The liver is the only site of metastatic disease in 30% of patients who develop CRLM. These patients are potential candidates for curative-intent resection of CRLM. Without treatment, the median survival for patients with CRLM is 6 to 12 months. With improvements in systemic therapy, the median survival for patients with unresectable metastatic disease has improved from 12 months to up to 28 months. Despite this, the survival of patients with CRLM who do not undergo complete resection remains low at about 5% to 10% at 5 years. Complete resection remains the only therapy for CRLM with the potential for long-term cure.

Risk factors for CRC include age, obesity, physical inactivity, alcohol consumption, diet high in red meat, and smoking. Hereditary and medical risk factors for CRC include a personal or family history of CRC or colorectal adenomas and a personal history of inflammatory bowel disease and genetic syndromes such as Lynch syndrome and familial adenomatous polyposis.

DIAGNOSIS

Diagnosis of CRLM is most common on staging cross-sectional imaging at the time of initial diagnosis or during surveillance after treatment of the primary. All patients who are being considered for surgery for CRLM should undergo thorough preoperative assessment to assess the extent of intrahepatic disease as well as to rule out extrahepatic metastases. Patients should be assessed with computerized tomography (CT) or magnetic resonance imaging (MRI) of the liver. Preoperative imaging of the liver should characterize the number of liver lesions, their location, and their proximity to major vascular and biliary structures. In addition, all patients should have imaging of the chest and a colonoscopy within the last 6 to 12 months to rule out extrahepatic metastatic disease and local recurrence or a metachronous primary tumor, respectively.

On contrast-enhanced CT scan, liver lesions typically appear hypodense and are best seen on the venous phase. Dual-phase helical CT has been reported to have a sensitivity of 69% to 71% and a specificity of 86% to 91% for detecting and characterizing CRLM. With newer multiple detector helical CT, the sensitivity of identifying liver metastases now approaches 80% to 90% as higher image resolution is achieved with the thin collimation possible with multidetector row CT. Thin-slice multidetector CT scan also provides excellent resolution of vascular and biliary structures to aid opera-tive planning. Limitations of CT scan are that sensitivity is low for CRLM less than 1 cm in diameter and for detecting peritoneal-based extrahepatic metastases. In addition, the sensitivity of CT for CRLM appears to decrease after patients receive preoperative chemotherapy—especially in the set-ting of steatosis or steatohepatitis, which can result in the background liver appearing darker. This results in less contrast between the liver paren-chyma and the hypovascular metastasis and can hinder detection of CRLM.

CT scan can detect extrahepatic metastases, such as lung metastases. At the very minimum, all patients with CRLM should undergo a chest x-ray prior to surgery. The role of chest CT in imaging patients with CRLM remains controversial among those patients with a normal chest x-ray. Two reports demonstrated a diagnostic yield of only 4% to 5% of CT chest in patients with a normal chest x-ray. Chest CT has high sensitivity but is hindered by low specificity in ruling out pulmonary metastases. Despite this, the NCCN rec-ommends that a staging CT of the chest be performed in patients with CRC.

Contrast-enhanced MRI with agents such as gadolinium and feru-moxide has an accuracy of detecting malignant liver tumors of 80% to 90%. Limitations of MRI are long scanning times and low sensitivity for detect-ing extrahepatic disease. MRI appears to be superior to CT in the setting of chemotherapy-induced steatosis or steatohepatitis. A number of fat-suppressing techniques including chemical shift imaging and fat saturation techniques can be used to compensate for steatosis in this setting.

Positron emission tomography (PET) and PET/CT have also been increasingly used to assess patients with CRLM for extrahepatic disease. In contrast to CT and MRI, PET offers information on the metabolic activity of the tumor based on the uptake of 18-F fluoro-2-deoxy-d-glucose (18-FDG). The superiority of PET in staging patients with suspected liver metastases for extrahepatic disease has been demonstrated in several meta-analyses. Use of PET has also been associated with decreased rates of nontherapeutic laparotomy and a change in treatment plan in up to one-third of patients. PET/CT merges images from PET with CT, which enhances the sensitivity from 75% to 89% when compared with PET alone. In one study, PET/CT identified additional lesions in 32% of patients and changed clinical man-agement in 24%. Several consensus statements have advocated for PET/CT in the preoperative staging of patients with CRLM. PET/CT is more effective in identifying metastatic disease prior to starting chemotherapy. Preoperative chemotherapy impairs glucose uptake in tumor cells due to diminished hexokinase activity, thereby decreasing the sensitivity of FDG-PET. Following the initiation of preoperative chemotherapy, a decrease in avidity on PET/CT has been demonstrated to be an independent predic-tor of long-term outcome. Complete metabolic response of a metastasis on FDG-PET after preoperative chemotherapy is, however, an unreliable indi-cator of complete pathologic response. In general, a baseline PET/CT prior to chemotherapy administration is recommended in order to accurately ascertain all metabolically active sites of disease.

In a meta-analysis comparing CT, MRI, and PET for detection of CRC metastases, PET was the most accurate and sensitive modality for detecting CRC metastases on a per-patient basis. On a per-lesion basis, CT, MRI, and PET were comparable in detecting CRC metastases. In contrast, MRI appears to be the best modality for detecting CRLM in patients who have received chemotherapy. In a recent meta-analysis, the diagnostic performance of MRI, CT, and PET/CT was compared in a pooled analysis of patients treated with preoperative chemotherapy. The pooled sensitivity of MRI for imaging CRLM after preoperative chemotherapy was 85.7% compared with a sensi-tivity of only 69.9% for CT, 54.5% for PET, and 51.7% for PET/CT.

A multimodality imaging strategy for preoperative staging of patients with CRLM, including FDG-PET and contrast-enhanced CT chest and abdomen, is probably the most common approach. Contrast-enhanced MRI should be considered over CT, especially among all patients who have had a significant amount of prior chemotherapy and have evidence of steatosis. MRI can also be useful as an adjunct to CT in patients with equivocal lesions seen on CT.

MANAGEMENT

Preoperative Considerations

Improvements in patient selection and perioperative management have resulted in improvement in the mortality after liver resection from 10% to 20% before 1980 to approximately 1% currently. Current estimates of mortality, however, often reflect single-institution experiences from high-volume centers and may be misleading. In a report looking at mortality after hepatic resection from the National Inpatient Sample, the adjusted perioperative mortality for hepatectomy was 5.6%. Patient selection is also critical in ensuring good postoperative outcomes. Patient comorbidities including coronary artery disease, renal failure, and heart failure as well as measures of physiologic fitness including the American Society of Anesthesia and the Acute Physiology and Chronic Health Evaluation scores are predictive of risk of postoperative complications. Age has not been shown to be an independent risk factor for increased complications in liver resection, and chronologic age alone should not be a contraindication to liver resection. The preoperative evaluation should aim to identify patients who do not have prohibitive operative risk for hepatectomy and to refer patients who have modifiable risk factors to appropriate providers to have these risk factors addressed preoperatively.

A number of clinicopathologic factors that are associated with patient survival after hepatectomy for CRLM have been identified. These include stage, nodal status of the primary, disease-free interval from the primary to development of CRLM, the number and distribution of CRLM, preoperative carcinoembryonic antigen (CEA), and the presence of extrahepatic disease. A number of these factors were combined to form a clinical prognostic score by Fong et al. using data derived from 1,001 patients undergoing liver resection for CRLM. The clinicopathologic factors that comprise the Fong score include node-positive primary disease, disease-free interval from primary to metastases less than 12 months, more than one hepatic metastasis, largest hepatic metastases greater than 5 cm, and CEA level greater than 200 ng/mL. In this scoring system, one point is assigned for each criterion, and the total score is predictive of patient outcome. Although these factors are predictive of patient outcome, patients with one or more poor prognostic factors can still derive a substantial survival benefit from hepatic resection. All patients with resectable CRLM should thus be considered as surgical candidates and be fully evaluated for resection.

The criteria for resectability of CRLM have changed significantly over the past 20 years. In the past, the presence of more than three hepatic metastases, bilobar disease, an anticipated surgical margin of less than 1 cm, hilar lymphadenopathy, or extrahepatic disease was considered either absolute or relative contraindications to resection for CRLM (Table 15.1). Each of these criteria has been challenged, and the current definition of resectability for CRLM is determined by the surgeon's ability to resect all sites of disease while leaving an adequate future liver remnant (FLR). Specifically, resectability is defined by four criteria:

1. An R0 resection of both the primary lesion and any extrahepatic disease sites must be technically feasible.
2. At least two adjacent liver segments need to be spared.

	Old	New
		Changing Definition of Resectability for Colorectal Liver Metastases
Number of metastases	<4	Any number, provided an R0 resection can be achieved
Distribution of metastases	Unilobar	Two contiguous segments of liver must be preserved
Size of metastases	<5 cm	Any size, provided an adequate FLR is preserved
Presence of extrahepatic disease	None	Allowed, provided all disease can be resected with an R0 resection

3. Vascular inflow and outflow and biliary outflow to the remaining liver segments must be spared.
4. The FLR must be of adequate volume to account for any underlying hepatic dysfunction.

With expanded criteria of resectability for CRLM, a number of strategies for improving resectability have emerged, with the goal of increasing the number of patients eligible for hepatic resection for CRLM. These strategies fall into three broad categories: increasing hepatic reserve, decreasing tumor size, and using combined modality local therapy.

Portal vein embolization (PVE) has been used to increase hepatic reserve in patients undergoing hepatectomy for CRLM (Fig. 15.1). In patients with normal hepatic function, an FLR of 20% to 30% is required to ensure adequate hepatic regeneration and function following resection. Patients with underlying hepatic dysfunction require a larger FLR: Patients

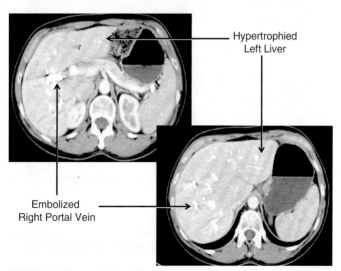

FIGURE 15.1 CT scan of the liver following PVE of the right portal vein; note the hypertrophy of the left liver.

with steatosis or steatohepatitis require an FLR of 30% to 40%, and patients with cirrhosis require a 40% to 50% FLR. FLR can accurately be measured on CT or MRI using volumetric assessment. This is the most commonly used method for measuring FLR in Western centers and is used to identify patients who may benefit from preoperative PVE. Indocyanine green retention at 15 minutes has also been demonstrated to predict postoperative liver failure and mortality; however, the availability of this technique in Western centers is limited. Preoperative PVE is a technique that involves embolization of the portal vein with cyanoacrylate, gelatin microspheres, polyvinyl alcohol, or coils. Embolization of the tumor-bearing liver induces hypertrophy of the contralateral liver and thus increases the FLR volume. PVE is well tolerated with a low complication rate (<5%) and normally results in an absolute increase in FLR of approximately 8% to 16% depending on the degree of underlying hepatic dysfunction. The timing and degree of hypertrophy in response to PVE may help guide patient selection for operation.

A two-stage hepatectomy is a surgical approach that may be used in patients with extensive disease involving both sides of the liver (Fig. 15.2). In a subset of patients, clearance of all disease is often not possible in one operation due to concerns of an inadequate FLR. When the CRLM are bilateral, PVE is often not ideal as embolization of the entire tumor-bearing liver is not feasible. In these circumstances, a two-stage approach may be possible. With the two-stage approach, the disease in one hemiliver is cleared and the contralateral portal vein is occluded either by portal vein ligation during this first operation or by PVE performed postoperatively. The remnant portion of the liver that has been "cleared" is then allowed to hypertrophy, and then the patient is brought back to the operating room 4 to 6 weeks later to resect the remaining disease in the liver. When performing a two-stage hepatectomy, most surgeons advocate initial resection of minor

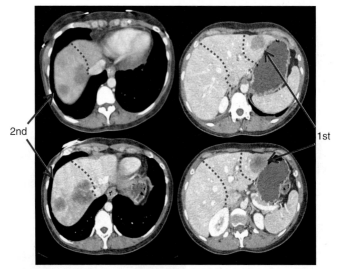

2nd

1st

FIGURE 15.2 Depiction of a two-stage hepatectomy. The first stage was a segmentectomy of the left lateral bisector; following PVE, the patient was brought back to the operating room 6 weeks later for the second stage, which was a right hepatectomy.

disease (three or fewer segments) followed by resection of major disease (greater than three segments) at the second operation. Doing the minor liver resection first will spare a subset of patients the morbidity of a major hepatic resection, as 20% to 30% of patients will never undergo the second stage due to disease progression or worsening performance status. Of note, patients undergoing a two-stage approach can safely be treated with chemotherapy between stages without impairing hypertrophy of the FLR.

Improvements in chemotherapy for patients with CRC have substantially improved tumor response rates in patients with CRLM (Fig. 15.3). Indeed, 12% to 33% of patients with initially unresectable disease can be downsized after receiving "conversion chemotherapy" to a point where curative intent resection is feasible. Average 5-year survival for these patients is 30% to 35%, which is significantly better than patients receiving chemotherapy alone (approximately 10%). In this subset of patients, multidisciplinary involvement including close collaboration between the medical oncologist and the surgeon is essential. Chemotherapy should be continued until the patient is resectable, not until maximal response is achieved. Prolonged chemotherapy beyond the point of resectability may increase rates of chemotherapy-associated hepatotoxicity and contribute to increased patient morbidity after hepatic resection. While the care of each patient must be individualized, in general, preoperative cytotoxic chemotherapy (e.g., FOLFOX or FOLFIRI) should be stopped about 4 to 6 weeks prior to surgery, while bevacizumab (Avastin) should generally be stopped 6 to 8 weeks prior to surgery.

Ablation can involve either radiofrequency ablation (RFA) or microwave ablation. Ablation either alone or in combination with resection can increase the number of patients eligible for liver-directed therapy for colorectal metastases. Ablation should not be viewed as a substitute for hepatic resection but as a complementary therapy in patients in whom complete resection is not possible. Often in patients with extensive disease,

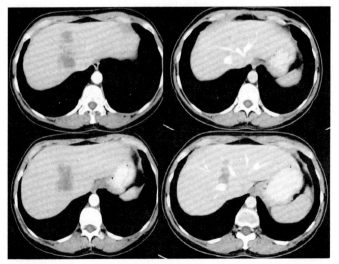

FIGURE 15.3 CT scan of a patient pre- and postreceipt of preoperative chemotherapy. Note the cytoreduction of the tumor and the decrease in the size of the masses following chemotherapy.

larger lesions can be resected, while smaller lesions are ablated. Ablation can be performed percutaneously, laparoscopically, or during laparotomy and can be used to successfully ablate tumors of up to 3 to 4 cm in diameter with a single application. Generally, a 1-cm "margin" of thermal necrosis is desired around the lesions. The efficacy of RFA in lesions adjacent to large blood vessels decreases due to a heat-sink effect, which is associated with higher local recurrence rates; microwave ablation may be less susceptible to this "heat-sink" effect. Ablation should generally be avoided with lesions near the hilum of the liver, as ablation may damage biliary structures and lead to subsequent stricturing. The combination of ablation with hepatic resection results in morbidity and mortality rates similar to those seen with resection alone. It is difficult to compare survival of patients undergoing ablation to those undergoing resection because patients who undergo ablation often have more extensive disease and medical comorbidities than those undergoing resection. Nonetheless, ablation can have an important role in the management of patients with hepatic metastases as an adjunct to the treatment plan in patients with unresectable disease.

Operative Strategy

At the time of hepatectomy, a thorough assessment for the extent of disease including full liver mobilization, visual inspection, palpation, and intraoperative ultrasound (IOUS) should be performed in all patients. IOUS is an important tool to identify lesions intraoperatively and to define the relationship of hepatic lesions to vascular structures. In several studies, IOUS has been demonstrated to be superior to intraoperative inspection and palpation for identification of hepatic neoplasms. A systematic approach should be used to perform IOUS in order to identify all hyper-, iso-, and hypoechoic lesions. All suspicious lesions should be scanned in the transverse and sagittal planes to define size and anatomic relationships. The IOUS characteristics of hepatic metastases tend to be similar within patients (as compared to between patients), and the echogenic appearance of the index lesion can be used to predict the appearance of additional lesions in the same patient, facilitating intraoperative identification of lesions. IOUS has been demonstrated in the literature to change the operative plan in up to 67% of patients undergoing hepatectomy. In addition, in 10% to 12% of patients, IOUS identifies at least one lesion not seen on preoperative imaging when routinely employed. IOUS should therefore be used in all patients undergoing surgery for CRLM to facilitate identification of all lesions and complete clearance of the liver.

Complete resection of CRLM with a microscopic negative margin should be the goal when undertaking hepatectomy for CRLM. Numerous studies have documented both a higher risk of recurrence and decreased overall survival in patients with positive resection margins. Historically, a 1-cm resection margin was considered mandatory based on data from a 1999 study by Cady et al., which demonstrated improved overall survival in patients with a 1-cm margin. A number of studies have subsequently demonstrated no difference in local recurrence or overall survival in patients with a subcentimeter R0 resection compared with those with margins greater than 1 cm. In a 2008 study, de Hass et al. demonstrated that while patients undergoing an R1 resection had increased risk of local recurrence, there was no difference in overall survival when compared with patients undergoing R0 resection. The authors attribute this change in outcome after R1 resection for CRLM to increasingly effective chemotherapeutic regimens. Thus, while the goal of surgery for CRLM remains an R0 resection and the surgeon should strive for at least a 1-cm margin, resection should be considered in patients where less than a 1-cm margin is obtainable as long as all macroscopic disease can be resected.

| | | | | 5-Year |
Author	Year	Number of Patients	Number of Patients with R0 Resection	Overall Survival
Fong	1999	1,001	895	37%
Choti	2002	133	NS	58%
Abdalla	2004	190	NS	58%
Fernandez	2004	100	100	58%
Wei	2006	423	407	47%
Rees	2008	929	833	36%
de Jong	2009	1,669	1,391	47%
Morris	2010	3,116	NS	44.2%

TABLE 15.2   Outcomes Following Resection for Colorectal Liver Metastases

NS, not specified.

OUTCOMES/FOLLOW-UP

The 5-year survival after curative intent hepatic resection for CRLM ranges from 40% to 58% (Table 15.2). The NCCN currently recommends surveillance with history, physical exam, CEA, and CT chest/abdomen/pelvis every 3 to 6 months for 2 years and then every 6 months for years 3 to 5. Over 60% of patients with resected hepatic disease will recur at some point during their disease course. If patients do recur with liver-only disease, repeat hepatectomy may be considered in a select group of patients. Several studies have demonstrated perioperative morbidity and mortality of repeat resection for CRLM similar to that for patients undergoing initial surgery. Five-year overall survival for patients undergoing hepatectomy range from 29% to 42%; thus, an aggressive approach to repeat resection is warranted in well-selected patients, as it may be the only chance for long-term cure.

CONCLUSION

Significant improvements in chemotherapeutic regimens, surgical technique, and patient selection have resulted in improved survival for patients undergoing hepatic resection for CRLM. Many patients with disease that was once considered unresectable are now able to enjoy the survival benefits of resection for CRLM due to expanded indications for hepatectomy, use of conversion chemotherapy, utilization of techniques to increase the FLR, and liver-directed therapies. Careful preoperative planning and multidisciplinary collaboration are essential to ensure optimal outcomes for these patients.

Suggested Readings

Adam R, Avisar E, Ariche A, et al. Five-year survival following hepatic resection after neoadjuvant therapy for nonresectable colorectal. *Ann Surg Oncol* 2001;8:347–353.

Asiyananbola B, Chang D, Gleisner AL, et al. Operative mortality after hepatic resection: are literature-based rates broadly applicable? *J Gastrointest Surg* 2008;12:842–851.

Charnsangavej C, Clary B, Fong Y, et al. Selection of patients for resection of hepatic colorectal metastases: expert consensus statement. *Ann Surg Oncol* 2006;13:1261–1268.

de Haas RJ, Wicherts DA, Flores E, et al. R1 resection by necessity for colorectal liver metastases: is it still a contraindication to surgery? *Ann Surg* 2008;248:626–637.

Fong Y, Fortner J, Sun RL, et al. Clinical score for predicting recurrence after hepatic resection for metastatic colorectal cancer: analysis of 1001 consecutive cases. *Ann Surg* 1999;230:309–318.

Mayo S, Pawlik T. Current management of colorectal hepatic metastases. *Expert Rev Gastroenterol Hepatol* 2009;3:131–144.

Pawlik TM, Abdalla EK, Ellis LM, et al. Debunking dogma: surgery for four or more colorectal liver metastases is justified. *J Gastrointest Surg* 2006;10:240–248.

16 Neuroendocrine and Noncolorectal Liver Metastases

Mark J. Truty and David M. Nagorney

NEUROENDOCRINE LIVER METASTASES

Introduction

Arguably, one of the greatest advances in solid tumor oncology in the early twentieth century has been the evolving treatment of liver metastases. Improvements in modern imaging modalities, refinement in surgical indications and techniques, more effective systemic therapies, and advancing technology in locoregional nonresectional strategies led to an increasing number of treatment options for patients with hepatic metastases. Although typically regarded as slow-growing neoplasms, neuroendocrine tumors vary widely in their clinical behavior and biologic activity, and the liver is the most common site of distant metastases. Various classification systems and nomenclature exist for the clinical staging and management of patients with primary neuroendocrine carcinoma (NEC). Herein, we will overview the management of hepatic metastases from well-differentiated NEC from various sites and summarize management options to provide an algorithm and overall treatment strategy to approach these complex patients. Importantly, although cure is rare, treatment typically leads to prolonged survival, significant palliation of symptoms, and improved quality of life (QOL) for patients with metastatic NEC.

After colorectal cancer, NEC is the second most common indication for liver-directed therapies in patients with metastatic disease. The relatively indolent growth of these lesions compared to hepatic metastases from other sites allows for a planned aggressive approach incorporating resection as a major component of treatment. Surgical treatment must balance the significant risk of treatment-related morbidity particularly if major hepatic or multivisceral resections are performed concomitantly. Although the operative morbidity and mortality of such resections may be significant, specifically with combined procedures, operation generally provides durable oncologic or symptomatic benefits and rarely precludes medical therapy.

NECs of the gastrointestinal tract and pancreas are rare and comprise less than 1% of all malignant disease. Recent prospective national tumor database studies suggest a linearly increasing overall incidence of NEC, with the second highest prevalence of all gastrointestinal cancers. Overall prognosis is dependent on the primary tumor type, site of origin, stage, and various pathologic features such as size, histologic differentiation, and proliferative activity. No single system of nomenclature and grading for all NECs has been universally accepted. Importantly, poorly differentiated or high-grade NECs are more frequently associated with distant metastases (liver and bone approximately 50% of cases) at initial diagnosis, and overall survival is poor regardless of therapy. Thus, these patients are rarely candidates for hepatic resection because of biologic aggressiveness. Overall, the therapeutic modalities for management of patients with hepatic metastases from NEC include surgical, chemo-/biotherapy, ablative, and nuclear medicine strategies. Given the heterogeneity of NEC, variable disease extent, and biologic behavior, the recommendations for therapy are based on the results of retrospective outcomes with sparse prospective high-level evidence.

Hepatic metastases from NEC are diagnosed either at the time of primary disease diagnosis (synchronous) or with disease progression (metachronous). In general, the primary and regional extent of the NEC should be resected before addressing hepatic metastases. Concomitant resection of the primary NEC and the hepatic metastases should be undertaken only after multidisciplinary assessment of the patient's disease stage. Staged resection of the primary NEC with subsequent hepatic resection of the metastases is performed typically, although data from referral centers suggest that concomitant resection can be performed safely in selected patients. Most frequently, concomitant resections are undertaken in patients requiring minor hepatic resections. In patients with clinical endocrinopathies, preoperative control is recommended. Preoperative octreotide therapy is essential in patients with the carcinoid syndrome to prevent intraoperative carcinoid crises (Fig. 16.1). Patients with carcinoid heart disease occasionally require cardiac surgery to address valvular right heart failure prior to hepatic resection (Fig. 16.2). Additionally, interval hepatic arterial embolization in selected patients with bulky functioning NEC metastases may be required in preparation for hepatic resection either to address residual endocrinopathies after resection of the primary NEC or to downsize intrahepatic metastases. Patients with pancreatic NEC generally should undergo staged resections of the primary and hepatic metastases to avoid excess morbidity from combined hepatic and pancreatic resection.

Diagnostic Evaluation

A comprehensive evaluation of patients with neuroendocrine liver metastases includes identification of the anatomic site of origin (whether in situ or previously resected), clinical and biochemical functional status,

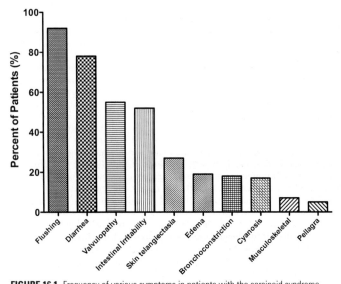

FIGURE 16.1 Frequency of various symptoms in patients with the carcinoid syndrome.

tumor histopathology and grade, and evaluation of extent and distribution of metastatic disease for resectability. Tumor site of origin is usually determined by endoscopy, contrast-enhanced enterography, radiolabeled scintigraphy, or cross-sectional imaging computed tomography (CT) or magnetic resonance imaging (MRI). NECs are termed functional if associated with a discrete clinical syndrome. The syndrome is confirmed biochemically through serum assays of respective neuroendocrine peptides. The clinical neuroendocrine syndrome is specific to the dominant functioning peptide. Not infrequently, multiple peptide levels are elevated but rarely do patients present with a combined clinical endocrinopathy. Nearly all NECs secrete chromogranin A; baseline concentration of this marker should be obtained regardless of clinical syndrome. Other secretory

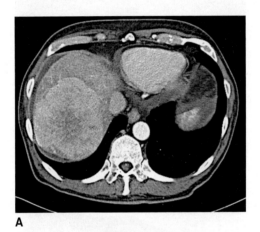

A

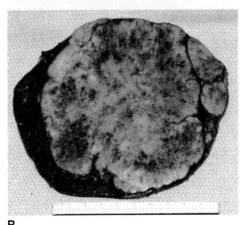

B

FIGURE 16.2 A. Contrast-enhanced CT with large right hepatic ileal carcinoid metastasis. The inferior vena cava is dilated, and the liver has a heterogenous appearance due to preexisting severe tricuspid valve regurgitation. **B.** Gross specimen of resected tumor—the patient underwent tricuspid/pulmonary valve replacement prior to liver resection.

(Continued)

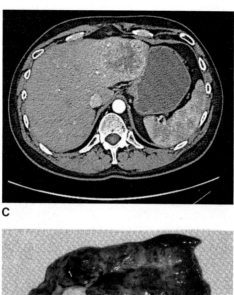

C

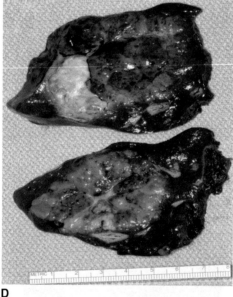

D

FIGURE 16.2 (Continued) C. Contrast-enhanced CT with low-density jejunal carcinoid metastasis in left lateral sector. **D.** Gross specimen of resected liver tumor.

peptides should be evaluated as clinically indicated. Pathologic confirmation of NEC by fine needle aspiration or core biopsy (either metastases or primary tumor) is essential for clinical management. Grade of NEC is defined by proliferative activity via the Ki-67 index and mitotic rate. These key features of grading are critically important for clinical management. Indeed, pathologic findings correlate, in part, with the malignant behavior of NEC. In general, patients with well-differentiated grade 1 NEC benefit the most from aggressive therapy because of typically indolent growth. Patients with moderately differentiated grade 2 NEC have a less predictable and more aggressive course though are often still candidates for operative treatment. Operative intervention in patients with poorly differentiated grade 3 NEC is rarely indicated as these NECs are typically highly aggressive and are characterized by rapid dissemination and resistance to most therapeutic interventions. Currently, NEC is most frequently staged by the AJCC TNM staging system. Staging is crucial for planning overall management. As patients with hepatic metastases harbor by definition stage IV disease, the site and extent of local–regional disease and the site, extent, and distribution of other distant metastases to the peritoneum, lung, and bone significantly influence treatment planning.

Imaging

Radiolabeled somatostatin receptor scintigraphy (SRS) is the most sensitive and accurate imaging modality for diagnosis and initial staging particularly for identification of occult extrahepatic disease. Positive scintigraphy is dependent upon the presence of active somatostatin receptors (SR) on the NEC (Fig. 16.3). Current agents do not bind to all SRS receptors nor do all NEC harbor all SRs. In addition, SRS also predicts response to somatostatin analog therapy. More recently, fludeoxyglucose positron emission tomography (18-FDG-PET) also has been used as an alternative staging adjunct. However, contrast-enhanced CT remains the primary imaging study for assessing resectability of hepatic metastases from NEC. Metastases are hypervascular and are best visualized during the arterial phase of contrast administration. In patients with iodinated contrast allergies or significant steatosis, gadolinium-enhanced MRI is indicated; the contrast-enhanced T2-weighed sequences are most sensitive (Fig. 16.4). In our experience, MRI is complementary to CT with particular utility in detection of very small hepatic metastases that may alter treatment strategies. Liver-specific contrast agents such as gadoxetate disodium (Eovist) increase the sensitivity for detecting small NEC hepatic metastases. Such agents preferentially are taken up by hepatocytes; thus, small contrast-negative metastases not visible on CT are more readily identified. Additionally, contrast-enhanced cross-sectional imaging is essential to assess resectability of the primary NEC, if present, and to assess residual or recurrent regional disease if previously

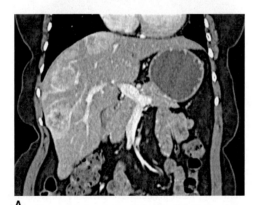

A

FIGURE 16.3 A. Computed tomography revealing numerous enhancing metastases in the liver.

(Continued)

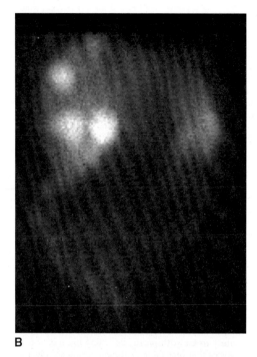

B

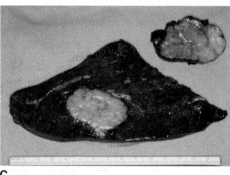

C

FIGURE 16.3 (Continued) B. In-111 octreotide scan revealing multiple large foci of intense radiotracer uptake in the liver as well as pancreatic tail, confirming metastatic (*arrow*) pancreatic NEC. **C.** Gross specimen of resected liver tumors.

resected. Most patients with hepatic metastases from NEC harbor multifocal bilobar disease, though 25% of patients have isolated lobar disease.

In potentially resectable patients, radiologic data should estimate the future liver remnant volume in patients considered for extended or complex hepatectomy or in patients with bulky parenchymal disease. Formal upper and lower endoscopy and endoscopic ultrasound are also important tools with which to identify primary NECs. Patients with carcinoid syndrome

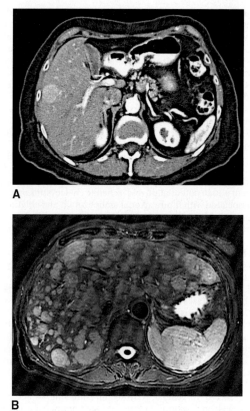

FIGURE 16.4 Neuroendocrine liver metastases. **A.** Enhancing right lobe mass on the arterial phase of computed tomography. **B.** Diffuse bilobar metastases on T2-weighted MRI imaging.

should have a formal cardiac evaluation including echocardiography to evaluate the extent of right heart valvular disease. If present, valvular disease should be corrected prior to any major liver resection.

Potentially Curative Resection

Although NEC is considered indolent, metastatic disease can be associated with severe, life-threatening endocrinopathies or symptoms from locally invasive nonfunctional NEC. The leading cause of mortality aside from hormonal complications is extensive hepatic progression and hepatic failure. The timing and type of treatment should be considered in a multidisciplinary setting. Ideally, the first-line treatment for well-differentiated hepatic metastases from NEC without extrahepatic spread and unilobar alone or unilobar and limited contralobar metastases is resection with or without concomitant ablation. Potentially curative resection (R0) is defined as resection/ablation of all gross disease with an adequate functional liver remnant. Fewer than 50% of patients undergoing hepatic resection of metastatic NEC with hepatic metastases have R0 resection due to the extent of hepatic metastases. The historical 5-year survival for unresected patients with NEC liver metastases is approximately 30%. In contrast, the expected 5-year survival for patients after R0 resection of hepatic metastases based on retrospective series ranges from 60% to 80%. Factors correlating with long-term survival include size and site of metastases, tumor grade, extent of hepatic resection and baseline hepatic disease, presentation with stage IV disease, and impact of endocrinopathy such as carcinoid heart disease. Importantly, regardless of the apparent completeness of resection, disease progresses in most patients, either extra- or intrahepatically. Most patients will manifest disease progression within 5 years; the median identification of disease progression is 18 months. Perioperative octreotide is recommended to prevent the carcinoid crisis in patients with the carcinoid syndrome and other patients with demonstrable clinical control of endocrinopathies. Additionally, cholecystectomy is performed routinely during hepatic resection to avert cholelithiasis associated with somatostatin analog treatment and to potentially avoid ischemic cholecystitis or gallbladder necrosis associated with future arterial embolization and ablation, respectively. Adjuvant systemic chemotherapy is not established as the standard of care, but participation in clinical trials where available is recommended.

Palliative Resection

QOL related to endocrinopathies can be improved significantly through appropriate hepatic resection provided that residual disease is minimized. In general, durable relief of endocrine symptoms is obtained when nearly all radiographic metastases are resected even in the presence of gross residual disease. Palliative cytoreductive resection should be considered primarily in patients with endocrinopathies, particularly in patients who have failed medical management. Whether survival in patients *without* endocrinopathies is improved by palliative resection remains unproven. The completeness and duration of response to palliative resection are primarily based on residual metastatic volume and not resected metastatic volume. Given the growth kinetics of NEC, at least 90% or more of the hepatic metastases should be resected. In general, R2 resections are single-stage operations and are parenchymal sparing because disease progression is inevitable. Resection of the primary NEC may be undertaken concomitantly or at a staged procedure (Fig. 16.5). Palliative resection has limited applicability in patients with high-grade NEC or those with unresectable extrahepatic

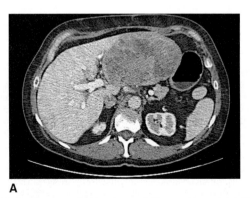

A

FIGURE 16.5 Synchronous carcinoid metastasis. **A.** Computed tomography of large atypical carcinoid metastases replacing the left lateral sector.

(Continued)

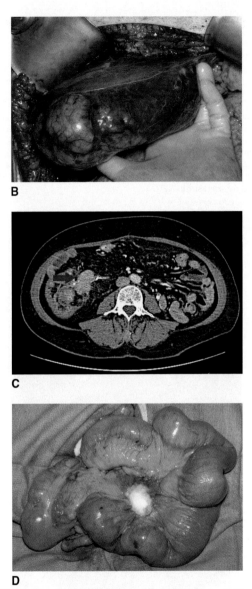

FIGURE 16.5 (Continued) B. Gross intraoperative photo of this lesion. **C.** CT with infiltrative primary carcinoid arising in the terminal ileum and involving the small bowel mesentery (*arrow*). **D.** Gross intraoperative photo of this ileum tumor and the sclerotic adjacent mesentery.

metastases. Importantly, no high-level evidence has shown that debulking improves survival or QOL compared to nonsurgical therapies. Palliative resection can be enhanced by subsequent percutaneous ablative therapies after hepatic regeneration. Notably, palliative resection does not preclude subsequent liver-directed therapies, antihormonal treatment, or chemotherapy.

Liver Transplantation

The role of liver transplantation for metastatic NEC is limited. As may be expected, complete resolution of endocrine symptoms is achieved after liver transplant, but disease progression is typical, and survival has not exceeded that of hepatic resection. Liver transplantation in patients harboring completely unresectable hepatic metastases who have controlled primary and regional disease is clearly reasonable; however, selection criteria are currently unclear. Patients who are young, have had resection of the primary NEC without progression of extrahepatic disease for at least 6 months, and have low-grade NEC may be potential transplant candidates (Fig. 16.6). Fewer than 1% of liver transplants in the United States are performed for metastatic NEC.

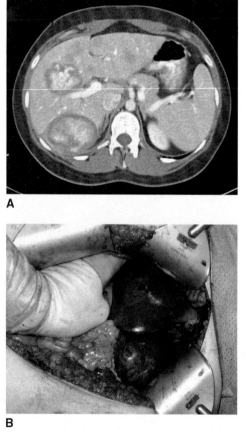

A

B

FIGURE 16.6 A. Contrast-enhanced CT with numerous bilobar ileal carcinoid metastases in a 26-year-old female. **B.** Intraoperative photos of liver lesions at the time of staged primary tumor resection.

(Continued)

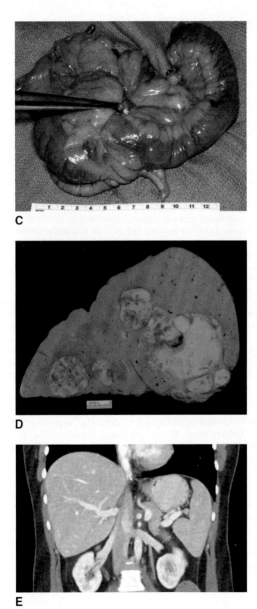

FIGURE 16.6 (Continued) C. Intraoperative photo of resected ileal carcinoid and mesentery during staged primary tumor resection. **D.** Gross photo of liver explant following liver transplantation 18 months after primary staged tumor resection and no evidence of interval extrahepatic disease. **E.** Computed tomography 3 years following transplantation showing no evidence of recurrent disease.

Ablative Therapy

Ablation as a single therapy is applicable in patients with limited unresectable hepatic NEC metastases. Ablation is most frequently employed as an adjunct during resection or for progressive disease following resection. Ablative techniques are either thermal—cryotherapy, radiofrequency ablation (RFA), microwave, or chemical—alcohol or acetic acid. Metastatic NEC is quite sensitive to ablative therapy. Ablation has been shown to effectively control disease progression and palliate symptoms whether performed during laparotomy, laparoscopically, or percutaneously with image guidance. In general, ablation should be considered as an adjunct to hepatic resection for deep-seated metastases during hepatic resection and as an adjunct to R2 hepatic resection postoperatively to further reduce residual disease. Ablation should be considered as a primary liver-directed therapy in patients with limited hepatic disease progression after prior hepatic resection and as the initial liver-directed therapy for limited deep small metastases to avoid major hepatic resection at the initial presentation of the NEC. Ablative therapy should be avoided in patients with numerous metastases, large metastases (>5 cm), or juxtahilar metastases or in patients with prior bilioenteric anastomoses because of the risk of chronic intrahepatic infection.

Transarterial Therapies

Because NECs are hypervascular, hepatic metastases from NEC are well suited for transarterial embolization therapies. This locoregional treatment should be considered in patients with hepatic dominant disease where resection and ablation are not tenable. Transhepatic arterial embolization (TAE) may either be "bland" or use particles loaded with various additional chemotherapeutic agents (transarterial chemoembolization—TACE). Both TAE and TACE effectively control symptoms for up to 1 year and result in significant decrease in biochemical markers and objective tumor responses in about 50% of patients. Response to TACE is greater for high-grade NEC; however, treatment of high-grade tumors is associated with greater toxicity. Selective peripheral percutaneous embolization has replaced proximal hepatic arterial embolization to minimize hepatic ischemia– and procedure–related liver failure. Moreover, embolization is frequently staged; the lobe harboring the dominant metastatic burden is embolized initially. Both TAE and TACE should be performed in experienced centers that have developed clear-cut treatment algorithms. The most common side effect of TAE/TACE is postembolization syndrome (PES), an inflammatory reaction triggered by tumor necrosis and/or hepatocellular injury. This reaction occurs in up to 80% of patients either immediately following the procedure or up to 2 weeks after the procedure. Typically, PES includes fever, pain, extreme fatigue and malaise, and nausea/vomiting. A chemical and/or ischemic cholecystitis may also occur if the cystic artery is inadvertently embolized. Contraindications to TAE/TACE include ipsilateral or complete portal vein thrombosis, hepatic insufficiency, and previous bilioenteric anastomoses such as after pancreaticoduodenectomy. Although embolization can be repeated, eventually the arterial supply to residual metastases becomes pruned with development of alternative arterial collaterals that become inaccessible to further embolization.

An alternative to TAE or TACE is selective internal radiation therapy (SIRT). In SIRT, radioactive ^{90}Yttrium is incorporated into microbeads that are delivered transarterially to lodge within the neovasculature of the metastases. This treatment delivers irradiation locally and concomitantly reduces tumor blood supply. Although embolic in concept, the major arterial supply remains intact, which permits subsequent TAE/TACE. Candidates for

SIRT must harbor hepatic dominant disease and have angiographic proof of limited extrahepatic arterial shunting. SIRTs should be considered in patients with miliary hepatic metastases in particular. Repeat SIRT is possible. Current data suggest that SIRT is equally efficacious as TAE in achieving symptom control.

Radiation Therapy

External beam irradiation for the treatment for hepatic metastases has been limited by the inability to deliver effective cytotoxic radiation doses to tumors without associated significant parenchymal damage. Because NECs have SRs that bind endogenous somatostatin, radiolabeled somatostatin analogs potentially can deliver radioactive compounds directly to the metastases. Peptide receptor radionuclide therapy (PRRT) combines octreotide with various radionuclides. Radiopeptides are typically delivered through selective arterial perfusion as in SIRT. The radioparticles are retained preferentially in the metastases due to selective receptor binding delivering high-dose local irradiation while sparing normal liver tissue. Radionuclides vary (^{90}Yttrium, ^{111}Indium, ^{177}Lutetium); each emits radiation of differing type and depth of tissue penetration. Although conceptually attractive, most agents are still investigational. Selective radiolabeled therapies have shown significant benefits, specifically in patients with recalcitrant tumor and symptoms after TAE/TACE. Objective response to PRRT has been seen in up to 50% of patients. Furthermore, PRRT has been shown to be effective treating the hypoglycemia of metastatic insulinoma and is recommended after failure of standard treatments. The overall role for radiolabeled receptor therapy in conjunction with other liver-directed therapies including surgery is evolving.

Hormonal Therapy

Somatostatin analog treatment is the gold standard medical therapy for patients with inoperable carcinoid cancer. In most patients with the carcinoid syndrome, control is often urgently required, and somatostatin analogs provide prompt relief. Treatment is initiated with short-acting analogs to confirm response because octreotide only binds to some SR. Once response is confirmed, long-acting analogs are used to maintain response with monthly injections. Randomized trial data support octreotide use for control of symptoms and improved QOL. Additionally, octreotide has an antiproliferative, apoptotic effect. Although used as a first-line treatment in patients with advanced, unresectable midgut NEC, response in this setting is frequently partial (< 10%) and typically stabilizing (50%). Other somatostatin analogs that bind with higher affinity to various SRs are emerging and will likely play a greater role in primary and adjuvant therapy in the future. Interferon alpha has also been utilized however carries significant and often poorly tolerated side effects. Somatostatin analogs are also typically used as adjuncts in combination therapy. Eventual treatment failures occur after 1 to 2 years due to tachyphylaxis from the larger doses that are required. Gastric antisecretory agents such as H2 blocker and PPI should be used in all patients with gastrin-secreting tumors; similar cumulative tachyphylaxis is also seen with these agents (Fig. 16.7).

Chemotherapy

The role of systemic chemotherapy for metastatic NEC is limited, though chemotherapy efficacy has been seen in well-differentiated NEC. Regardless of agents, response to chemotherapy is dependent on the site of NEC origin and tumor grade. Chemotherapy is considered second-line therapy for midgut NEC because response rates are typically only 10% to 15%.

In contrast, various combinations of streptozocin and doxorubicin/5-FU, temozolomide and thalidomide, or single-agent dacarbazine may be considered in patients with advanced unresectable or progressive low-grade metastatic pancreatic NEC. Objective response rates approach 30%, and overall survival is improved compared to no therapy. More than 50% of patients with poorly differentiated NEC (regardless of origin) respond to combinations of etoposide and cisplatin. Systemic treatment failure in

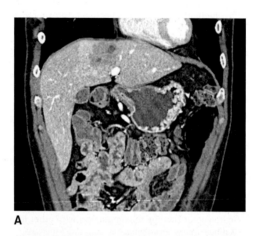

A

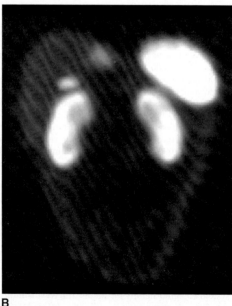

B

FIGURE 16.7 A. Computed tomography of a hypodense duodenal gastrinoma metastasis. **B.** In-111 octreotide scan revealing left medial sector gastrinoma metastasis with normal physiologic uptake of indium-111 in the gallbladder, spleen, and kidneys.

(Continued)

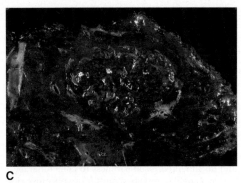

C

FIGURE 16.7 (Continued) C. Gross specimen of resected liver tumor.

poorly differentiated NEC is typically associated with rapid progression and death.

Numerous targeted agents have been used to treat patients with metastatic NEC. Typically, NECs express vascular endothelial growth factor (VEGF) and its receptor (VEGFR) making them candidates for antiangiogenic agents such as sunitinib (tyrosine kinase inhibitor with activity against VEGFR) or bevacizumab (a VEGF antibody). Trials have demonstrated either disease stability (in most patients) or objective partial regression (in a minority) with anti-VEGF therapy. The mTOR pathway is altered in some NECs, particularly those pancreatic in origin. Everolimus, an orally active mTOR inhibitor, has shown efficacy in low- to intermediate-grade NEC as demonstrated in the multicenter RADIANT Trial. Everolimus has been less effective in nonpancreatic NEC. Other agents (gefitinib, imatinib temsirolimus, bortezomib, etc.) have been used to treat NEC patients, but significant and durable tumor responses are rarely obtained (< 10%) with targeted agents alone. Thus, targeted agents are not typically considered first-line therapy and may be more effective as a chemotherapy adjunct.

Treatment Follow-up Evaluation

Current data show that despite surgical and medical therapy, disease progression occurs in more than 80% of patients with NEC hepatic metastases. Given the high rate of recurrence following potentially curative resection or progression following palliative procedures, continued surveillance is warranted. Typically, follow-up is based on serial abdominal imaging with CT or MRI and serum biomarkers (chromogranin A, neuron-specific enolase, and other specific neuroendocrine peptides [if functional NEC]) approximately every 3 to 6 months for low-grade NEC and every 2 to 3 months for high-grade NEC or in patients with documented symptom recurrence or progression. Functional (SRS) whole body imaging is performed only if the extent of the metastatic disease would affect liver-directed therapy.

HEPATIC METASTASES FROM NONCOLORECTAL, NONNEUROENDOCRINE MALIGNANCIES

As a common site for metastatic spread of most solid tumors, metastases apparently confined to the liver will frequently arise from noncolorectal, nonneuroendocrine malignancies. Given the benefits realized after resection of colorectal and neuroendocrine metastases, hepatic resection may be appropriate for some patients with noncolorectal, nonneuroendocrine metastases. The low frequency of liver-limited disease and the wide variation of underlying histopathology and tumor biology make outcome prediction difficult in this patient group as a whole. In general, resection of hepatic metastases from noncolorectal, nonneuroendocrine malignancies may be considered if the primary and regional malignancy has been resected, whole body imaging excludes extrahepatic metastases, and the performance status of the patient permits resection. Resection of such metastases should be undertaken only as one component of a multidisciplinary treatment approach with discussions among various cancer and procedural specialists. Favorable selection factors for operation related to the tumor include metachronous presentation of the hepatic metastasis, long recurrence interval, number of metastases, extent of hepatic resection, and documented responsiveness to chemotherapy. Clearly, the potential survival benefit of resection must offset operative risk. The entire supportive data for hepatic resection in such patients are based on limited series of retrospective studies in highly selected patients. In general, resection of liver metastases from primary gastrointestinal tumors (esophageal, pancreatic, gastric, and biliary) is unlikely to lead to meaningful survival benefit. In contrast, resection of duodenal and small bowel liver metastases (more similar to colorectal cancer in biology) may have more favorable outcomes. Other highly selected patients with nongastrointestinal liver metastases may potentially benefit from an aggressive approach. For example, although less than 5% of metastatic breast cancer is limited to the liver, the overall prevalence of the disease in the general population makes this scenario relatively frequent. Patients with hormone receptor–positive tumors have the best outcomes after attempts at curative liver resections; however, most breast cancer liver metastases do not express receptors (triple negative). Thus, the overall median survival after hepatectomy for breast cancer metastases is typically 12 months, and development of extrahepatic disease is common after resection. Resection of hepatic renal cell carcinoma metastases results in a good prognosis similar to outcomes for colorectal metastases resection. The best outcomes in renal cell metastasis patients occur in those with a prolonged disease-free interval. Resection of sarcoma liver metastases remains the only potentially curative option given the limited effective systemic therapies. Outcomes appear to be improving for metastatic gastrointestinal stromal (GIST) tumors due to development of effective targeted chemotherapy agent. Melanoma, specifically ocular in origin, harbors one of the worst prognoses after liver resection due to either occult or metachronous development of disseminated disease soon after liver resection.

The standard approach to hepatic resection for malignancy should be employed when considering atypical indications. Important planning includes evaluating the margins of resection and adequate functional liver remnant. The operative approach may be laparoscopic or open depending on individual surgeons' experience preference. Patients with noncolorectal, nonneuroendocrine liver metastases may also be treated with percutaneous ablation. Some noncolorectal, nonneuroendocrine metastases such as renal cell cancers or melanomas are quite vascular, and this feature may predict responsive to transarterial therapy. Based on the experience of isolated limb perfusion for melanoma and sarcoma, isolated hepatic perfusion is a potential option at specialized centers for highly selected patients with liver-only unresectable disease. This regional treatment allows higher doses of chemotherapy to be delivered directly to the tumor, limiting systemic toxicity.

Suggested Readings

Adam R, et al. Hepatic resection for noncolorectal nonendocrine liver metastases: analysis of 1,452 patients and development of a prognostic model. *Ann Surg* 2006;244(4):524–535.

Ahmed A, et al. Midgut neuroendocrine tumours with liver metastases: results of the UKINETS study. *Endocr Relat Cancer* 2009;16(3):885–894.

Ercolani G, et al. The role of liver resections for noncolorectal, nonneuroendocrine metastases: experience with 142 observed cases. *Ann Surg Oncol* 2005;12(6): 459–466.

Glazer ES, et al. Long-term survival after surgical management of neuroendocrine hepatic metastases. *HPB (Oxford)* 2010;12(6):427–433.

Gupta S, et al. Hepatic arterial embolization and chemoembolization for the treatment of patients with metastatic neuroendocrine tumors: variables affecting response rates and survival. *Cancer* 2005;104(8):1590–1602.

Gurusamy KS, et al. Palliative cytoreductive surgery versus other palliative treatments in patients with unresectable liver metastases from gastro-entero-pancreatic neuroendocrine tumours. *Cochrane Database Syst Rev* 2009;(1):CD007118.

Gurusamy KS, et al. Liver resection versus other treatments for neuroendocrine tumours in patients with resectable liver metastases. *Cochrane Database Syst Rev* 2009;(2):CD007060.

Knox CD, et al. Survival and functional quality of life after resection for hepatic carcinoid metastasis. *J Gastrointest Surg* 2004;8(6):653–659.

Leblanc F, et al. Comparison of hepatic recurrences after resection or intraoperative radiofrequency ablation indicated by size and topographical characteristics of the metastases. *Eur J Surg Oncol* 2008;34(2):185–190.

Mayo SC, et al. Surgical management of hepatic neuroendocrine tumor metastasis: results from an international multi-institutional analysis. *Ann Surg Oncol* 2010;17(12):3129–3136.

Pavel M, et al. ENETS Consensus Guidelines for the management of patients with liver and other distant metastases from neuroendocrine neoplasms of foregut, midgut, hindgut, and unknown primary. *Neuroendocrinology* 2012;95(2):157–176.

Que FG, et al. Hepatic resection for metastatic neuroendocrine carcinomas. *Am J Surg* 1995;169(1):36–42; discussion 42–43.

Reddy SK, et al. Resection of noncolorectal nonneuroendocrine liver metastases: a comparative analysis. *J Am Coll Surg* 2007;204(3):372–382.

Sarmiento JM, et al. Surgical treatment of neuroendocrine metastases to the liver: a plea for resection to increase survival. *J Am Coll Surg* 2003;197(1):29–37.

Strosberg J, Gardner N, Kvols L. Survival and prognostic factor analysis of 146 metastatic neuroendocrine tumors of the mid-gut. *Neuroendocrinology* 2009;89(4): 471–476.

Touzios JG, et al. Neuroendocrine hepatic metastases: does aggressive management improve survival? *Ann Surg* 2005;241(5): 776–783; discussion 783–785.

Vinik AL, Perry RR. Neoplasms of the gastroenteropancreatic endocrine system. In: Holland JF, Bast RC, Morton DL, et al. (eds.), *Cancer medicine.* Baltimore, MD: Williams & Wilkins, 1997:1605–1641.

Benign Liver Tumors

Jason B. Liu and Marshall S. Baker

Liver lesions are being detected incidentally with increasing frequency on imaging done as part of the evaluation of vague abdominal symptoms. The primary question regarding these lesions is to distinguish benign from malignant. Radiologic imaging broadly characterizes hepatic lesions as solid or cystic. Patient history and radiographic patterns can further aid in determining risk of malignancy and characterizing the lesion as either benign or malignant. For instance, risk factors for significant hepatic disease including a history of alcoholism, viral hepatitis, autoimmune hepatitis, primary biliary cirrhosis, hemochromatosis, hemosiderosis, or primary sclerosing cholangitis aid the clinician in assessing risk of malignancy. Long-term oral contraceptive (OCP) or anabolic steroid use confers increased risk of adenomatous change in the liver. This chapter focuses on the presentation, diagnosis, and management of benign liver lesions.

BENIGN CYSTIC LESIONS OF THE LIVER

Simple Cyst

Presentation

Simple hepatic cysts are found in 2.5% to 18% of the population. They may be single or multiple. These cysts are serous fluid-filled sacs lined by cuboidal biliary-type epithelium without communication to bile ducts. They are typically less than 1 cm in diameter and are most commonly detected as incidental findings on diagnostic imaging. Simple cysts tend to occur more commonly in the right hepatic lobe and are more prevalent in women with a peak in the fifth decade of life. Large cysts can be symptomatic due to mass effect. Most commonly, large cysts will be associated with right upper quadrant pain (Glisson capsule stretch), early satiety, or nausea. Rarely, simple cysts will become large enough to cause compression of the vena cava or biliary obstruction. Patients may also develop pain from hemorrhage into the cyst, bacterial superinfection of intracystic blood products, or free rupture. Approximately 5% of patients will require intervention due to symptoms.

Diagnosis

Ultrasonography is the most useful diagnostic test for simple cysts, which appear as anechoic fluid-filled spaces without septations and with posterior acoustic enhancement indicating a well-defined fluid–tissue interface. Computed tomography (CT) imaging demonstrates a well-demarcated cystic lesion with water attenuation and without contrast enhancement. Similar features are seen on magnetic resonance imaging (MRI). Fine needle aspiration is typically not required for diagnosis because the radiographic appearance is definitive. Recently, microbubble contrast-enhanced ultrasound (CEUS) has been used to confirm the absence of vascular flow within simple cysts.

Treatment

Most simple cysts do not require treatment or follow-up. Giant simple cysts (≥6 cm) that become symptomatic warrant operative management. Cysts that are noted to be increasing in size raise concern for a cystadenoma or cystadenocarcinoma and also warrant operative management. For patients in whom imaging is not definitive or patient history raises suspicions for possible hydatid disease, *Echinococcus* should be ruled out with serology prior to surgical intervention. Methods for treatment of simple cysts include percutaneous aspiration with or without a sclerosant (e.g., alcohol, minocycline, or tetracycline), laparoscopic or open marsupialization ("unroofing"), or laparoscopic or open resection. Simple aspiration typically leads to guaranteed recurrence. The recurrence rate is moderately decreased with the addition of a sclerosant following aspiration, but minor complications such as nausea, vomiting, or increased pain can occur. Repeated treatments may also be necessary for large cysts. Laparoscopic marsupialization with fulguration of the cyst epithelium remains the treatment of choice for giant, symptomatic cysts with a reported recurrence rate as low as 2% in published series. Recurrence is associated with incomplete unroofing and location within the posterior liver segments. An omental pedicle flap placed within the cyst bed may decrease recurrence by adhesion formation. Formal cystectomy or segmentectomy has also been performed but is associated with increased morbidity and mortality.

Polycystic Liver Disease

Presentation

Polycystic liver disease (PLD) occurs in association with autosomal dominant polycystic kidney disease (ADPKD) or as an isolated form of autosomal dominant polycystic liver disease (ADPLD). The development of polycystic liver occurs over time in patients with ADPKD, while renal cysts are rarely associated with isolated ADPLD. The increased prevalence of polycystic livers in ADPKD is attributed to the improved life expectancy of these patients. Hepatic involvement is also associated with female gender and severity of renal disease.

PLD is discovered commonly during the fourth or fifth decade of life. Patients are typically asymptomatic, but symptoms associated with hepatic enlargement can occur. Abdominal pain in the setting of PLD is usually associated with cyst hemorrhage or infection. Infection of hepatic cysts carries a 2% mortality rate and should be treated aggressively with intravenous antibiotics and percutaneous drainage. Liver function is preserved, and laboratory values typically only demonstrate a mild elevation in γ-glutamyl transpeptidase (GGT) and alkaline phosphatase when symptoms are present.

Diagnosis

The same modalities used to diagnose simple hepatic cysts are used to diagnose PLD (Fig. 17.1). Ultrasound remains the preferred diagnostic tool due to its accuracy and low cost. Three types of PLD have been suggested based upon CT characterization of the number and size of cysts as well as the amount of hepatic parenchyma between cysts. Type I patients have a limited number of large cysts with large areas of normal hepatic parenchyma. Type II patients have multiple medium-sized cysts isolated to certain segments. Type III patients are characterized by near replacement of the hepatic parenchyma with diffuse cysts. Surgical intervention for PLD is grossly reflective of these three categories.

Treatment

Therapy for PLD is aimed at minimizing the proportion of hepatic cysts while maximizing hepatic parenchyma, thereby relieving symptoms associated

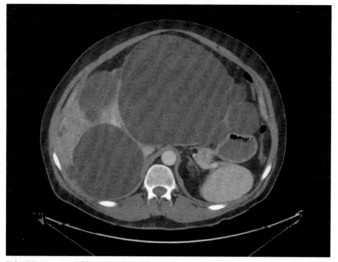

FIGURE 17.1 Axial CT imaging for a 54-year-old male presenting with epigastric pain. He was found to have isolated PLD and underwent laparoscopic left hepatic lobectomy and marsupialization of the dominant right hepatic cyst. He is currently asymptomatic 3 years postresection.

with mass effect while avoiding the risk for liver failure. Strategies are identical to the management of simple hepatic cysts except for the addition of orthotopic liver transplantation in diffuse type III disease. Patients with type I disease are approached with marsupialization or percutaneous drainage with sclerotherapy. No significant differences in morbidity, mortality, or recurrence rates have been seen using laparoscopic versus open approaches. Hepatic resection becomes applicable in patients with type II or type III disease whereby removal of multiple segments that are grossly affected can be beneficial in volume reduction. Transplantation is reserved for patients who have severely impaired quality of life, are in intractable pain and for whom there are no other surgical options for management. Candidates usually have cachexia, significant weight loss, malnutrition, recurrent cyst infections, portal hypertension, and ascites. The decision to pursue liver transplantation requires weighing the high mortality rates (12% to 30%) associated with transplant against the potential improvement in quality of life.

Cystadenoma

Presentation
Cystadenoma is the most common primary cystic neoplasm of the liver with an associated malignant potential. The incidence is limited to case reports and small case series. These cysts occur most commonly in women between 40 and 60 years of age, are discovered incidentally on diagnostic imaging, and are generally asymptomatic. Patients may develop symptoms of right upper quadrant pain and anorexia due to mass effect from cyst growth.

Diagnosis
Diagnosis of cystadenoma is based primarily on ultrasonographic findings. These include irregular borders, hypoechoic cyst with hyperechoic

septations, solid components, papillary projections, wall enhancement, and dorsal shadows demonstrating calcified areas. Difficulty arises when differentiating between cystadenoma, cystadenocarcinoma, complex cysts (i.e., simple cysts with resolved internal hemorrhage), and hydatid cysts. Multiphase CT or diffusion weighted MRI imaging may reveal vascularity of the septa perhaps suggesting cystadenocarcinoma. Hydatid cysts demonstrate similar patterns on imaging, and *Echinococcus* should be ruled out with serology. CEUS can be helpful to rule in cystadenoma and cystadenocarcinoma as this modality may detect vascular flow, which is absent in complex cysts. Analysis of cyst fluid nearly always shows elevated CA 19–9 concentration.

Treatment

Surgical resection with clear margins is the definitive treatment for cystadenoma due to the risk of malignant transformation, which is generally reported to be 10% to 15%. Some authorities consider enucleation effective therapy for cystadenoma.

Hydatid (*Echinococcus*) Cyst: Cystic Echinococcosis and Alveolar Echinococcosis

Hydatid cysts arise from infection with the tapeworm *Echinococcus granulosus* that live in the small intestines of canines and sheep. Humans are accidental intermediate hosts due to ingestion of eggs via the fecal–oral route. Other virulent species include *E. multilocularis, E. vogeli,* and *E. oligarthus.* Echinococcal disease is endemic in many Mediterranean countries, Eastern Europe, the Middle East, East Africa, East Asia, Australia, and South America. In the United States, most cases occur in immigrants from endemic regions. Infection with *E. granulosus* causes cystic echinococcosis (CE), while infection with *E. multilocularis* causes alveolar echinococcosis (AE).

Cystic Echinococcosis (CE)

Presentation. *E. granulosus* has an annual incidence of 1 to 200 per 100,000 and is endemic to temperate climates such as the Mediterranean, Central Asia, Australia, and South America where pastoral communities are prominent. Cyst growth is slow and can remain asymptomatic for years. Cysts can be found throughout the body with the liver (approximately 80%) most commonly affected followed by the lung (approximately 20%). Symptoms occur due to either mass effect (e.g., cholestasis, portal hypertension, Budd-Chiari syndrome) or rupture. Severe presentations include bacterial superinfection/hepatic abscess formation, secondary cholangitis due to rupture into the biliary tree, or peritonitis and anaphylaxis due to intra-abdominal rupture.

Diagnosis. CE is diagnosed based upon patient history, clinical findings (e.g., abdominal pain, fever, chest pain, and dyspnea), ultrasonography, and positive serology. Eosinophilia is rarely present unless there is already leakage of antigen into the circulation. Ultrasonography has a sensitivity of 90% to 95% and is the imaging modality of choice (Fig. 17.2). The World Health Organization (WHO) classification bases treatment decisions on ultrasound findings, which differentiate cysts into active, transitional, and inactive states (Table 17.1). MRI or magnetic resonance cholangiopancreatography (MRCP) can be used to evaluate any lesions that may involve the biliary tree or for preoperative planning. The diagnosis is further corroborated with detection of serum antibodies, which has a sensitivity range between 85% and 98%.

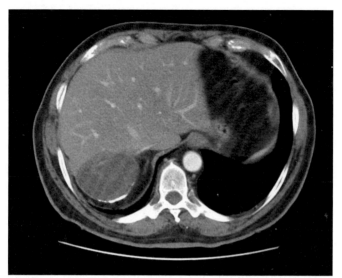

A

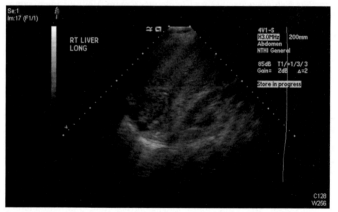

B

FIGURE 17.2 Computed tomography **(A)** and ultrasound **(B)** imaging of an echinococcal cyst in a 74-year-old male of Greek origin. This cyst demonstrates ultrasound features typical of a CE4 type cyst. It is heterogeneous with degenerative contents and no daughter cysts. On CT the wall is thickened and partially calcified. These findings are characteristic of inactive cysts. The patient was managed with observation and has been asymptomatic over 3 years of follow-up.

Treatment. There have been no randomized trials regarding the treatment of CE. Treatment decisions are made based upon the standardized WHO ultrasound-based classification as well as the available medical and surgical expertise in the endemic region. Surgery, percutaneous treatments, and antiparasitic drug therapy are the mainstays.

TABLE 17.1 Classification of World Health Organization

	Phase	Characteristics	Surgery	Percutaneous Therapy	Drug Therapy	Suggested Initial Therapy
CE1	Active	Unilocular, simple cyst with visible cyst wall and hydatid sand, "snowflake sign"	No	Yes	Yes	PAIR + albendazole
CE2	Active	Multiseptated daughter cysts within mother cyst; "wheel-like," "rosette-like," "honeycomb-like" structures	Yes	Yes	Yes	Other percutaneous therapy + albendazole
CE3a	Transitional	Detached laminated membrane from cyst wall, "water-lily" sign	No	Yes	Yes	PAIR + albendazole
CE3b	Transitional	Solid with daughter vesicles, "complex mass"	Yes	Yes	Yes	Other percutaneous therapy + albendazole
CE4	Inactive	Heterogeneous, degenerative contents, "ball of wool" sign	No	No	No	None
CE5	Inactive	Calcified cyst wall, cone-shaped shadows	No	No	No	None

Surgery is indicated for the treatment of WHO class CE2-CE3b (active cysts with multiple daughter vesicles), single liver cysts situated superficially in the liver, infected cysts when percutaneous therapy is unavailable, cysts communicating with the biliary tree, and cysts compressing adjacent vital organs. The primary goal is to remove the entirety of parasitic material while avoiding spillage and secondary echinococcosis. Total cystectomy can be performed using open or laparoscopic techniques although the frequency of spillage has not been compared. Total cystectomy is ideally performed in a "closed" manner whereby the cyst is removed by means of a partial hepatectomy without opening the cyst. Cystectomy done "open" whereby the cyst is injected with protoscolicidal agents (i.e., 20% hypertonic saline), unroofed, and the pericystic tissue is excised has also been described but is believed to carry increased risk of dissemination. Involvement of the biliary tree is more commonly found in large cysts greater than 7.5 cm. Biliary communication can be detected intraoperatively by using dye or fluoroscopy, and the communication can be simply suture ligated. Perioperative benzimidazoles (e.g., albendazole, mebendazole) are recommended to minimize the risk of perioperative dissemination.

Percutaneous treatment including PAIR (puncture, aspiration, injection, reaspiration) and modified catheterization techniques is indicated for inoperable patients, recurrent disease, or cysts that fail to respond to benzimidazoles only. Communication with the biliary tree must be ruled out prior to performing PAIR to avoid the risk of chemically induced sclerosing cholangitis. Success is associated with many of the types of CE except for CE2 and CE3b, which tend to relapse after PAIR. These types are treated with surgical resection, as discussed above, or with modified catheterization techniques that involve large-bore catheters, sclerosing agents, and curettage.

Cyst types CE4 and CE5 (inactive or heavily calcified cysts with no daughter cysts) can be simply surveyed without treatment. These are generally of limited clinical significance and unlikely to cause biliary complications or symptoms.

Alveolar Echinococcosis (AE)

Presentation. Infection with *E. multilocularis* has an annual incidence of 0.03–1.2 per 100,000 and is isolated to regions of central and eastern Europe, Russia, China, and northern Japan. It has been noted that the frequency of cases in Western Europe has increased with the popularity of fox hunting. Interestingly, AE affects the liver primarily and does not form cysts like CE. The larvae invade locally or spread hematogenously akin to malignancy. The disease is chronic with an average incubation period of 5 to 15 years. Symptoms include cholestatic jaundice, abdominal pain, fatigue, weight loss, and hepatomegaly.

Diagnosis. Diagnosis of AE is based on patient history, clinical presentation, ultrasonography, and positive serology. Cross-sectional imaging including CT and MRI/MRCP are used to further evaluate the local extent of the disease particularly during preoperative planning. Classification of AE is based upon the WHO PNM staging system analogous to the TNM staging of malignancy.

Treatment. After diagnosis is confirmed and the extent of disease delineated, the PNM staging system is used to direct therapy. Treatment involves surgical resection, orthotopic liver transplantation, antiparasitic drug therapy, or endoscopic or percutaneous interventions. The primary goal of treatment is complete surgical excision whenever possible. Endoscopic or percutaneous interventions should be employed as palliative procedures when surgery is not feasible. Benzimidazoles are always indicated and, in the setting of surgical resection, given as lifelong adjuvant therapy.

Liver transplantation can be considered in the setting of patients who have severe liver insufficiency secondary to biliary cirrhosis or Budd-Chiari syndrome, recurrent cholangitis, inability to perform radical liver resection (i.e., lack of hepatic reserve), and the absence of extrahepatic disease. As of 2003, 45 liver transplantations have been performed for AE with variable success.

Pyogenic Liver Abscess

Presentation

Pyogenic (bacterial and fungal) liver abscesses (PLA) were once complications from inadequately treated appendicitis, diverticulitis, or other intra-abdominal infections. Biliary sources are now the primary causes of PLA. The incidence is estimated at 20 cases per 100,000 hospital admissions with the average patient between 50 and 60 years of age and of male predominance. The incidence of PLA is not associated with ethnicity or geographic location.

Abscesses can be divided into six categories based upon the route of infection listed in order of descending frequency: (1) biliary (60%), (2) cryptogenic (17%), (3) hepatic artery (10%), (4) portal vein (7%), (5) penetrating trauma (5%), and (6) direct extension (3%). Iatrogenic causes include biliary–enteric anastomoses, liver-directed therapies for malignancy, and transplantation. *Escherichia coli* and *Klebsiella pneumoniae* are the most common pathogens followed by *Staphylococcus aureus*, *Enterococcus* spp., *Streptococcus viridans*, and *Bacteroides*. The incidence of *Klebsiella* as the primary pathogen in liver abscesses has increased recently, particularly in those with diabetes mellitus. PLA have become a unique complication associated with patients undergoing chemotherapy with hepatotoxic drugs, such as oxaliplatin (sinusoidal obstruction syndrome) and irinotecan (steatohepatitis), for treatment of hepatic metastases. Drug-induced liver injury is postulated to cause increased susceptibility to liver abscess formation.

Fever, right upper quadrant abdominal pain, nausea, vomiting, malaise, chills, and weight loss are common presenting symptoms. Elevated transaminases and/or obstructive jaundice can be present on laboratory evaluation. Leukocytosis is frequently but not always present. Bacteremia is present 50% to 95% of the time. Severe complications such as intraperitoneal or pericardial rupture, empyema, and broncho–pleural–hepatic fistulae are rare.

Diagnosis

The diagnosis of PLA is dependent on imaging studies, where they can be solitary or multiple. The right hepatic lobe is most often involved, although a miliary presentation can occur. CT imaging with intravenous contrast is the preferred modality with a diagnostic accuracy of 93% to 96%. Imaging reveals a hypodense lesion, uni- or multiloculated, without contrast enhancement surrounded by rim enhancement with or without the presence of gas (Fig. 17.3). Cross-sectional imaging can also demonstrate a likely cause in approximately 70% of cases.

Treatment

Treatment primarily involves parenteral antibiotics and percutaneous drainage, which has a success rate of 60% to 90%. Antibiotics are usually

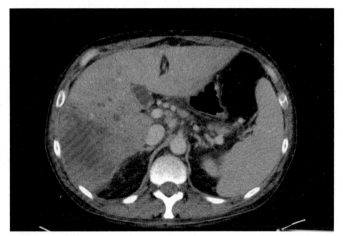

FIGURE 17.3 Axial CT imaging of a pyogenic liver abscess presenting in a 49-year-old male alcoholic. The abscess presented in the context of an acute bout of alcohol-inducted hepatitis associated with portal vein thrombosis and was managed by percutaneous drainage and antibiotic administration.

continued for 4 to 6 weeks and tailored to culture results. Repeated percutaneous aspiration without drain placement can be considered in those with solitary, unilocular abscesses 1 to 3 cm in diameter. No randomized controlled trial has compared percutaneous aspiration versus drain placement. Percutaneous drainage carries a 5% to 6% mortality rate.

Surgical drainage is reserved for patients who fail percutaneous drainage. In patients with a biliary source of pyogenic liver abscess, failure of percutaneous drainage is associated with biliary fistula. In these patients, endoscopic biliary decompression should be combined with percutaneous drainage to resolve the abscess without requiring surgical intervention. Surgical drainage can be approached laparoscopically or with formal hepatic resection. No studies have compared the effectiveness of these approaches.

Amebic Liver Abscess

Presentation

Liver abscess is the most common extraintestinal site of amebic infection but occurs in less than 1% of *Entamoeba histolytica* infections. *E. histolytica* is endemic to tropical and temperate climates, such as Mexico, India, Indonesia, sub-Saharan Africa, and Central and South America. It most commonly affects men between 20 and 40 years of age.

The disease is contracted via ingestion of contaminated water or food, which typically results in dysentery. However, the trophozoite can burrow through the colonic mucosa in certain hosts to enter the portal circulation and form an abscess within the liver. Clinical presentation usually occurs within 8 to 20 weeks. Signs and symptoms most commonly include right upper quadrant abdominal pain, high fever (>38.5°C), and tenderness to liver palpation. Amebic dysentery and liver abscess rarely occur together.

Laboratory evaluation demonstrates leukocytosis without eosinophilia, elevated alkaline phosphatase, and occasional transaminitis.

Diagnosis

Imaging and serology remain the cornerstones of accurate diagnosis. Enzyme-linked immunoabsorbent assay (ELISA) has a sensitivity of 99% and a specificity of 90% for amebic liver abscess. This test should be repeated in 7 days if the initial result is negative due to the delayed formation of antibodies. Furthermore, patients from endemic regions may have positive serology due to previous infection. Serum antigen detection assays can also be used to aid in diagnosis.

It is difficult to distinguish between pyogenic and amebic liver abscess on imaging as they demonstrate similar features (e.g., rim enhancement). Percutaneous aspiration of an amebic abscess typically yields an odorless, reddish-brown "anchovy paste" fluid composed of necrotic hepatocytes. Trophozoites are seen in less than 20% of aspirates. Superinfection of amebic abscesses with enteric bacteria may occur.

Treatment

Amebic abscesses are treated with an amebicidal agent and a luminal agent. Metronidazole for 7 to 10 days and either paromomycin or iodoquinol for 7 days provide adequate treatment. Percutaneous aspiration or surgical drainage is rarely necessary in amebic liver abscesses except when abscesses are greater than 6 cm. Intracavitary injection of metronidazole during percutaneous aspiration is an effective strategy for larger abscesses (Table 17.2).

BENIGN SOLID LESIONS OF THE LIVER

Hemangioma

Presentation

Cavernous hepatic hemangiomas are the most common solid benign liver tumor with an overall prevalence of 5% to 20%. Hemangiomas occur predominantly in females (2–6:1) between 30 and 50 years of age. They are thought to arise from congenital hamartomas due to progressive ectasia. No causal link to estrogen therapy has thus far been identified. Hemangiomas are most often asymptomatic and are discovered incidentally on abdominal imaging. Symptoms occur in approximately 12% of patients, usually due to capsular stretch or compression of adjacent structures. Symptoms include right upper quadrant pain, palpable midepigastric mass, nausea, early satiety, or dyspepsia. Rarely, patients may present with Kasabach-Merritt syndrome, a consumptive coagulopathy manifesting with thombocytopenia, hypofibrinogenemia, and systemic bleeding. Hemangiomas have no malignant potential and rarely if ever rupture.

Diagnosis

Ultrasonography yields a sensitivity of 60% to 70% and specificity of 60% to 90% for identification. Multiphase CT and MRI are more accurate than is ultrasound. Peripheral nodular contrast enhancement with centripetal filling is the classic presentation of hemangioma on multiphase imaging. Magnetic resonance imaging has reported sensitivity and specificity of 95% in identifying hemangiomas. Because of this, excellent accuracy angiography or biopsy is no longer used to diagnose hemangiomas. Surveillance imaging is generally not recommended unless there is uncertainty regarding the diagnosis or symptoms develop.

Treatment

Most hemangiomas remain asymptomatic and stable over time. Intervention to prevent future complications is not justified. Rare case reports of hemangioma rupture associated with large size or trauma are not enough

TABLE 17.2 Management of Benign Cystic Liver Lesions

	Risk Factors or Associations	Potential Complications	Malignant Potential	Initial Diagnostic Modality	Initial Therapy	Follow-up
Simple Cyst	Age > 60 y, Female gender	Portal hypertension, hemorrhage, biliary obstruction, bacterial superinfection, rupture	None	Ultrasound	None unless symptomatic	None required regardless of intervention
Polycystic Liver Disease	Intracranial aneurysms, mitral valve prolapse, mitral valve regurgitation, pancreatic cysts, renal cysts	Portal hypertension, hemorrhage, biliary obstruction, bacterial superinfection, rupture	Rare	Ultrasound	None unless symptomatic	None unless symptoms recur
Cystadenoma	Female gender	Obstructive jaundice, chronic cholecystitis, cholelithiasis	Yes	Ultrasound/MRI	Surgical resection	None
Cystic Echinococcus	Endemic regions	Portal hypertension, cholestasis, Budd-Chiari syndrome, bacterial superinfection, rupture, anaphylaxis	None	Ultrasound and serology	Depends on WHO classification	Depends on WHO classification
Alveolar Echinococcus	Endemic regions	Cholestasis	None	Ultrasound and serology, Multiphase CT	Depends on WHO classification	Depends on WHO classification
Pyogenic Liver Abscess	Iatrogenic (biliary-enteric anastomosis, liver direct therapies, transplantation)	Rupture, empyema, broncho–pleural–hepatic fistula, septic shock	None	Ultrasound and serology	Antibiotics ± percutaneous drainage	None unless symptoms recur
Amebic Liver Abscess	Endemic regions, immunocompromise, history of splenectomy	Rupture, empyema, broncho–pleural–hepatic fistula, septic shock	None	Ultrasound and ELISA	Pharmacologic	None unless symptoms recur

to warrant prophylactic surgery. Surgical resection can be considered in patients with symptoms, in lesions in which malignancy cannot be excluded, or to treat complications. Enucleation is the operation of choice due to a significantly lower rate of perioperative morbidity compared to hepatic lobectomy. Radiofrequency ablation (RFA) and cryotherapy have also been used in select situations.

Focal Nodular Hyperplasia

Presentation

Focal nodular hyperplasia (FNH) is the second most common benign solid hepatic lesion after hemangiomas. The reported incidence of FNH is 0.3% to 3%, though only 0.03% have clinical significance. They are associated with female gender (8:1) and occur between 30 and 50 years of age. Concurrent adenomas are diagnosed in up to 3.6% of patients and concurrent hemangiomas in up to 23% of patients with FNH. FNH is not associated with OCPs or pregnancy. Lesions are typically found incidentally, and symptoms are associated with capsular stretch or compression of adjacent structures. No malignant potential and no potential to rupture spontaneously have been associated with FNH.

Diagnosis

The classic description of FNH is a lobular mass with homogeneous arterial enhancement, radiating fibrous septa, and a central, nonenhancing scar. This pattern is detected, however, in only 40% to 50% of cases. The diagnosis of FNH must be differentiated from that of hepatocellular adenoma as these two entities are managed differently. Multiphase MRI with liver-specific contrast agents has been shown to have a sensitivity and specificity of 97% and 100%, respectively, in differentiating FNH from adenoma. In addition, FNH should also be distinguished from fibrolamellar hepatocellular carcinoma (HCC), which also demonstrates a central scar. Characteristics of fibrolamellar HCC include large size greater than 10 cm, heterogeneous enhancement, presence of calcifications, and hypointensity of the central scar on T2-weighted MRI imaging compared to the hyperintensity seen with FNH.

Treatment

Symptoms or the inability to exclude malignancy are the indications for intervention. Hepatic enucleation or lobectomy remains the procedure of choice, although interventional procedures involving embolization and RFA have also been used.

Hepatocellular Adenoma

Presentation

HCA is a benign neoplasm composed of hepatocyte proliferation. These lesions occur in the population with a female:male ratio of 11:1, and usually present between 30 and 40 years of life. Risk factors for HCA development include OCP use and pregnancy in females and anabolic steroid use in males. A subset of patients with glycogen storage diseases type Ia and type III can develop HCA, typically with a male:female 2:1 predominance. Patients with HCA present with pain 25% to 50% of the time or are otherwise asymptomatic with the lesion incidentally discovered on axial imaging. They are isolated lesions located commonly within the right hepatic lobe. Liver adenomatosis occurs when more than 10 lesions are present (see below). Lesions greater than 5 cm, OCP use, and pregnancy are risk factors for rupture or hemorrhage with the classic presentation of sudden-onset right upper quadrant pain followed by hypotension. Rupture and hemorrhage are relatively rare events. HCAs carry a potential for malignant transformation in up to 11% of lesions. Adenomas occurring in men, lesions greater than 5 cm, those associated with androgen steroid use, and those associated with beta-catenin gene mutations are more likely to be malignant.

HCAs are classified into three histopathologic varieties: (1) Steatotic HCA caused by hepatocyte nuclear factor 1a (HNF1α) mutation, (2) inflammatory HCA caused by IL-6 signal transducer (IL6ST) mutation, or (3) HCAs associated with β-catenin mutation. Inflammatory HCA is the most common variant representing 35% to 50% of HCAs. The specific subgroup of HCA involving β-catenin mutations may have a greater risk for malignant transformation compared to those with HNF1α or IL6ST mutations. Further investigation is needed to determine the benefit of histopathologic diagnosis. Core needle biopsy itself carries a risk of sampling error, bleeding, and the theoretical risk of biopsy tract seeding.

Diagnosis

The confirmatory diagnosis of HCA is challenging because of its heterogeneous imaging features, particularly in the setting of necrosis, old or recent hemorrhage, and calcific foci. Ultrasound has no utility in diagnosis of HCAs unless contrast enhancement is used. Contrast enhanced ultrasound reveals a centripetal enhancement during arterial phase compared to a centrifugal filling pattern in FNH. Multiphase CT scan is more useful than ultrasound to diagnose HCA, but its utility lies in its ability to identify FNH and hemangiomas to rule out HCA. Multiphase MRI with liver-specific contrast agents provides the best definitive diagnosis and can be used to suggest the subtype. Steatotic adenomas display diffuse signal dropout on T1-weighted chemical shift sequence associated with their high fat density, and are moderately enhancing in the arterial phase without persistent enhancement in the portal venous and delayed phases. This pattern yields a sensitivity and specificity of 86% and 100%, respectively. Inflammatory adenomas display high-intensity signal on T2-weighted MRI and lack of signal dropout of fat suppression images and have strong arterial enhancement with persistent enhancement of portal venous and delayed phases. This pattern yields a sensitivity and specificity of 85% and 87%, respectively. Unfortunately, no particular MRI pattern has been associated with β-catenin mutated lesions, which carry the greatest potential for malignant transformation.

Treatment

Patients who take OCPs or anabolic steroids should be advised to discontinue these medications as this may lead to regression of the lesion. Treatment modalities include RFA, transarterial embolization (TAE), and hepatic resection. Hepatic resection, either anatomic segmentectomy/lobectomy or enucleation, is preferred. To date, no clinical trial has compared RFA or TAE against surgical resection. Surgical resection is indicated in all adenomas occurring in men, those that cause symptoms or hemorrhage, and those greater than 5 cm in women. Adenomas that have ruptured should be managed initially with resuscitation followed immediately by TAE. Resection during acute rupture has a reported mortality of 8% to 10%. In addition to hemorrhage control, TAE has been shown to cause tumor shrinkage. Lesions that are smaller than 5 cm in size should be surveyed for growth. A typical regimen includes ultrasound examination every 3 months for 6 months and extending the duration thereafter if no growth or suspicious features are detected. Patients who develop symptoms should be offered resection.

Women with adenomas greater than 5 cm in size are advised to undergo resection prior to conception. Women who are diagnosed with adenomas during pregnancy are advised to undergo elective resection

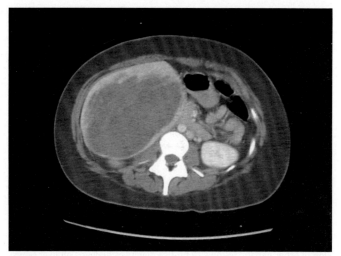

FIGURE 17.4 Axial CT imaging demonstrating a large hepatic adenoma in a 55-year-old woman presenting with hypotension and anemia. The scan demonstrates evidence of hemorrhage into the tumor. This patient was managed with selective embolization to the right hepatic lobe mass and interval right hepatic lobectomy.

during the second trimester for lesions greater than 5 cm in size. Lesions that are discovered in the third trimester should be monitored with serial ultrasound exams as the rare risk of spontaneous rupture exists (Fig. 17.4).

Hepatic Adenomatosis

Presentation
Liver adenomatosis refers to the patient with arbitrarily defined greater than 10 HCAs. The presentation is identical to that of isolated HCAs. It has been argued that adenomatosis is not a separate entity from solitary HCAs.

Diagnosis
Histologic and radiographic features of adenomatosis are identical to that of isolated HCA.

Treatment
The optimal mode of treatment has not been defined due to the rarity of presentation and the difficulty of isolated lobectomy. Treatment options include a combination of surgical resection, RFA, and TAE. Orthotopic liver transplantation has been performed in rare cases. The number of adenomas is not associated with increased risk of malignant transformation or hemorrhage. Treatment should be aimed at the lesion greater than 5 cm in size with close surveillance of the remaining lesions.

Nodular Regenerative Hyperplasia

Presentation
Nodular regenerative hyperplasia (NRH) occurs when normal hepatic parenchyma is transformed into 1- to 3-mm regenerative nodules separated by atrophic areas without the presence of perisinusoidal fibrosis as seen in cirrhosis. This condition is thought to occur due to altered blood

flow causing hepatocyte hyperplasia in regions with adequate blood flow and atrophy in regions with ischemia. NRH is a rare condition with autopsy studies demonstrating an overall incidence between 0.7% and 2.6%. Our understanding of the condition is limited to case reports with only approximately 350 cases reported from 1975 to 2011. It most commonly presents in middle age and increases in frequency with age. There is no association with gender or ethnicity. It is felt that NRH occurs in response to other systemic perturbation including immunologic, hematologic, medication-associated, cardiac, or pulmonary conditions.

Patients with NRH are usually asymptomatic and detected on workup of the underlying systemic condition. When symptoms do occur, they are the result of portal hypertension. Differentiation should be made between NRH and large regenerative nodules (LRN), which occur in the presence of hepatic outflow obstruction, such as in Budd-Chiari syndrome.

Diagnosis

Suspicion for NRH usually occurs during the evaluation of portal hypertension especially in the patient without evidence of cirrhosis. Imaging studies in the diagnosis of NRH cannot readily distinguish LRN from the regenerative nodules of cirrhosis. Imaging subsequently is most useful for the exclusion of other hepatic lesions. Definitive diagnosis depends on liver biopsy with histopathologic analysis.

Treatment

Treatment of NRH is geared towards management of the underlying condition and the management of portal hypertension when it occurs. Standard therapies for portal hypertension should be employed, including dietary changes, medical management of ascites, endoscopic intervention for varices, and surgical shunting procedures or transjugular intrahepatic portosystemic shunts (TIPS). Orthotopic liver transplantation can be considered in the patient with hepatic failure. Mortality from NRH is most commonly due to variceal bleeding.

Angiomyolipoma

Presentation

Angiomyolipomas (AML) are rare, benign mesenchymal tumors most often found in the kidney. Only approximately 300 cases of hepatic AML have been reported between 1976 and 2012. These lesions are well-circumscribed, soft masses composed of mature fat cells, blood vessels and smooth muscle. Their pathogenesis is unknown, and lesions are usually incidentally identified on diagnostic imaging. Both renal and hepatic AML are associated with tuberous sclerosis complex. Patients reporting symptoms usually have large AML causing capsular stretch or compression of adjacent structures. Spontaneous rupture has been reported rarely.

Diagnosis

The accurate diagnosis of AML depends upon the proportion of fat, smooth muscle, and blood vessels within the lesion. Generally, lesions that contain predominantly fat are more accurately diagnosed with imaging and those lesions containing less fat are commonly mistaken for malignancy (e.g., HCC, metastasis, liposarcoma). In general MRI with hepatic-specific contrast agents remain the best imaging modality for diagnosis, though the overall accuracy of MRI is still poor. In a recent series of 79 patients undergoing surgical resection for presumed AML, 48% were diagnosed incorrectly preoperatively with imaging or angiography.

TABLE 17.3	Management of Benign Solid Liver Lesions					
	Risk Factors or Associations	Potential Complications	Malignant Potential	Initial Diagnostic Modality	Initial Therapy	Follow-up
Hemangioma	Female gender	Kasabach-Merritt syndrome, rupture	None	Multiphase CT	None unless symptomatic	None unless symptomatic
Focal Nodular Hyperplasia	Female gender	None	None	Multiphase MRI	None unless symptomatic or cannot exclude malignancy	None unless symptoms recur
Hepatocellular Adenoma	Female gender, OCPs, pregnancy, glycogen storage disorders, anabolic steroids	Rupture, hemorrhage	Yes	Multiphase MRI	Surgical resection if >5 cm	Surveillance for growth
Hepatic Adenomatosis	Same as hepatocellular adenoma					
Nodular Regenerative Hyperplasia	Secondary to other systemic conditions	Portal hypertension	None	Tissue biopsy	Management of underlying condition	None unless symptomatic
Angiomyolipoma	Tuberous sclerosis	Rupture rarely	Rarely	Multiphase MRI	Surgical resection if >6 cm or cannot exclude malignancy	Surveillance for growth

Treatment

The preferred treatment of AML is controversial due to the rarity of the condition. In general, AML has been treated as a benign liver lesion; however, case reports of malignant transformation presenting as vascular invasion or metastatic disease have been published. Because of these observations, surgical resection is recommended in lesions greater than 6 cm, lesions that demonstrate rapid growth during surveillance, or lesions in which malignancy cannot be definitively excluded. Patients who have undergone percutaneous biopsy should be considered for surgical resection if vascular invasion, atypical epithelioid component, or p53 immunoreactivity is found on histopathologic examination (Table 17.3).

Suggested Readings

Chun YS, House M, Kaur II, et al. SSAT/AHPBA joint symposium on evaluation and treatment of benign liver lesions. *J Gastrointest Surg* 2013;17:636–644.

Devaney K, Goodman ZD, Ishak KG. Hepatobiliary cystadenoma and cystadenocarcinoma. A light microscopic and immunohistochemical study of 70 patients. *Am J Surg Pathol* 1994;18:1078–1091.

Ding G, Liu Y, Wu M, et al. Diagnosis and treatment of hepatic angiomyolipoma. *J Surg Oncol* 2011;103:807–812.

Farges O, Ferreira N, Dokmak S, et al. Changing trends in malignant transformation of hepatocellular adenoma. *Gut* 2011;60:85–89.

Filice C, DiePerri G, Strosselli M. Outcome of hepatic amoebic abscesses managed with three different therapeutic strategies. *Dig Dis Sci* 1992;37:240–247.

Hartleb M, Gutkowski K, Milkiewicz P. Nodular regenerative hyperplasia: evolving concepts on underdiagnosed cause of portal hypertension. *World J Gastroenterol* 2011;17:1400–1409.

Huang C, Pitt HA, Lipsett PA, et al. Pyogenic hepatic abscess: changing trends over 42 years. *Ann Surg* 1996;223:600–607.

Karkar AM, Tang LH, Kashikar ND, et al. Management of hepatocellular adenoma: comparison of resection, embolization and observation. *HPB (Oxford)* 2013;15:235–243.

Lambiase RE, Deyoe L, Cronan JJ, et al. Percutaneous drainage of 335 consecutive abscesses: results of primary drainage with 1 year follow up. *Radiology* 1992;184:167–179.

Lantinga MA, Gevers TJG, Drenth JPH. Evaluation of hepatic cystic lesions. *World J Gastroenterol* 2013;19:3543–3554.

Mazza O, Fernandez DL, Pekolj J, et al. Management of nonparasitic hepatic cysts. *J Am Coll Surg* 2009;209:733–739.

Mezhir JJ, Fong Y, Jacks L, et al. Current management of pyogenic liver abscess: surgery is now second-line treatment. *J Am Coll Surg* 2010;210:975–983.

Russell RT, Pinson CW. Surgical management of polycystic liver disease. *World J Gastroenterol* 2007;13:5052–5059.

Semelka RC, Martin DR, Balci C, et al. Focal liver lesions: comparison of dual-phase CT and multisequence multiplanar MR imaging including dynamic gadolinium enhancement. *J Magn Reson Imaging* 2001;13:397–401.

Shaked O, Siegelman E, Olthoff K, et al. Biologic and clinical features of benign solid and cystic lesions of the liver. *Clin Gastroenterol Hepatol* 2011;9:547–562.

Vachha B, Sun MR, Siewert B, et al. Cystic lesions of the liver. *AJR Am J Roentgenol* 2011;196:W355–W366. PMID: 21427297.

Van Vledder MG, Van Aalten SM, Terkivatan T, et al. Safety and efficacy of radiofrequency ablation for hepatocellular adenoma. *J Vasc Interv Radiol* 2011;22:787–793.

WHO-Informal Working Group on Echinococcus. International classification of ultrasound images in cystic echinococcosis for application in clinical and field epidemiological settings. *Acta Trop* 2008;85:253–261.

Complications of Liver Surgery Including Postoperative Hepatic Insufficiency

Ching-Wei D. Tzeng and Thomas A. Aloia

INTRODUCTION

Until the most recent two decades, hepatectomies were considered high-risk operations with frequent hemorrhagic events and high rates of morbidity and mortality that would be unacceptable by current standards. Even as surgeons have become more aggressive with the extent and radicality of hepatectomies, the overall mortality rate has decreased dramatically from historical rates of 10% to 20% to around 2.5%. This mortality improvement is due to better patient risk stratification and selection, optimization of the future liver remnant (FLR), using portal vein embolization (PVE), limiting preoperative chemotherapy toxicity, more advanced surgical techniques, more experienced perioperative care, novel multidisciplinary sequencing strategies, and improved capabilities to rescue patients who develop complications.

Although the hepatectomy mortality rate has decreased dramatically, the rates of any morbidity (30% to 45% by retrospective analyses) and of major morbidity (20% by the American College of Surgeons National Surgical Quality Improvement Program, ACS NSQIP, analysis) still remain clinically significant. Major posthepatectomy complications include those typical for major general surgery operations, such as bleeding, infected fluid collections, bile leaks, wound infections, cardiopulmonary events, organ system failure, sepsis, and venous thromboembolism (VTE). Complication rates often correlate with the extent of hepatectomy, making reports of overall complication rates uninformative without specification of the types of hepatectomy examined in these studies (Table 18.1).

Three complications specific to liver surgery are bleeding (intraoperative and early postoperative), bile leak (and associated organ space infection), and postoperative hepatic insufficiency (PHI, or liver failure) with liver-related mortality. Generally, PHI can be split into "early" and "late" phases, in which the late phase often leads to an irreversible cascade toward liver-related mortality that can happen well past 30 postoperative days. Late PHI mandates that surgeons look beyond the typical postoperative interval of 30 days to completely capture all liver-related morbidity and mortality. In fact, up to one-third of posthepatectomy deaths occur between 30 and 90 postoperative days.

Predictors of major complications can be divided into three categories—patient comorbidities, biochemical abnormalities, and perioperative risk factors (including magnitude of operation). These factors generally include the American Society of Anesthesiologists (ASA) class, smoking, elevated alkaline phosphatase, low albumin, elevated partial thromboplastin time (PTT), extent of hepatectomy, intraoperative or postoperative transfusions, and prolonged operative time. The last three factors are closely related, and thus surgeons should be cautious about pairing major simultaneous operations with major hepatectomies. While not all risk factors are

	All	Partial	Left	Right	Extended
Organ space infection[a]	6.0%	4.5%	5.2%	7.8%	10.9%
Pneumonia[a]	4.0%	3.1%	3.5%	5.5%	7.0%
Ventilator >48 h[a]	4.4%	3.2%	3.0%	6.7%	7.4%
Acute renal failure	1.5%	1.0%	0.4%	3.1%	2.2%
DVT[a]	2.0%	1.3%	1.7%	2.7%	5.2%
PE[a]	1.6%	1.2%	0.4%	2.5%	3.5%
Sepsis[a]	6.7%	5.7%	5.2%	8.4%	9.6%
Cardiac arrest	1.1%	0.7%	0.4%	2.0%	1.7%
Myocardial infarction	0.3%	0.4%	0%	0.4%	0.4%
Return to OR	4.8%	3.4%	4.8%	7.3%	7.9%
Death	2.5%	1.8%	0.9%	3.7%	5.2%

Common 30-Day Posthepatectomy Complications

[a]Complication rates increased with the extent of hepatectomy ($p < 0.05$)
Columns divided by magnitude of hepatectomy; DVT, deep venous thrombosis; PE, pulmonary embolus; OR, operating room.

completely reversible, certainly many are potentially modifiable through preoperative optimization of comorbidities and choosing operations of lesser extent when oncologically feasible.

Besides the typically reported surgical quality outcomes of postoperative complications and death, surgeons should also understand and further study the secondary implications of major morbidity—failure to return to preoperative performance status and failure to achieve intended oncologic therapy. The long-term benefits of the most extraordinary and aggressive hepatectomy may be completely negated if the patient loses his or her independence and becomes bound to a nursing home, is unable to return to his or her previous functional state, or is unable to complete his or her planned adjuvant cancer therapy.

The goal of this chapter is to describe the diagnosis, management, and risk factors for three major liver-related complications specifically associated with hepatic resection.

INTRAOPERATIVE AND POSTOPERATIVE HEMORRHAGE

Definition
Historically, hemorrhage has been the most feared complication of hepatectomy. "Bleeding" broadly encompasses a range of complications including catastrophic intraoperative hemorrhage, intraoperative bleeding requiring intraoperative and recovery room transfusions, postoperative hemorrhage requiring transfusions or even return to the operating room, symptomatic anemia requiring postoperative transfusions, or small drops in hemoglobin with no clinical sequelae.

Based on retrospective institutional reports, the posthepatectomy hemorrhage (PHH) rate ranges from 1% to 8%. Because of its broad definition, the International Study Group of Liver Surgery (ISGLS) attempted to define PHH based on transfusion requirement and clinical severity. The proposed definition is a hemoglobin drop greater than 3 g/dL after completion of surgery and/or transfusion for any postoperative hemoglobin drop and/or invasive intervention (interventional radiology [IR] or surgery) to stop bleeding (Table 18.2). Detection of hemorrhage can be via frank blood loss apparent in perihepatic drains (drain fluid hemoglobin >3 g/dL), examination consistent

TABLE 18.2 International Study Group on Liver Surgery Definitions of Posthepatectomy Complications

	Definition	Grade A	Grade B	Grade C
Post-hepatectomy hemorrhage (PHH)	>3 g/dL fall in hemoglobin or any postoperative transfusion for bleeding or reintervention for bleeding	≤2 units PRBC	>2 units PRBC	Requires intervention (IR or surgery)
Posthepatectomy bile leak	Drain bilirubin 3× serum bilirubin on or after POD3 or biloma requiring radiologic or operative intervention or bile peritonitis	No change from routine care plan	Requires nonoperative invasive intervention	Requires surgical intervention
Posthepatectomy liver failure or Postoperative hepatic insufficiency (PHI)	Impairment of liver synthetic, excretory, and detoxifying abilities on or after POD5 or elevation in INR or bilirubin	No change from routine care plan	Clinical care deviates from routine course	Requires intervention (IR or surgery)

PRBC, packed red blood cells; IR, interventional radiology; POD, postoperative day; INR, international normalized ratio.

with intra-abdominal hematoma, or active bleeding with any radiographic diagnosis. The ISGLS definition of PHH is specific to the postoperative period and does not include patients who receive up to 2 units packed red blood cells (PRBC) immediately after surgery in the recovery room. Functionally, PHH is split into three grades, A to C. Grade A PHH is defined as transfusion of ≤2 units PRBC with no significant change in clinical management. Grade B PHH corresponds to transfusion of greater than 2 units PRBC, often with changes in management including further radiographic evaluation. Bleeding that requires any invasive intervention is categorized as grade C. Importantly, grades B and C PHH can be associated with mortality rates as high as 17% and 50%, respectively.

The ACS NSQIP defines major postoperative transfusion as administration of greater than 4 units PRBC after leaving the operating room. Currently, the national rates of any intraoperative transfusion, greater than 4 units intraoperative PRBC transfusion, and major postoperative transfusion greater than 4 units PRBC are 26.4%, 9.0%, and 0.8%, respectively. This nationwide sample suggests that a significant intraoperative use of blood products exists, but the major PHH seems to be rare.

Diagnosis and Management

The diagnosis of bleeding or hemorrhage involves clinical evaluation supplemented by laboratory data, drain output (if available), and radiographic imaging when indicated. Clinically, the patient may first develop tachycardia (unless beta-blocked) and/or oliguria, with hypotension and diaphoresis only coming later as worsening hypovolemic shock ensues. As it is atypical for a postoperative liver surgery patient to need a large volume of intravenous fluid, if a patient has required several fluid boluses in the early postoperative period, a necessary workup into reasons for hypotension or low urine output is required. While ruling out extrinsic causes (excessive narcotics or epidural anesthesia) and cardiovascular events, bleeding should be high in the differential. As bleeding becomes more likely, the question turns to clinical significance.

The abdominal examination may not be helpful as most patients will have incisional tenderness. The exception is with massive hemoperitoneum that should be readily apparent and warrants urgent measures. A change in the character of the abdominal drain fluid to a more sanguineous consistency may be a sign of bleeding that can be confirmed with serum and drain hemoglobin measurement. While the ISGLS PHH definition includes drain hemoglobin of greater than 3 g/dL, in many cases when active bleeding is apparent, no fluid sample is needed to secure the diagnosis. The criteria for transfusion depend on the severity of anemia (serum hemoglobin <7 g/dL or relative drop that is hemodynamically relevant), the degree of coagulopathy, and the patient's overall condition. Given the evidence that transfusions may be associated with postoperative complications, which may in turn be detrimental to oncologic outcome, routine transfusions should be discouraged unless warranted by hemodynamic compromise with end-organ dysfunction. A contained hematoma does not require immediate intervention if tamponade stops further bleeding. In a stable patient with clinical evidence of bleeding, radiographic imaging with angiography (either by IR angiogram or by computed tomography [CT], angiogram) may allow for diagnosis and therapeutic intervention. However, if the patient is unstable or if IR cannot arrest the bleeding, then a return to the operating room is necessary. Laboratory values including platelet count, prothrombin time (PT), PTT, and fibrinogen help guide the resuscitation and replacement of deficient coagulation factors.

Preoperative and Intraoperative Considerations

Preoperative risk factors for major postoperative transfusion needs (defined by ACS NSQIP as >4 units PRBC) include preoperative bleeding disorder, ASA class ≥3, low albumin, and preoperative anemia. Right and extended hepatectomies are also at greater risk for PHH. One of the key reasons mortality from hemorrhage is now less common is better understanding of hepatic vascular anatomy and more advanced parenchymal transection techniques, either with or without inflow control. The numerous methods of parenchymal dissection and transection are discussed in Chapter 13. A few salient technical issues are reviewed here. Although the general use of stapling devices for parenchymal transection may be associated with higher bleeding rates, the targeted use of endovascular staplers to control vascular pedicles may increase the speed and safety of liver surgery. Newer tissue dissectors, including ultrasonic and water-jet devices, facilitate precise parenchymal dissection to identify vascular and biliary structures, which can be clipped or tied precisely rather than blindly transected without ligation. Tissue-sealing devices, borrowed from minimally invasive surgery, also aid in coagulation of the parenchymal before division.

Good planning and communication with the anesthesia team before and during surgery facilitate the safety of hepatectomy. During the time-out process, a discussion among the surgeon, nursing staff, and anesthesia team, of the extent of hepatectomy, plan for inflow clamping (Pringle maneuver), predicted blood loss, and blood product availability and antibody status, can decrease intraoperative surprises.

The concept of "low central venous pressure (CVP) anesthesia" is recommended for liver resections. This concept is critical to reducing intraoperative hemorrhagic events. However, accurate monitoring of CVP does not require a central venous catheter. Regardless of the method of intravascular volume monitoring, intravenous fluid administration should remain low (the surgeon can aid in monitoring this by examining the inferior vena cava) until the transection is completed. Keeping the CVP low significantly reduces venous bleeding during the parenchymal transection. Laparoscopic liver surgery has been associated with decreased blood loss because the required pneumoperitoneum decreases venous oozing from the parenchymal surface. The use of stay stitches to elevate the liver out of the abdominal cavity (with laparotomy pads behind the mobilized liver) may elongate and compress hepatic veins, decreasing venous bleeding during transection.

Regardless of the parenchymal dissection and transection technique, after the resection, the liver edge should be carefully inspected for vessels or bile ducts that were not adequately ligated. A gentle Valsalva maneuver by the anesthesia team can expose hepatic vein tributary bleeding, which may require suture ligation. The role of topical hemostasis to the liver transection bed with cautery, coagulant sheets, or fibrin glue is frequently debated. With no overt bleeding sites, some surgeons leave the surface alone, arguing that a viable liver edge may help decrease postoperative bile leak. Others cauterize the entire cut surface with or without placement of a hemostatic agent (fibrin glue or cellulose netting/gauze) applied to the surface. Others take the time to develop and place an omental flap to cover the raw liver surface.

Although the elements that contribute to major bleeding events in liver surgery are complex, an operative strategy that identifies and controls major hepatic vein tributaries and portal triad branches before and during the parenchymal dissection is the best way to avert major bleeding (and not coincidentally bile leak as well). Such a strategy is facilitated by careful preoperative planning that includes a thorough understanding of the patient's liver anatomy including the relationship of the liver vasculature to the target lesion(s). High-quality three-phase liver protocol CT scan or high-resolution magnetic resonance imaging (MRI) is important. General abdominal CT scans (such as those ordered during emergency room evaluation for abdominal pain) are inadequate and may be dangerous if used as a guide. Intraoperative ultrasound is also essential to permit exact dissection along the correct planes. This precise dissection balances adequate oncologic margins with maximal parenchymal sparing when possible, dividing only the necessary vessels and biliary pedicles. While bleeding risk cannot be fully eliminated, with adequate understanding of the patient's liver anatomy, good communication with the entire operating room team, and proper use of available intraoperative surgical technology, the risk of intraoperative and postoperative hemorrhage can be purposefully reduced to minimal rates.

BILE LEAK AND ORGAN SPACE INFECTIONS

Definition

Despite an overall decrease in posthepatectomy complications during the past two decades, the problem of bile leak still remains unsolved. In modern series, the incidence of postoperative bile leak ranges from 2% to 33%, depending on the reported series, definition, and extent of hepatectomy. Like high-grade PHH, high-grade bile leak remains a major cause of associated morbidity, often leading to longer hospitalization, increased health care costs, prolonged disability with abdominal drains, and the need for additional procedures. The mortality associated with bile leak can be as high as 39%. Data on rates of bile leak are varied because like PHH, a variety of bile leak definitions have been used. Some perihepatic fluid collections remain undrained and are treated with antibiotics only, further limiting the ability to accurately label them as "bilomas" in retrospective series. However, after liver resection, most organ space infections can be presumed to be bilomas or bile leaks.

The ISGLS convened an expert panel to define three grades of bile leak after hepatectomy. Mirroring the trend to grading surgical complications based on clinical sequelae rather than arbitrary laboratory values of bilirubin or international normalized ratio (INR), the ISGLS divided bile leaks into three categories. Bile leak was globally defined as a drain bilirubin at least three times the serum bilirubin on or after postoperative day 3, a biloma requiring radiologic or operative intervention, or clinically evident bile peritonitis. Grade A bile leak does not affect clinical management. Grade B requires a deviation in typical postoperative management such as a percutaneous drainage, but does not require surgery. Grade C bile leaks require a return to the operating room and are associated with extremely high mortality rates.

Diagnosis and Management

The management of a bile leak can be summarized by the singular importance of timely diagnosis and drainage if needed. Delays in diagnosis and drainage only feed the inflammatory cascade by allowing sepsis to trigger a systemic inflammatory response syndrome. In general, with proper external drainage and control of infection with antibiotics, bile leaks will heal with time as the surgical bed recovers from operative trauma. When left unattended and discovered late, bile leaks can be highly morbid requiring longer hospitalizations, more interventions, and transfers to higher-acuity beds. Bile leaks with high mortality rates are typically from associated complications. As an example of its significant downstream effects, organ space infection is the risk factor most strongly associated with posthepatectomy VTE.

Bile leak, also known as biloma or biliary fistula, can be diagnosed by several methods depending on the timing, severity, and presence or absence of an intraoperatively placed surgical drain. In the presence of a drain, the character of the fluid, which, if necessary, can be tested for bilirubin, can readily diagnose bile leak. By the ISGLS definition, a fluid bilirubin three times the serum bilirubin constitutes a bile leak. If the drain works well and there is no evidence of sepsis from an undrained biloma, then no further imaging is necessary. The drain is simply left in place when the patient is discharged from the hospital until the fluid output drops to a minimum. Antibiotics are not necessary in the absence of sepsis, abdominal wall infection, or undrained organ space infection. If the drain output does not decrease with short-term outpatient management, then either an endoscopic retrograde cholangiopancreatogram (ERCP) or percutaneous transhepatic cholangiogram (PTC) is warranted to study where the leak is coming from (central vs. peripheral bile ducts) and to place a biliary stent to increase preferential bile drainage toward its natural outflow tract (duodenum or enteric anastomosis). Neither ERCP nor PTC needs to be reflexively ordered when bile leak is first diagnosed and drain output has not yet been defined, because both ERCP and PTC have their associated risks.

If no surgical drain is present or if the bile leak is diagnosed after the drain has been removed, then CT is warranted to identify the location of the fluid collection. Because these bile leaks have been undrained for several days, the patients will often present with pain, fever, leukocytosis, nausea, ileus, and/or abdominal discomfort. Associated right pleural effusions may also occur. With systemic symptoms and leukocytosis, antibiotics are usually necessary. Antibiotics may be quickly tailored based on culture data. The CT allows the surgeon to determine if IR can access the presumed biloma and place a percutaneous drain. CT is important because it can help differentiate infected fluid collections with a rind or air bubbles versus benign fluid collections that are likely seromas not requiring drainage. In some cases, liver compression by a perihepatic fluid collection can be appreciated and helps to identify an ongoing bile leak "under pressure" (Fig. 18.1). Because of their later diagnosis, these patients usually require a short inpatient admission for CT, percutaneous drainage, and antibiotics. After the sepsis is controlled, they can be discharged and managed in a similar fashion as patients who had a bile leak diagnosed by a surgically placed drain. Treatment of bile leak includes timely diagnosis, control of sepsis through adequate drainage, and confirmation (clinically or radiologically) of preferential anatomic flow of bile toward the duodenum or through an enteric anastomosis.

Preoperative and Intraoperative Considerations

Perioperative risk factors for bile leak include bile duct resection/reconstruction, extended hepatectomy, repeat hepatectomy, need for *en bloc* diaphragm resection, and intraoperative transfusion. The surgeon should utilize a preoperative high-quality CT or MRI to define the planned extent of resection. Part of the resection plan should include the strategy for extrahepatic versus intrahepatic bile duct division. Using hilar cholangiocarcinoma as an example, the extent of biliary resection, the level of reconstruction, and the type of anastomosis should be anticipated. Preoperative planning can help prevent both unplanned division of the contralateral hepatic duct and accidental injury of hepatic duct tributaries, which can lead to catastrophic postoperative bile leaks.

After the resection, the transected liver surface and the hepatic duct division line are visually inspected for any bile staining. The liver itself should also be inspected for areas where the capsule has been sheared off or for areas with lacerations from retraction injury, as these can be the sites

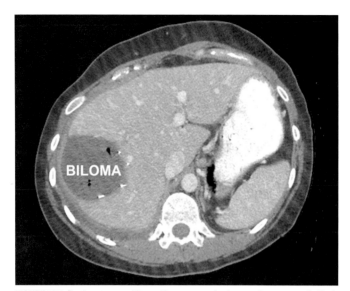

FIGURE 18.1 Posthepatectomy biloma. Liver compression by a posthepatectomy fluid collection can be appreciated and helps to identify an ongoing bile leak "under pressure."

of subsequent bile leaks. A number of posttransection cholangiogram techniques have been described in the literature. These methods include intraductal injections of fluoroscopic contrast (conventional cholangiography), saline, methylene blue, "white" fat emulsion, indocyanine green (ICG), or air (at our institution) for the intraoperative detection and repair of potential postoperative bile leaks. As with PHH prevention, some surgeons use various forms of hemostatic agents to "seal" the transection surface, and omental flaps can be used, although little evidence exists to support either practice in the prevention of bile leaks. There is also no consensus on the role of surgical drain placement. Some surgeons routinely place drains, even for partial hepatectomies. Others reserve drains for higher-risk operations such as major/extended hepatectomies or those with biliary–enteric anastomoses, while others do not routinely drain any hepatectomies. When drains are placed, they should be removed at the earliest possible time when they no longer function as a reliable indicator of bleeding or bile leak (usually 2 to 4 days). In summary, because bile leak remains a major source of potentially preventable morbidity, mortality, cost, and disability, surgeons should strive to develop a systematic preventative approach to the intraoperative identification of bile leaks and to be vigilant about the early detection of bile leaks in the postoperative setting.

POSTOPERATIVE HEPATIC INSUFFICIENCY AND LIVER-RELATED MORTALITY

Definition

After liver resection, the least reversible complication in the recovery period is PHI, or posthepatectomy liver failure. Its clinical consequences range from mild biochemical derangements with no change in routine postoperative course to irreversible liver failure with death. Ultimately, PHI is related to inability of the FLR to perform the functions of protein synthesis, biliary drainage, and filtration. But, PHI can be divided into early and late postoperative manifestations, each with its own risk factors. Early PHI is from insufficient FLR volume or acute liver injury that prevents the FLR from tolerating the immediate surgical and postoperative stress. This injury can include intraoperative liver ischemia from long inflow occlusion intervals without adequate reperfusion, perioperative major blood loss, and/or perioperative systemic hypotension, which combined with marginal FLR volume can lead to early liver failure. Beyond the acute phase of recovery, late failure is associated with insufficient FLR regeneration. Most commonly, this phenomenon is related to intrinsic parenchymal injury from preoperatively underrecognized cirrhosis, steatohepatitis, and/or extended-duration chemotherapy.

In general, PHI is defined by the ISGLS as the impairment of the liver's synthetic (INR), excretory (bilirubin), and detoxifying functions. The ISGLS avoided the use of arbitrary serum laboratory values in their definition, focusing instead on three grades of clinical sequelae. Grade A causes no change in routine postoperative care. These patients might have mild cholestasis, which does not affect their activities of daily living or their discharge planning. Grade B PHI requires some deviation from the routine clinical course. Grade C PHI requires invasive intervention.

A more clinically relevant definition of PHI was proposed in a retrospective international study of over 1,000 patients from three institutions undergoing hepatectomy of ≥3 segments. PHI was defined as a peak total bilirubin greater than 7 mg/dL, which had a sensitivity and specificity of greater than 93% and an odds ratio of 10.8 for predicting 90-day mortality. The authors found this cutoff to be a better predictor of liver-related mortality than previous combinations of hyperbilirubinemia with elevated PT.

Diagnosis and Management

There are a limited number of effective therapies to rescue patients from severe liver failure after hepatectomy. If PHI is suspected, the management includes ruling out biliary obstruction and biloma as reasons for increased serum bilirubin. If the serum bilirubin remains high despite a patent bile duct or biliary anastomosis, then cholestasis from PHI is the diagnosis. In this state, patients are especially tenuous and unlikely to tolerate further physiologic insults such as sepsis. As liver regeneration is dependent on nutrition and a lack of sepsis, nutritional support and timely treatment of any infections are especially important for recovery. Burdened by ascites, many patients will need diuresis to control their abdominal symptoms and to facilitate their ability to participate in activities of daily living. If there is no sepsis and no further need for inpatient management, these patients can be followed as outpatients. Labs every few days to weekly are sufficient to measure the trends, but it may take weeks to months for the late PHI to resolve. If the liver function tests and bilirubin do not eventually plateau, then death from liver failure is inevitable.

Preoperative and Intraoperative Considerations

Given the limited ability to reverse PHI, the best management of this complication is prevention. To avoid this complication, the surgeon must focus on preoperative planning and intraoperative considerations in choosing the extent of hepatectomy based on the FLR size and functional capacity. The FLR is the predicted volume of liver after resection, and adequate size, synthetic function, biliary drainage, and regenerative capacity are the keys to avoiding both early and late PHI. Based on a patient's calculated total liver volume (TLV) standardized to body surface area (BSA)

(TLV cm^3 = −794.41 + 1,267.28 × BSA m^2), the predicted FLR is compared as a ratio to this standardized TLV calculation to yield the standardized FLR. Generally, the required minimum standardized FLR is greater than 20% for normal livers, greater than 30% for livers with limited parenchymal injury such as from chemotherapy, and greater than 40% for permanently damaged livers such as those with cirrhosis. A number of modifiable risk factors may decrease PHI from inadequate FLR.

Arguably, the greatest advance in preventing early and late PHI in the past decade has been greater utilization of PVE before a major/extended hepatectomy. With increased availability of CT volumetry, the FLR volume can be accurately calculated down to the decimal point, and "eyeballing" a CT scan to estimate FLR is now discouraged. Up to 10% of patients at initial presentation have insufficient FLR for a right hepatectomy, and as many as 75% will have an inadequate FLR for an extended right hepatectomy. In practice, the real number is higher for both, because these calculations were based on patients with normal liver parenchyma and normal FLR volume requirements.

One may think of PVE as a functional test of the FLR that allows assessment of regenerative capacity prior to committing to hepatic resection. During the time between PVE and hepatectomy, surgeons can study both the degree of hypertrophy (DH, needs to be >5% points) and the kinetic growth rate (KGR = DH divided by time in weeks) of the FLR. Importantly, the technical aspects of PVE should be carefully considered to achieve maximum hypertrophy. With complete PVE of the right portal vein and segment IV branches with spherical microparticles and coils, an FLR hypertrophy of up to 69% can be expected.

In some cases with bilateral and/or multifocal disease, safe hepatectomy cannot be accomplished with a single operation. In this setting, the two-stage approach, with first-stage partial left hepatectomy, followed by percutaneous PVE, and second-stage extended right hepatectomy, has achieved excellent oncologic outcomes. As it facilitates extensive liver resection while limiting PHI, it is important to add the two-stage approach to the surgeon's armamentarium.

A major modifiable risk factor for late PHI is the duration of preoperative chemotherapy given to patients with liver tumor. The goal of preoperative chemotherapy should not be "optimal response" with complete disappearance of the liver lesions because extended-duration chemotherapy (>8 cycles) can increase the risk of chemotherapy-associated liver injury (CALI) and postoperative complications. Steatohepatitis from irinotecan (usually in patients with metabolic syndrome phenotype) is particularly important as it is the only CALI associated with increased mortality from PHI. This may be a key consideration when choosing neoadjuvant treatment with between FOLFOX and FOLFIRI. All of the aforementioned modifiable factors require preoperative planning by the surgeon in the context of a multidisciplinary discussion with medical oncologists, pathologists, hepatologists, and radiologists.

OUTCOMES/FOLLOW-UP

Posthepatectomy complications have significant short-term and long-term consequences. Certainly, the most impactful short-term complication is death, but fortunately, mortality from hepatectomy is infrequent. Early mortality from PHH is rare because of improved knowledge of liver anatomy, better preoperative imaging, intraoperative ultrasound, and better parenchymal dissection/transection tools. Late PHI-related mortality is better understood, and the necessary preoperative preventative steps (patient selection, CT volumetry ± PVE, and limiting chemotherapy) are being used more often.

As hepatectomy becomes more routine, outcome studies should move beyond 30-day metrics to include collection of data on return to intended oncologic therapy and return to preoperative functional status. Both measures more completely describe the downstream effects of complications beyond the mortality rate, and both measures may account for some of the data that link transfusions and major complications with decreased survival in cancer patients undergoing hepatectomy. Improvement in the diagnostic methods and the management of posthepatectomy complications have dramatically increased the rescue rate of patients from mortality after complicated hepatectomy. The next step in progress is to further optimize preoperative and intraoperative measures to prevent postoperative complications.

Suggested Readings

Abdalla EK, Denys A, Chevalier P, et al. Total and segmental liver volume variations: implications for liver surgery. *Surgery* 2004;135(4):404–410.

Abdalla EK, Hicks ME, Vauthey JN. Portal vein embolization: rationale, technique and future prospects. *Br J Surg* 2001;88(2):165–175.

Aloia TA, Fahy BN, Fischer CP, et al. Predicting poor outcome following hepatectomy: analysis of 2313 hepatectomies in the NSQIP database. *HPB (Oxford)* 2009;11(6):510–515.

Aloia TA, Zorzi D, Abdalla EK, et al. Two-surgeon technique for hepatic parenchymal transection of the noncirrhotic liver using saline-linked cautery and ultrasonic dissection. *Ann Surg* 2005;242(2):172–177.

Brouquet A, Abdalla EK, Kopetz S, et al. High survival rate after two-stage resection of advanced colorectal liver metastases: response-based selection and complete resection define outcome. *J Clin Oncol* 2011;29(8):1083–1090.

Dindo D, Demartines N, Clavien PA. Classification of surgical complications: a new proposal with evaluation in a cohort of 6336 patients and results of a survey. *Ann Surg* 2004;240(2):205–213.

Kishi Y, Abdalla EK, Chun YS, et al. Three hundred and one consecutive extended right hepatectomies: evaluation of outcome based on systematic liver volumetry. *Ann Surg* 2009;250(4):540–548.

Kishi Y, Zorzi D, Contreras CM, et al. Extended preoperative chemotherapy does not improve pathologic response and increases postoperative liver insufficiency after hepatic resection for colorectal liver metastases. *Ann Surg Oncol* 2010;17(11):2870–2876.

Koch M, Garden OJ, Padbury R, et al. Bile leakage after hepatobiliary and pancreatic surgery: a definition and grading of severity by the International Study Group of Liver Surgery. *Surgery* 2011;149(5):680–688.

Kooby DA, Stockman J, Ben-Porat L, et al. Influence of transfusions on perioperative and long-term outcome in patients following hepatic resection for colorectal metastases. *Ann Surg* 2003;237(6):860–869; discussion 869–870.

Madoff DC, Abdalla EK, Gupta S, et al. Transhepatic ipsilateral right portal vein embolization extended to segment IV: improving hypertrophy and resection outcomes with spherical particles and coils. *J Vasc Interv Radiol* 2005;16(2 Pt 1):215–225.

Mullen JT, Ribero D, Reddy SK, et al. Hepatic insufficiency and mortality in 1,059 noncirrhotic patients undergoing major hepatectomy. *J Am Coll Surg* 2007;204(5):854–862; discussion 862–854.

Rahbari NN, Garden OJ, Padbury R, et al. Post-hepatectomy haemorrhage: a definition and grading by the International Study Group of Liver Surgery (ISGLS). *HPB (Oxford)* 2011;13(8):528–535.

Rahbari NN, Garden OJ, Padbury R, et al. Posthepatectomy liver failure: a definition and grading by the International Study Group of Liver Surgery (ISGLS). *Surgery* 2011;149(5):713–724.

Ribero D, Abdalla EK, Madoff DC, et al. Portal vein embolization before major hepatectomy and its effects on regeneration, resectability and outcome. *Br J Surg* 2007;94(11):1386–1394.

Tzeng CW, Aloia TA. Colorectal liver metastases. *J Gastrointest Surg* 2013;17(1): 195–201.

Tzeng CW, Katz MH, Fleming JB, et al. Risk of venous thromboembolism outweighs post-hepatectomy bleeding complications: analysis of 5651 National Surgical Quality Improvement Program patients. *HPB (Oxford)* 2012;14(8):506–513.

Zimmitti G, Roses RE, Andreou A, et al. Greater complexity of liver surgery is not associated with an increased incidence of liver-related complications except for bile leak: an experience with 2,628 consecutive resections. *J Gastrointest Surg* 2013;17(1):57–64.

19 Multidisciplinary Approach to Liver Oncology

Mary A. Maluccio

MULTIDISCIPLINARY APPROACH TO LIVER ONCOLOGY

Liver oncology has expanded over the past decade to include not only the primary liver malignancies for which treatment paradigms have been established but also the secondary malignancies for which treatment paradigms are in evolution. Unlike other multidisciplinary oncology programs that have three major physician-based pillars, medical oncology, surgical oncology, and radiation oncology, adequate care of the liver oncology patient requires considerably broader physician engagement including input and commitment from organ transplant, hepatology, interventional radiology, abdominal imaging, and nuclear medicine. As we move into a health care environment that will expect well-defined treatment algorithms based on best practices, practitioners will need to move away from institutional-specific paradigms and embrace a more uniform approach that takes into consideration both effectiveness of treatment, quality outcomes, utilization of health care resources, and cost. An understanding of the advantages and disadvantages of treatment platforms and how patient- and tumor-specific variables weigh into medical decision making is the objective of this chapter.

PRIMARY LIVER CANCER (HEPATOCELLULAR CARCINOMA AND CHOLANGIOCARCINOMA)

Primary liver cancer presents unique challenges for which a multidisciplinary approach to patient care is considered imperative and without which quality outcome parameters will be difficult to reach. Hepatocellular carcinoma (HCC) is one of the few cancers with increasing incidence. As such, there has been a focus on safe and accurate diagnosis and the development of treatment algorithms that take into consideration the unique complexities of this patient population. The past decade has seen improvements in nonsurgical treatment platforms and better standardization with respect to the diagnosis and eligibility for liver transplant. How to navigate patients through the challenges of treatment is difficult and depends on several factors: (1) patient-related variables such as comorbid conditions that influence treatment eligibility; (2) liver-related variables such as Child-Pugh score; and (3) tumor-related variables such as size, number, pattern of spread within the liver, and vascular involvement.

Five-year survival rates for HCC in the United States have improved modestly to approximately 26%; felt to be associated with improved surveillance in identifiable high-risk patients (i.e., hepatitis B and C) and surgical intervention (i.e., resection or transplant) for early-stage disease. The vast majority of HCC occurs in the setting of chronic liver disease from viral hepatitis, alcohol abuse, and/or nonalcoholic steatohepatitis (NASH). Prevention of HCC must therefore focus on the prevention of hepatitis B and C transmission and the institution of guidelines to reduce the prevalence of obesity.

Consensus guidelines have been published by several organizations including the American Association for the Study of Liver Disease (AASLD), National Comprehensive Cancer Network (NCCN), and European Association for Study of Liver (EASL) to standardize the approach to diagnosis and treatment. As is true with the most disease processes, HCC is more effectively treated when it is diagnosed at an early stage. The best chance for prevention and/or early diagnosis comes from attempts to eliminate viral hepatitis and the surveillance of patients known to be at high risk. This includes patients with cirrhosis from any cause and hepatitis B carriers. The 2012 NCCN guidelines recommend screening high-risk patients with serum AFP and liver ultrasound every 6 to 12 months. A rising AFP associated with a liver nodule greater than 1 cm raises suspicion for HCC and warrants evaluation with cross-sectional imaging. Better biomarkers of cancer risk would improve our ability to stratify patients into more cost-effective surveillance programs, chemoprevention trials, and/or treatment algorithms.

Criteria for the diagnosis of HCC have evolved over the past decade. In order to minimize the use of percutaneous biopsy and its inherent risks in patients with underlying liver disease (tract seeding, bleeding, etc.), the AASLD, NCCN, and EASL working groups have adopted imaging criteria that predict cancer with acceptable accuracy. Dedicated abdominal imagers are necessary to protocol and read the cross sectional imaging such that the reports are in keeping with what is required to appropriately characterize the lesions. On contrast-enhanced images using CT and MRI, the typical enhancement pattern of HCC is early arterial enhancement and venous phase washout, related to the fact that these are hypervascular lesions supplied predominantly by branches of the hepatic artery. In the setting of chronic liver disease, lesions larger than 1 cm that demonstrate these imaging characteristics on triple-phase CT *or* contrast-enhanced MRI are considered to be HCC. This is a change from previous guidelines where lesions between 1 and 2 cm required characteristic enhancement on both imaging modalities (CT and MRI) to define HCC. Despite changes in the imaging criteria, only lesions greater than 2 cm with characteristic enhancement are eligible for model of end-stage liver disease (MELD) exception points for liver transplant. Some centers have adopted MRI with a novel contrast agent, gadoxetate disodium (EOVIST), to better define lesions that do not meet criteria on arterial and venous-phase imaging alone. Lesions suspicious for HCC appear darker than background liver on T1- (hepatocyte-phase) weighted imaging. To date, EOVIST has not changed the diagnostic paradigm currently used to determine treatment eligibility despite reports of improved imaging specificity.

Several clinical staging systems, including the Cancer of the Liver Italian Program (CLIP) and the Barcelona Clinic Liver Cancer (BCLC), have emerged to predict prognosis and stratify patients for treatment. The goal of each staging system is the same: to better define the prognostic weight of clinical variables on outcome in HCC patients being considered for treatment or clinical trials. The CLIP system includes Child-Pugh score, tumor morphology (uninodular, multinodular, or extensive), AFP, and the presence or absence of portal vein thrombosis. The BCLC system includes the Child-Pugh score, clinical performance status, and tumor stage (solitary, multinodular, vascular invasion, or extrahepatic spread) and categorizes patients. Early HCC (BCLC A1-A4) includes well-compensated (Child A) liver reserve with an excellent performance status and limited tumor burden. Intermediate HCC (BCLC B) includes moderate liver reserve (Child A and B), excellent performance status, and multinodular tumors. Advanced HCC (BCLC C) includes patients with moderate liver reserve (Child A and B), vascular invasion or extrahepatic spread, and a vulnerable performance status (PST 1–2). The difference in estimated survival at

Treatment Options for HCC
Liver transplant
Liver resection
Ablation
Thermal (radiofrequency, microwave, etc.)
Chemical (ethanol, acetic acid)
Transarterial therapy
Bland embolization
Chemoembolization
Radioembolization
SBRT
Chemotherapy

3 years in untreated BCLC A versus C patients was 50% versus 8%, respectively. The impact of any given treatment on patients with more advanced disease is unclear. Modifications of these staging systems with the addition of plasma-based tumor markers like vascular endothelial growth factor or insulin-like growth factor-1 have been proposed to improve prognostic stratification of patients with advanced HCC and better select patients for treatment or clinical trials.

Multiple treatment options are available for patients with HCC (Table 19.1).

Liver Transplant

Liver transplant is considered the most effective method to treat both the cancer and the underlying liver disease from which most HCC develop. Therefore a productive relationship between oncology (surgical and medical) and transplant is required to maximize this option for appropriate patients. Transplant eligibility is based on the size and number of tumors, and criteria have been established to optimize cancer-specific outcomes. Most commonly used worldwide are the Milan criteria in which patients with up to three foci of HCC less than 3 cm or one tumor less than 5 cm are eligible for liver transplantation. These patients experienced 5-year overall survival (75%) that paralleled survival observed in patients transplanted without cancer at that time. Other centers, such as The University of California San Francisco (UCSF), have broadened criteria (one tumor <6.5 cm or two to three tumors, none >4.5 cm, with the total tumor diameter not to exceed 8 cm) for eligibility based on outcome-based evidence that less strict parameters do not adversely affect overall survival with the development of more sophisticated liver-directed therapies (LDTs) for HCC, and down-staging of patients into either Milan or UCSF criteria has emerged as a reasonable approach to select patients. What has become apparent is that progression of disease despite LDTs identifies cancers that are at high risk for recurrence after transplant. Demonstration of a response to LDTs prior to transplant in combination with surveillance over a period of time prior to committing to transplant allows centers to select out more favorable biology and broaden patient eligibility without compromising cancer-specific survival.

Surgical Resection

Liver resection remains the gold standard for patients with resectable HCC that develops in the setting of normal liver. However, most patients with HCC have diseased liver parenchyma, and resection in this population is more fraught with potential for complications. For this reason, preservation of liver parenchyma is critical, and treatment requires a balance between the effect of any surgical intervention short of transplant and the potentially detrimental effect of this treatment on a vulnerable and "high-risk" remnant. Most published resection series focus on patients with single tumors or limited disease burden up to a certain size and well-preserved (Child A) function. As LDTs have improved, the gap in overall survival between LDT and resection in patients with underlying liver disease has narrowed substantially. This is in part due to the high rate of recurrence or de novo tumor emergence in the liver remnant. The recurrence rate after resection is approximately 50% at 2 years and 75% at 5 years in most series. Institutional treatment paradigms with respect to resection versus transplant should be established with input from both transplant and surgical oncology since transplant eligibility may come into play with either recurrence after resection or in the event that the patient struggles with liver insufficiency postoperatively.

In regions of the world where hepatitis B is the dominant risk factor for cancer, resection is employed more commonly for several reasons including the following: (1) cadaveric organ availability is limited; (2) centers outside the United States rely more on living related donor pools where the human investment in the process is greater; and (3) a higher proportion of patients with hepatitis B have preserved liver function making resection safer. Therefore, to minimize unnecessary risk to a living donor and help select patients whom would most benefit from a liver transplant, resection is used up front with transplant reserved as a salvage option in the event that the cancer recurs or the liver function worsens over time.

The natural history of HCC in the background of NASH would suggest a higher proportion of noncirrhotic patients and a lower rate of recurrence (or de novo tumor emergence) than either hepatitis B or hepatitis C. For this reason, resection may emerge as a reasonable option in this patient population as well. Resection versus transplant in NASH patients must be evaluated based on underlying liver reserve.

Embolization

Most patients are not candidates for resection or transplantation at the time of diagnosis because of either the extent or the distribution of tumor, underlying liver function, or medical comorbidities. Interventional radiology has played a central role in the treatment of HCC for decades. For this reason, engagement of interventional radiology is critical to adequately address the range of HCC patients within a robust liver oncology program. The dual blood supply to the liver has allowed the development of hepatic artery–based therapies over the past 30 years. Whereas non–tumor-bearing liver parenchyma receives nutrient supply predominantly from the portal vein, most HCC are supplied predominantly by the hepatic artery. Catheter-based techniques take advantage of this unusual architecture to deliver intra-arterial therapy directly to tumor bed. Several different treatments have been administered by catheter via the artery to treat HCC, including bland embolization, transarterial chemoembolization (TACE), chemoembolization with drug-eluting beads (DEB), and radioembolization. To date, there have been no prospective or randomized trials defining any of the available options as superior in terms of survival. Centers around the world have therefore gravitated toward the technique that works best in their hands. Complications common to all catheter-based therapies for HCC include postembolization syndrome (fever, nausea, and pain), nontarget embolization (stomach, gallbladder, duodenum, pancreas), and liver failure (<2% in well-selected patients).

Bland Particle Embolization

Bland particle embolization is based on the unique dependence of HCC on the hepatic artery. Small particles (40 to 120 μm) are injected into the tumor arterial supply to cause terminal vessel blockade and resultant ischemic necrosis. The 5-year data on response and survival suggest comparable cancer-specific outcomes to other catheter-based techniques. The results of bland embolization are essentially immediate, and radiologic evidence of tumor necrosis is seen within hours of the procedure. This is a particularly useful feature in patients who present with significant tumor burden where further progression may render them untreatable. Other theoretical advantages of bland embolization include (1) the particles come in a range of sizes that can effectively address unique vascular characteristics of the tumor, including intrahepatic portal–systemic shunting; (2) lower periprocedural cost; (3) no delay between initial arteriogram and treatment delivery; (4) no chemotherapy or radiation-related side effects; (5) the ability to retreat due to better preservation of intrahepatic arteries after treatment; and (6) less institutional infrastructure requirements such as radiation safety.

Chemoembolization/Drug-Eluting Beads

Doxorubicin-eluting beads are another catheter-based LDT. The use of an eluting bead is considered an improvement on conventional chemoembolization (TACE) in which hydrophilic chemotherapeutic agent(s) (with or without Lipiodol) was injected into the liver via the hepatic artery. To prevent washout of the chemotherapy from the tumor bed and thereby allow prolonged contact between chemotherapeutic agent(s) and tumor cells, the feeding artery was then occluded with particles or Gelfoam. Conventional TACE has largely been replaced by embolization with DEBs. DEBs are preformed deformable microspheres that are loaded with doxorubicin up to 150 mg per treatment. The pharmacokinetic profile of the DEB is significantly different from that seen with conventional TACE, with evidence that the peak drug concentration in the serum is an order of magnitude lower for DEBs compared to TACE. Objective response by EASL criteria has been reported to be 70% to 80%. One- and 3-year survival rates of 89.9% and 66.3%, respectively, have been reported in a heterogeneous cohort of Barcelona Clinic Liver Cancer (BCLC) A–C patients. The advantages of DEB overlap with those related to bland embolization: (1) the ability to treat multiple tumors in different regions of the liver during the same procedure; (2) the use of superselective techniques limits toxicity to normal liver substance; and (3) the ability to repeat the procedure several times over the lifetime of the patient.

Radioembolization

Yttrium-90 (Y90) is a beta-emitter that can be loaded into glass or resin microspheres and administered via a microcatheter in the hepatic artery. The TheraSphere™ glass microspheres are approved by the U.S. Food and Drug Administration (FDA) for treating HCC. The spheres are preferentially taken up by tumor vasculature and, as such, deliver a high dose of radiation directly to the tumor bed. The half-life of the bead allows for treatment over weeks with the theoretical advantage of an improvement in durability of response. Other advantages of Y90 include (1) better tolerability in patients with vulnerable liver reserve (Child B) when used in a selective manner; (2) because of the size and number of particles, there is little embolic effect; (3) the effect of radiation is less acute than any of the embolic techniques, and there is less postembolization syndromes commonly seen after TACE, DEBs, or bland particle embolization. Y90 is delivered in the outpatient setting. The objective response rate is comparable to other catheter-based modalities and depends on several factors including size of the lesion, pattern of spread within the liver (unilobar vs. bilobar), and vascularity of the lesion noted on planning arteriogram. In patients with limited liver reserve (Child C), some centers will still consider treatment but usually as a bridge to a timely transplant. There are disadvantages specific to radioembolization: (1) the need for a mapping procedure to embolize potential nontarget vasculature arising from or near the target vessels (i.e., right gastric artery, falciform artery, gastroduodenal artery); (2) the risk of shunting radioactive particles into the lung resulting in pulmonary fibrosis; and (3) radiation-induced liver toxicity (approximately 1% to 3%). Nontarget radioembolization to the lung or GI tract can be particularly devastating compared to TACE or bland embolization.

Tumor evaluation after any catheter-based treatment is difficult. Instead of decrease in the size and volume of tumor as seen after response to chemotherapy, a change in enhancement from early arterial to no enhancement is widely accepted as response. Therefore, the modified RECIST criteria (mRECIST) have been established for this purpose. mRECIST reports the percentage of tumor that has imaging findings consistent with necrosis rather than absolute size measurements. After radioembolization, 1-month response rates are difficult to measure because there are often radiation-induced changes in the treated liver. In cases in which AFP is elevated, changes in AFP may provide better insight into early response. A 3-month time point is a far better judge of maximal response to treatment. Continued response to Y90 even after 3 months has also been observed.

Stereotactic Body Radiation Therapy

Stereotactic body radiation therapy (SBRT) is a type of targeted radiation therapy whereby computer modeling is used to delineate the treatment area. Historically radiation therapy for HCC has been limited to the palliation of pain in surgically unresectable disease. Based on contemporary data, SBRT now enters the most recent NCCN guidelines as a reasonable up front treatment in select patients. For this reason, finding one or more radiation oncologists interested in participation in the multidisciplinary physician network will improve the breadth of treatment options available at a given institution. Using an immobilization device, respiratory variation is limited during treatment. SBRT is noninvasive, delivered in the outpatient setting, and very well tolerated. It has been studied in single lesions up to 6 cm or up to three tumors, none greater than 3 cm. There must be at least 700 mL of liver volume outside the treatment field. The phase I data escalated dosage up to 16 Gy in three fractions. For the Child A patients, there was no dose-limiting toxicity. In Child B patients, dose-limiting toxicities were encountered and the protocol changed to a protracted 5-fraction course with the same total dose. This diminished the toxicity to levels seen in Child A patients. The phase II data from the same cohort of patients showed a 2-year tumor control rate of 90%. In patients with larger tumors treated off protocol, the response rates are still excellent although the long-term control rate is lower with increasing tumor size (unpublished data).

Ablation

Ablation is a potentially curative treatment option for patients with early-stage disease. Depending on institutional infrastructure, ablative techniques will reside with either the interventional radiologists or the abdominal imagers. The success of ablation is highest with lesions less than 2 to 3 cm and decreases significantly in tumors larger than 3 cm. For larger or pauci-focal tumors, ablation may be performed in combination with embolization. In solitary tumors up to 7 cm, this combination has shown to provide 5-year survival on par with surgical resection. Both thermal ablation (RFA, microwave, etc.) and chemical ablation (ethanol, acetic acid) have been used to treat HCC. HCC is the ideal target for ablation because it is a soft tumor surrounded by a fibrotic liver in most cases. This is the source of the so-called "oven effect" where heat applied to the tumor is insulated by the cirrhotic liver. The soft tumor–hard liver combination is also beneficial in chemical ablation, because the ethanol or acetic acid can diffuse easily in the soft tumor, but is kept from escape by the cirrhotic liver. Which ablative technique is appropriate depends on the location and size of the target tumor. For example, radiofrequency ablation is susceptible to the "heat-sink" effect, in which large vessels close to tumor can take the heat away in flowing blood and prevent complete ablation. For a tumor close to a large vessel, microwave ablation may be a better choice because it is not as susceptible to this effect. The long-term efficacy for either technique drops substantially with increasing size and number of lesions.

Chemotherapy

Sorafenib is FDA approved for the treatment of HCC. Since its approval, there has been a surge in the number of HCC patients being treated with the drug regardless of tumor stage. The use of sorafenib is based on phase II and phase III data in patients with advanced metastatic HCC; the treatment group showing close to a 3-month survival advantage over the nontreated group. The objective response rate rests at around 2% with most of the effect associated with the 35% to 71% stable disease rate noted in the phase II and phase III trials, respectively. Over 80% of the patients in the phase III study had been previously treated with LDTs (chemoembolization) prior to entry. The response rate to LDTs remains above 70%, and therefore, sorafenib must be considered in the context of all treatment options currently available. Sorafenib has been used in combination with LDTs with reasonable toxicity profiles and slight improvement in efficacy. Dose delays and/or reduction have been required in the vast majority of patients. Recent phase III data investigating the benefit of sorafenib in the adjuvant setting after embolization are less convincing. Short of a small series, sorafenib has not been studied in the neoadjuvant setting before LDT, resection, or transplant. Using lessons learned from other antiangiogenic compounds used in the neoadjuvant setting, this introduces potential periprocedural or perioperative complications that would compromise either the ability to deliver therapy successfully or patient/graft survival. For example, with catheter-based techniques, the arterial pruning associated with antiangiogenic agents may impact the delivery of the small micron particle into the tumor bed.

Cholangiocarcinoma

Cholangiocarcinoma (CCA) is commonly defined by the location of the tumor into intrahepatic CCA, hilar CCA, or distal. The treatment of CCA has historically hinged with surgical oncology, medical oncology, and radiation oncology, and treatment paradigms rested mainly on whether the patient was deemed resectable. The definition of resectable often rested primarily with the surgeon. As nonsurgical LDTs have emerged and liver transplant became an option for highly select patients, the importance of multidisciplinary input grew as did the use of neoadjuvant protocols of chemotherapy and/or combination chemoradiation.

Liver Transplant

The rationale for liver transplant for CCA centers on the relationship between margins of resection and outcome. In hilar CCA, the intrahepatic bile duct margin of resection is close in the majority of cases and local recurrence most often drives outcomes. This has established medical oncology as a more central figure in the multidisciplinary management of HCC. With the overall response rate low, medical oncology will also be pressed to contribute clinical trials of novel systemic agents. Most centers providing transplant as an option for these patients will have surgical oncology, medical oncology, radiation oncology, hepatology, and organ transplantation providing some aspect of patient care. Some form of neoadjuvant treatment is required prior to transplant consideration, and most centers will follow the Mayo Clinic protocol closely, including some method to document that lymph nodes in the porta hepatis are not involved. The natural history of intrahepatic CCA is not well defined, and therefore, the role of liver transplant is currently unknown.

Yttrium-90 Microspheres

Unresectable patients with intrahepatic CCA were often treated with external beam radiation therapy and radiation-sensitizing doses of chemotherapy. With the familiarity of Y90 microspheres (radioembolotherapy) in HCC, many centers have initiated protocols using combination Y90 with gemcitabine for intrahepatic CCA with reasonable local control rates. The theoretical advantage of this approach is improved delivery of the radioactivity into the tumor bed and diminished parenchymal toxicity. There are no established "best practices," and the use of this approach is best served under the direction of a clinical trial.

SECONDARY MALIGNANCIES INVOLVING THE LIVER

Many of the techniques described above have been integrated, to some extent, into the treatment of secondary cancers such as metastatic colorectal cancer. Unlike HCC, we are still trying to define where these techniques fit into established standards of care. The following is a description of how our multidisciplinary liver tumor group has approached their use in metastatic colorectal cancer.

Chemotherapy

Any decision about LDT must take into account the fact that the standard of care for metastatic colorectal cancer remains a complete course of systemic chemotherapy. Most of the improvements in survival in this disease have been linked to the introduction of more effective systemic agents. As patients progress from first-line treatment to second-line systemic options, the response rate to chemotherapy drops substantially. For this reason, I feel that LDTs may play a role either alone or in combination with second-line chemotherapy in patients with stable disease or progression after first-line treatment.

Resection

There are ample data in large retrospective and smaller prospective series on liver resection for metastatic colorectal cancer. Memorial Sloan Kettering published a nomogram that will predict the 5-year survival depending on one or more predictors. This nomogram may be useful to gauge the risk/benefit of resection for any given patient. Survival benefit with resection is limited to patients with liver-only disease in whom a margin-negative resection is possible and in whom all measurable disease is removed in a single operation. Small single-institution series have suggested a role for staged bilobar liver resections in select patients; however, repeat hepatectomy is associated with higher than average liver morbidity (liver insufficiency or failure) and diminished ability to tolerate additional systemic therapy for extrahepatic progression postresection. With the emergence of LDTs for secondary cancers, a clear potential advantage lies in buying potential time before committing to resection, thereby helping select patients for surgery who are most likely to benefit long term.

Stereotactic Body Radiation Therapy

The data using SBRT in secondary cancers, including metastatic colorectal cancer, are quite good. The multi-institutional data in secondary cancers from a number of primary organ sites (lung, colon, breast) showed a 93% 2-year tumor control rate. Single-institution prospective data in a larger cohort of patients have corroborated that result. In patients with colorectal lesions less than 3 cm, the 2-year tumor control rate approaches 100%. The eligibility criteria for these trials were the same as for HCC: solitary lesions up to 6 cm or up to three lesions (none larger than 3 cm). SBRT is an excellent choice in patients with unpredictable disease (synchronous metastatic disease) or significant comorbid conditions making resection more risky. Again, its advantage lies in buying considerable time to determine the inherent cancer biology.

Yttrium-90

Y90 is also FDA approved for metastatic colorectal cancer. The response rates are much lower than with HCC (40% vs. 70%). Some of this decreased response is most likely due to the tumors being less vascular. However, the response rate of 40% is higher than the established response rate to second-line systemic chemotherapy. With current pressure to justify cost of treatment and define objective measures of benefit, clarifying the role of Yttrium 90 in metastatic colorectal cancer will become increasing more important, more a multidisciplinary liver oncology group. For patients in whom surgical resection is less likely to improve survival (multifocal and/or bilobar disease), clinical trial data will define how Y90 therapy integrates into treatment paradigms for secondary colorectal cancer.

Drug-Eluting Beads

The DEB used in metastatic colorectal cancer includes irinotecan. The elution kinetics are quite variable and, as such, the toxicity is variable as well. Our experience with irinotecan-eluting beads has been subpar, compared with Y90, and for this reason, Y90 remains our platform of choice.

Ablation

The results of radiofrequency ablation or microwave ablation in treating hepatic colorectal cancer metastases are disappointing when compared to SBRT. However, when used in combination with resection, ablation can help eliminate all measurable disease in select patients. When used percutaneously under image guidance, the recurrence rate in the treated area is moderately high (20% to 30%).

CONCLUSION

A strong, multidisciplinary panel of invested physicians from HPB surgery, transplant surgery, hepatology, interventional radiology, radiation oncology, medical oncology, nuclear imaging, and abdominal imaging is ideal to develop, standardize, and continuously evaluate institutional treatment strategies for primary and secondary liver malignancy.

Suggested Readings

Andolino DL, Johnson CS, Maluccio M, et al. Stereotactic body radiotherapy for primary hepatocellular carcinoma. *Int J Radiat Oncol Biol Phys* 2011;81(4):447.

The Cancer of the Liver Italian Program (CLIP) Investigators. A new prognostic system for hepatocellular carcinoma: a retrospective study of 435 patients. *Hepatology* 1998;28:751–755.

Cardenes HR. Price TR, Perkins SM, et al. Phase I feasibility trial of stereotactic radiation therapy for primary hepatocellular carcinoma. *Clin Transl Oncol* 2010;12(3):218.

European Association for Study of Liver. EASL-EORTC clinical practice guidelines: management of hepatocellular carcinoma. *Eur J Cancer* 2012;48(5):599.

Kudo M. Diagnostic imaging of hepatocellular carcinoma: recent progress. *Oncology* 2011;81(Suppl 1):73–85.

Llovet JM, Bru C, Bruix J. Prognosis of hepatocellular carcinoma: the BCLC staging classification. *Semin Liver Dis* 1999;19(3):329–338.

Llovet JM, Ricci S, Mazzaferro V, et al. Sorafenib in advanced hepatocellular carcinoma. *N Engl J Med* 2008;359:378.

Maluccio M, Covey AM, Gandhi R, et al. Comparison of survival rates after bland arterial embolization and ablation versus surgical resection for treating solitary hepatocellular carcinoma up to 7 cm. *J Vasc Interv Radiol* 2005;16(7):955–961.

Maluccio MA, Covey AM, Schubert J, et al. Transcatheter arterial embolization with only particles for the treatment of unresectable hepatocellular carcinoma. *J Vasc Interv Radiol* 2008;19(6):862–869.

Mazzaferro V, Regalia E, Doci R, et al. Liver transplantation for the treatment of small hepatocellular carcinomas in patients with cirrhosis. *NEJM* 1996;334(11):693–699.

Salem R, Lewandowski RJ, Kulik L, et al. Radioembolization results in longer time to-progression and reduced toxicity compared with chemoembolization in patients with hepatocellular carcinoma. *Gastroenterology* 2011;140(2):497.

Shiina S, Tateishi R, Arano T, et al. Radiofrequency ablation for hepatocellular carcinoma: 10-year outcome and prognostic factors. *Am J Gastroenterol* 2012; 107(4):569–577.

Yoshitaka T, Kazuhiro N. Nonalcoholic steatohepatitis-associated hepatocellular carcinoma: Our case series and literature review. *World J Gastroenterol* 2010; 16(12):1436.

Laparoscopic Liver Surgery

Juan M. Sarmiento and Edward Lin

INTRODUCTION

Liver resection is the final frontier yet to be conquered by laparoscopy. In spite of the fact that it has been 20 years since the description of the first laparoscopic liver resection (nonanatomic wedge resection), there is no universal application of the laparoscopic technique. In fact, laparoscopic major hepatectomy is still done sparsely around the world and in the United States. There are some explanations for the lack of enthusiasm for adopting this technique. First, some of the maneuvers currently utilized in open surgery are not available laparoscopically (mobilization, palpation, compression, etc.) with the consequent fear of torrential or uncontrollable bleeding. Second is the continuous fear of air (gas) embolism with hemodynamic disturbances, including cardiac collapse. Third, tumors located near the major vessels or biliary structures. Finally a natural learning curve that is less tolerant to surgical mishaps due to the potentially catastrophic consequences of hemorrhage. Fear of oncologic in adequacy of the laparoscopic technique is less of an issue nowadays after the publication of the COST trial for laparoscopic colectomy.

Up until 2009, there have been about 3,000 reported cases of laparoscopic liver operations, most of them minor resections (<3 segments). Still, the morbidity (10%) and mortality (<1%) rates of such series remain low. These numbers compare favorably with the open approach and call for a renewed enthusiasm on the application of laparoscopic techniques to liver surgery. Even though the use of this relatively new technique is somewhat in its infancy, and therefore a scientifically proven evaluation is in order, the hope for a randomized trial is quickly fading. Those who think laparoscopy offers real value consider it unethical to submit patients to a more aggressive form of therapy, and those who are not laparoscopic experts do not have the skills to mount a comparable series to their open technique experience. Therefore, the knowledge we can acquire in this situation is driven from retrospective studies and from relatively small series coming from major centers with experienced laparoscopic surgeons.

Another limitation to the use of laparoscopic hepatectomy has to do with surgeon training. A classically trained hepatobiliary surgeon (from any track) is focused on open resections with exposure to operations done through large incisions. On the other hand, the laparoscopic expert is seldom trained in liver resections, as the focus of their technical expertise is hollow viscus, bariatric surgery, and small solid organs such as the adrenal glands and spleen. The point of confluence remains to be defined as the practice setting is also completely different and the referral of patients limited. The best route to overcome such limitation is the fusion of both disciplines and the intimate collaboration by those surgeons coming from their respective tracks.

By 2007, the majority of the experience came from small case series of mostly minor liver resections. Koffron in 2007 presented the largest series then from a single institution of 300 cases, with a very good number of major hepatectomies. This series is probably responsible for changing the landscape on the feasibility and application of this technique.

The need to standardize this technique came to realization in 2008 after the international conference on laparoscopic liver surgery in Louisville, KY. This conference brought together expert hepatobiliary surgeons, both with and without experience in laparoscopic liver resection, and produced a document with the following recommendations:

- The group cautioned on the expansion of the application of the laparoscopic technique for benign lesions that were not offered resection otherwise.
- There was a concern for patient safety due to a rapid and indiscriminate growth of programs offering this technique without adequate training of surgeons and paramedical personnel and minimal standards of quality.
- There was clarity in defining laparoscopic surgery ("pure laparoscopy") and hand-assisted (for obvious reasons) and hybrid technique (laparoscopy for mobilization and dissection but transection performed via an open approach).
- There was a definition for the ideal candidate for laparoscopic hepatectomy: patients with solitary small (<5 cm) lesions, located peripherally (segments II through VI). Also, it was stated that left lateral sectionectomy should be done laparoscopically as the standard of practice.
- Need for expeditious recognition of conversion to an open approach due to safety or lack of progress.
- Need for a cooperative registry for all laparoscopic liver resections to monitor outcomes, especially in high-risk resections (major hepatectomy, living donors). A randomized trial was probably impractical, and this registry would serve as an alternate source of information and follow-up.
- Definition that resection, either open or laparoscopic, is the gold standard for the treatment of colorectal metastases. Caution was given to the need of keeping comparable rates of negative-margin resections and the avoidance of missing occult lesions.
- Definition of how laparoscopic resection is still a valuable tool in the treatment of hepatocellular carcinoma (HCC), and no specific distinction was made between ablation and transplantation.

One of the realities in dealing with laparoscopic liver resections is the great variance of operations fitting the definition. If we somewhat simplify the term, and call it major resection, we can describe at least five operations that fit this term: right lobectomy, extended right lobectomy, left lobectomy, extended left lobectomy, and central hepatectomy. If we add the caudate lobe, technically a minor liver resection but operatively demanding, and also add combined liver and biliary resection, there is a whole spectrum of "major" resections to be mastered laparoscopically. Other subspecialized areas like Whipple procedures or colectomies really encompass two to three operations that are more reproducible and amenable to standardization. Like any other operation, the surgeons' comfort grows with experience in the procedure; laparoscopic wedge resections are tackled at first, then progressing to the laparoscopic left lateral sectionectomy, and then to subsegmentectomy/segmentectomy II to VI. With the progressive experience, the confidence of the surgeon and dexterity will increase, and at some point, the surgeon will be ready to take on laparoscopic major hepatectomy, resembling the learning process of the open liver resection.

The hand-assisted technique could even bridge that transition as it applies principles of both the open and the laparoscopic approach. The hand is particularly useful for the mobilization of the liver, the palpation of structures, the compression of the liver parenchyma for hemostatic purposes, as well as the rapid and secure control of bleeding from major vascular structures. In addition, the hand port is used for specimen extraction, an incision that is unavoidable for major liver resection. Along the same lines, rapid conversion to an open approach early in the experience and implementation of the hybrid technique are also valid strategies to reach the degree of confidence necessary to achieve competence in laparoscopic liver resections.

As Cherqui points out, laparoscopic liver resection should be based upon the foundation of open liver surgery, being that laparoscopy is most difficult of the two major skill sets necessary for this technique. The surgeon collaboration is mutually enriching and, based on the maturity of the surgeons, will serve as the basis for independent criticism of their own technique and the development of proficiency and standardization of these cases. Doubling the experience to two surgeons with a single case is another perk in a field with limited number of cases. Finally, the application of production quality measurement tools adopted from the manufacturing industry has helped with the refinement of the final product, in this case laparoscopic hepatectomy.

LAPAROSCOPIC MAJOR HEPATECTOMY

Dagher et al. published an international registry study collecting information on 210 patients undergoing laparoscopic major hepatectomy, 57% being hand-assisted approaches. They reported a mortality of 1% and a morbidity of 8% with a conversion rate of 12%. Experience over time showed that operative time, blood loss, portal triad clamping time, conversion rate, and length of stay were improved. Martin et al. from the University of Louisville more recently showed in a matched study of laparoscopic major liver resection a mortality of 1% with a morbidity of 23% and a conversion rate of 4%. Blood loss, use of the Pringle maneuver, length of stay, complication rate, operative time, and blood transfusion were significantly better than the matched open group. These two studies show that laparoscopic major liver resection can be achieved with acceptable results in terms of complications and, that with enough experience, all the feared events (i.e., hemorrhage, increased operative time, need for transfusion) not only are manageable but result in better outcomes.

Two recent meta-analyses (including both minor and major laparoscopic liver resections) have shown similar results to the two studies mentioned above, with the exception that operative time was longer with the laparoscopic method. However, blood loss, morbidity rate, and length of stay were significantly better for the laparoscopic group with similar margin-negative rates. Taking into account the inherent bias in the selection of patients submitted to laparoscopic resection, there is at least a comparable outcome profile for the laparoscopic technique, with a trend toward lower blood loss and decreased hospital stay.

ONCOLOGIC APPLICATIONS

Colorectal Metastases

The fact that no randomized trial has been done for liver resection as the treatment of colorectal metastases basically defines the impossibility of doing one for laparoscopic versus open resection. After the COST trial for surgical resection of colorectal cancer, where no oncologic differences were found between the two approaches (laparoscopic vs. open), there is sufficient approval of laparoscopy as a technique for resection, if feasible, for colorectal cancer. The other issue is that most of these patients have prior abdominal operations (colectomy) and adhesions could be difficult to overcome for a definitive liver resection. An international multicenter study of 109 patients was reported by Nguyen et al. in 2009. Almost 40% of the resections were a full lobectomy; 95% of patients had negative margins with a 5-year disease-free survival of 43% and an overall survival at 5-year of 50%. Another study from Europe of about 150 patients showed a 93% margin-negative rate, though major resection accounted for less than 20% of the patients in that series. Although the follow-up was short, the disease-free survival was similar to that seen in open resection. The above-cited studies were descriptive in nature and basically, they both justify per se the laparoscopic approach, when feasible, for resection of colorectal metastases to the liver. Another important article from France was done with case–control methodology, including 60 patients in each group and having comparable incidence of major hepatectomy (about 40% in each group). Important differences shown in this paper include a higher R0 resection rate (87% vs. 72%) in the laparoscopic group. In terms of survival, the 5-year recurrence free rate was similar (35% laparoscopic vs. 27% open) as well as the overall survival (64% laparoscopic vs. 56% open). It is perfectly valid to assume after studying all these series that the oncologic safety of the laparoscopic procedure is acceptable and that the administration of pneumoperitoneum does not increase the recurrence of the tumor in these patients.

Hepatocellular Carcinoma

The higher number of studies in laparoscopic resection for HCC probably speaks more of the higher incidence of this condition than the comfort of the surgeons with this technique. Ninety percent of HCC patients have accompanying cirrhosis, and the implications of this association are diverse. First, the manipulation of the liver with cirrhosis is more complex, with a higher tendency to tear and bleed, and also the hard consistency of the fibrotic liver complicates parenchymal transaction. Second, pneumoperitoneum increases the abdominal pressure creating ischemia to the liver and the kidneys, with a further decrease of glomerular filtration (a common occurrence in cirrhosis) and possible renal decompensation. Third, portal hypertension and coagulopathy, again a common occurrence in cirrhotic patients, increase intraoperative bleeding and obscure the limited laparoscopic field; this coupled with the fact that manual compression/manipulation is not readily available theoretically could alert the surgeon to be more cautious when submitting these patients to laparoscopy. In spite of the above considerations, there are more data on HCC than on colorectal metastases, although for obvious reasons, the rate of major hepatectomy is consistently low for the HCC series. Two matched studies (Belli et al. and Sarpel et al.) have shown comparable results between laparoscopic and open techniques for resection of HCC. The first one shows a similar mortality rate but a lower morbidity rate for the laparoscopic approach. Interestingly, overall survival at 3 years was similar (67% lap, 62% open) as well as the disease-free survival (52% lap, 59% open). Furthermore, the survival statistics are in accordance with traditional series on survival for the open approach. The second matched study confirmed the similar rates of overall survival and disease-free survival as the first study, without difference in perioperative results but a lower hospital stay favoring the laparoscopic group. Hence, matched studies show again the oncologic safety of the laparoscopic approach.

A meta-analysis of nine studies performed by Fancellu in 2011 compiled 600 patients, 40% of them performed laparoscopically. Among the differences found, the laparoscopic group had a higher R0 resection rate, shorter hospital stay, lower operative blood loss and need for transfusions, lower rates of liver failure and ascites, and a trend for lower perioperative mortality without increase in operative time.

A last point is worth mentioning: When the liver resection is used as a bridge to transplantation or the patient needs a rescue liver transplant, the laparoscopic approach has proved to create fewer adhesions and decreases the complexity of the procedure as demonstrated by lower operative time, blood loss, and need for transfusion during the hepatectomy phase of the liver transplant.

Overall, all the results of the laparoscopic technique are at least comparable to the open approach in managing HCC and do not alter the recurrence and survival rates compared to open resection. Obviously, these operations are more challenging due to the reasons explained above but experienced laparoscopic HPB surgeons can approach these patients with confidence in both perioperative and long-term results.

ANATOMIC RESECTIONS

In an effort to make comparisons more realistic, as all the series mentioned above contain a great range of the type of liver resections, it is important to include in this analysis a direct comparison of patients undergoing both techniques for the same type of hepatectomy.

Left Lateral Sectionectomy

In an analysis by Cherqui's group in 2003, which includes patients with any type of disease, operative blood loss and hospital stay were lower in the laparoscopic group, with no differences in morbidity but an increase in operative time. This study was presented early in the development of the laparoscopic technique. Another study performed at Pittsburgh compared 29 laparoscopic cases with 40 open; again, the length of stay was lower in the laparoscopic group, and the morbidity rate was also lower. Interestingly, adding these two factors to an economic model, they determined that laparoscopy saved between 1,500 and 3,000 US dollars per patient. Overall, as determined by the international conference in 2008, this specific type of liver resection should now be approached laparoscopically as the primary option.

Right Hepatectomy

This is the most common major hepatectomy done, and it is probably the best model to establish the standard results and also to compare with the open approach. Right hepatectomy is very well defined traditionally, is done routinely in major centers, and is the most common major resection of the liver. On the other hand, as surgeons become facile with the laparoscopic approach while other experienced members of the team continue performing the traditional open approach, this creates a setting for comparative studies over the same time period. The two largest published studies represent that scenario. Even in that setting, laparoscopic right hepatectomy accounted for 22 patients in a French study and 36 in another. In the first study by Dagher et al., patients were matched by demographics and risk factors (comorbidities). The results showed similarity in operative times (an improvement, as traditionally laparoscopic cases take longer) and liver-specific complications, but lower blood loss, shorter hospital stay, and lower overall morbidity rate for laparoscopy. In the second paper by Hilal et al., also case-matched, operative times were longer in the laparoscopic group, with similar morbidity rates and blood loss, but with a significantly shorter hospital stay. The authors of this review also have shown with a comparative study of about 50 laparoscopic right hepatectomies that all the perioperative parameters are improved including operative time (unpublished data). Also, we found a significantly lower morbidity rate and a significantly shorter hospital stay for the laparoscopic cases. Even though operative costs were increased, they were compensated by early dismissal and lower complications resulting in a similar overall cost for both procedures.

Laparoscopic right hepatectomy should also serve as a tool to establish standards of quality for major HPB centers. This operation is easily deconstructed in steps, amenable to measurement (each one of them), and is done frequently enough to produce data from each center. We have done this structured comparison and have found consistency for each of the steps (i.e., low standard deviation) except for the parenchymal transaction. We have observed that liver-specific features such as size and presence of steatosis or cirrhosis (all of them beyond the surgeon's control) account for some of these variances. By defining these steps and identifying the variance, we can measure costs associated with these differences and predict complication rates and associated costs.

Overall, laparoscopic right hepatectomy and, by extension, major hepatectomy in general are associated with shorter hospital stay and comparable blood loss/transfusion rates. The morbidity is probably lower as well, and operative times, which tend to improve with experience and standardized protocols, will be amenable to improvement with this technique. We predict that laparoscopic major hepatectomy will become as routine as left lateral sectionectomy is today and certainly could potentially be the main indication for laparoscopic liver resection.

Other Major Resections

There is interest for other types of anatomic resections but with sparse data. Living donor left lateral sectionectomy was reported in the last decade for 17 cases with overall good results. Some data have been included also on donor right hepatectomy (this one mostly with the hybrid approach), again with comparable results to the open technique. The authors of this chapter have presented a small series of caudate resection and combined major hepatectomy with bile duct resection/reconstruction, which are technically demanding but are almost unexplored in the field of laparoscopic resections. These patients so far have had good results and show promise as this technique is further developed.

ROBOTIC LIVER SURGERY

Robotic surgery is an extension of minimally invasive liver resection. Through the experience in prostatectomy and other abdominal operations, there has been a proven benefit with emphasis on shorter hospital stay, better cosmetic results, and lower postoperative pain. Advantages of tridimensional view (resembling the human eye), greater articulation, and overall resemblance of the surgeon's physical approach to these operations engender enthusiasm toward applying this technique to liver surgery. However, the learning curve, the high level of dexterity needed, and the overall enhanced technical skills make the robotic technique less available for widespread use. With better devices to control bleeding and approach parenchymal transactions, some centers are starting to reexplore the robot's use in liver surgery. The robotic technique is so young that it was not discussed at the international conference in 2008.

It is important to point out certain potential benefits of robotic liver surgery. Biliary reconstructions are theoretically ideal for the dexterity and "wrist" articulation of the robot. There are case reports of robotic Kasai procedures, choledochal cyst resection, and biliary reconstruction. It offers advantages in this setting over laparoscopy in terms of better ergonomics, increased dexterity, and higher degree of needle rotation. This improvement for biliary anastomosis is also applied to combined liver/biliary resections, even if the liver resection only uses laparoscopy and not the robot. The addition of the third robot arm is critical here to set-up the anastomosis, to keep gentle retraction (i.e., the base of segment IV), and to facilitate the formation of the anastomosis or even facilitate hemostasis.

There is also interest in combined robotic abdominal resections. Since rectal surgery is really going in the direction of robotics, and about 20% of the patients present with simultaneous liver metastases, there is a renewed interest in combining these two resections robotically. Like in any other cancer operation, the hope with this technique is to improve the recovery of the patient and make the patient fit for timely start of chemotherapy.

There is no question that robotic liver surgery is in its infancy. Most series are very low in number and mostly done by single surgeons who developed focused interest in this practice. The difficult learning curve and the challenge of new instruments will select the surgeons who want to take advantage of the robot platform. Even after conquering the laparoscopic phase of liver surgery, few surgeons will be prepared to advance to the robotic phase. We must remember that there was also fear that came at the beginning of the laparoscopic era, but laparoscopy is the standard of practice for many abdominal procedures nowadays. With the improved ergonomics of the robot and the incorporation of haemostatic and transecting devices to the robot platform, the challenges of hepatic surgery are ready to be conquered.

TECHNIQUE OF LAPAROSCOPIC LIVER RESECTION

This technique should follow both the indications and the initial steps of the open procedure. The surgeon should master laparoscopic intraoperative ultrasound and should follow the initial inspection of the abdominal cavity as the first stages of the operation. For wedge resections, the surgeon should triangulate as three trocars usually suffice: the camera being placed in direct ("perpendicular") view of the segment to resect and the other two ports at a variable distance that allows for freedom of movement with comfortable distance to the target area. Most wedges can be done with regular hemostatic devices like bipolar energy, ultrasonic scalpel, and radiofrequency ablation. Use of staplers is not necessary for the most part.

Laparoscopic left lateral sectionectomy is very straightforward. The camera is placed in the umbilicus or slightly higher. Then the other two ports are placed above the level of the umbilicus, close to the midclavicular line (Fig. 20.1). We use 10- to 12-mm trocars in all the ports to exchange stapling devices and large graspers on both sides of the midline. The transection is started to the left of the umbilical fissure with any hemostatic device after "hanging" the liver from the round ligament (approached from the right trocar). After thinning out the liver parenchyma and identifying the portal pedicles, an endovascular stapler is fired from the left trocar; usually two loads are necessary to take both the pedicle for segment 3 and the one for segment 2. The rest of the transection is done with the energy device, and care must be taken in the posterior area to avoid an injury to the left hepatic vein. Upon identification of the left hepatic vein, dissection is done around it, and then, the stapler is fired this time from the right-sided trocar. Then, parenchymal transection is completed, and the triangular ligament is transected as the last step of the resection. The specimen is removed via an extended incision over the umbilical trocar.

Laparoscopic Right Hepatectomy. We follow the same technique as the open approach. The advantages of laparoscopy are better visualization,

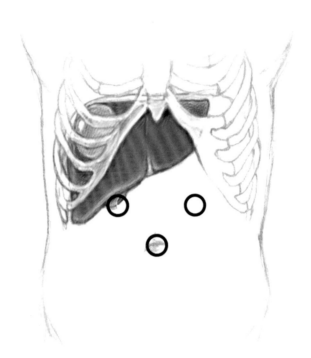

FIGURE 20.1 Trocar placement for left lateral sectionectomy.

especially of the areas behind the liver, over the inferior vena cava (IVC), over the right hepatic vein, etc. Also, the increased pressure of the pneumoperitoneum keeps the operative field relatively bloodless as small venules on the transection line are collapsed. Since the patient will need an incision for specimen extraction, a hand-assisted technique has been developed with an additional advantage for liver mobilization, compression, and urgent management of major vascular bleeding. We place the trocars as shown in Figure 20.2. No mobilization of the liver is done after the ultrasound, and the gallbladder is kept in situ for traction. The right hepatic artery is visualized after taking the cystic artery and is ligated and transected. The right portal vein is transected with endovascular staplers. This is important as the space to the area of the right portal pedicle "opens up" with traction and moves away allowing for a more lateral transection, thus avoiding injury to the contralateral bile duct (or the common hepatic duct). The right bile duct is transected within the liver. Mobilization is done all the way up to the right hepatic vein, and then we use energy devices to take all the small vessels of the anterior surface of the IVC until identification of the IVC ligament, which is taken with staplers. After this, the right hepatic vein is dissected and stapled. With the line of demarcation now present, we score the capsule of the liver and then start transecting with energy devices, which is done blindly for the first 2 to 3 cm in depth as the vessels lying in that area are within the hemostatic capabilities of these devices. With further dissection, we take smaller bites on

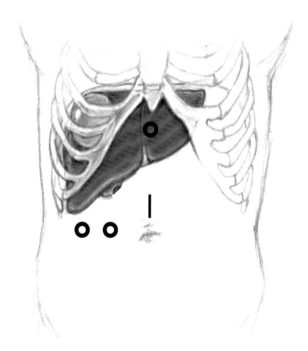

FIGURE 20.2 Trocar placement for laparoscopic right hepatectomy.

the transection area, making sure not to injure major tributaries of the hepatic veins. These will be taken with staplers. When the transection is finished, the specimen is removed through the hand port and pneumoperitoneum is reinstated to secure hemostasis and repair any bile leaks. No drains are placed.

We have found that the Pringle maneuver is not necessary for any of these major hepatectomies and that the blood loss is minimal. In fact, our blood transfusion rate is less than 5%.

Laparoscopic liver resection is a technique that will be used more frequently in the future. Established advantages like decreased blood loss and shorter hospital stay will make it even more attractive in the era of cost containment and bundled payments. Other possible advantages like decreased complication rates with similar operative times will put this technique even more in the forefront of the liver surgery armamentarium. Robotic liver surgery is still very undeveloped, but it has great promise not only to achieve similar results to laparoscopy but also to overcome the limitations of the latter technique.

Suggested Readings

Buell JF, Cherqui D, Geller DA, et al. The International position on laparoscopic liver surgery. The Louisville statement, 2008. *Ann Surg* 2009;250:825–830.

Dagher I, Belli G, Fantini C, et al. Laparoscopic hepatectomy for hepatocellular carcinoma: a European experience. *J Am Coll Surg* 2010;211:16–23.

Kluger MD, Vigano L, Barroso R, et al. The learning curve in laparoscopic major liver resection. *J Hepatobiliary Pancreat Sci* 2013;20:131–136.

Koffron AJ, Auffenberg G, Kung R, et al. Evaluation of 300 minimally invasive liver resections at a single institution. Less is more. *Ann Surg* 2007;246:385–394.

Nguyen KT, Gamblin TC, Geller DA. World review of laparoscopic liver resection. *Ann Surg* 2009;250:831–841.

Nguyen KT, Laurent A, Dagher I, et al. Minimally invasive liver resection for metastatic colorectal cancer. *Ann Surg* 2009;250:842–848.

21 Liver and Biliary Anatomy

Steven M. Strasberg

This chapter is an overview of hepatobiliary anatomy. It covers the prevailing, that is, commonest anatomic patterns and common anomalies, with emphasis on surgically important anomalies.

ANATOMY AND NOMENCLATURE OF THE LIVER

The Brisbane 2000 Terminology of Hepatic Anatomy and Resections used throughout this chapter is the official nomenclature adopted by the International Hepato-Pancreato Biliary Association.

Ramification of the Hepatic Artery

The primary (first-order) division of the proper hepatic artery is into the right and left hepatic arteries (Fig. 21.1). These branches supply arterial inflow to the *right and left hemilivers or livers* (Fig. 21.2). The border or watershed of the first-order division is the *midplane of the liver*. It intersects the gallbladder fossa and groove for the inferior vena cava (IVC) (Fig. 21.2). The right liver usually has a larger volume than the left liver (60:40), although this is variable.

The second-order branches (Figs. 21.1 and 21.2) of the hepatic artery supply the four hepatic *sections*. The right liver has two sections, the *right anterior section* and the *right posterior section,* supplied by the right anterior sectional hepatic artery and the right posterior sectional hepatic artery, respectively (Fig. 21.1). The plane between these sections is the *right intersectional plane*, which does not have surface markings to indicate its position (Fig. 21.2). The left liver also has two sections, the *left medial section* and the *left lateral section*, which are supplied by the left medial sectional hepatic artery and the left lateral sectional hepatic artery (Fig. 21.1). The plane between these sections is referred to as the left intersectional plane. It does have surface markings indicating its position—the umbilical fissure and the line of attachment of the falciform ligament to the anterior surface of the liver.

The third-order branches of the hepatic artery divide the right and left hemilivers into *segments* 2 to 8 (Figs. 21.1 and 21.2). Each of the segments has its own feeding segmental artery. The left lateral section is divided into Sg2 and Sg3. The pattern or ramification of vessels within the left medial section does not permit subdivision of this section into segments, each with its own arterial blood supply. Therefore, the left medial section and Sg4 are synonymous. However, segment 4 is arbitrarily divided into superior (4a) and inferior (4b) parts. The right anterior section is divided into two segments, Sg5 and Sg8. The right posterior section is divided into Sg6 and Sg7. The planes between segments are referred to as intersegmental planes. *The ramifications of the bile ducts are identical to that described for the arteries as are the zones of the liver drained by their respective ducts.*

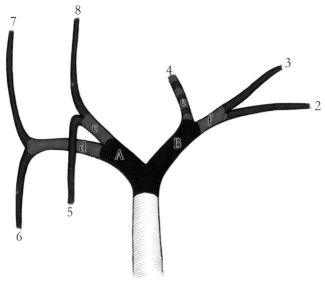

FIGURE 21.1 Three orders of ramification of the proper hepatic artery are shown color coded. First order (*red*) is division into right (*A*) and left (*B*) hepatic arteries. The second order is division into sectional arteries (*green*), including the right anterior (*c*), the right posterior (*d*), the left medial (*e*), and the left lateral (*f*) sectional arteries. The third-order division (*blue*) is into segmental arteries that are numbered and correspond to the Couinaud segments. The three orders supply the hemilivers or livers, sections, and segments. Note that the second order and third order for the left medial sectional artery and artery to segment 4 are identical (*banded green* and *blue*). Segment 1, which is separate from the two hemilivers, is supplied by the arteries that arise from the right and left hepatic arteries (not shown). Ramification of the bile ducts is identical to that of the arteries. (From Strasberg SM, Philips C. Use and dissemination of the Brisbane 2000 nomenclature of liver anatomy and resections. *Ann Surg* 2013;257(3):377–382.)

Segment 1 (caudate lobe) is a distinct portion of the liver, separate from the right and left hemilivers. It has three parts: the bulbous left part (spigelian lobe); the paracaval portion, which lies anterior to the vena cava; and the caudate process (or right part), on the right (Fig. 21.3). The caudate lobe is situated posterior to the hilum and the portal veins. The caudate receives vascular supply from both right and left hepatic arteries (and portal veins). Caudate bile ducts drain into both the right and left hepatic ducts. The caudate lobe is drained by several short caudate veins that enter the IVC directly. These veins enter the IVC on either side of the midplane of the vessel, an anatomical feature that normally allows the creation of a tunnel behind the liver on the surface of the IVC without encountering the caudate veins.

Resectional Terminology
Anatomic liver resections are hemihepatectomies (or hepatectomies), sectionectomies, or segmentectomies. The nomenclature for specific resections is described in Figures 21.4 to 21.8.

Resection of segment 1 is usually called a caudate lobectomy.

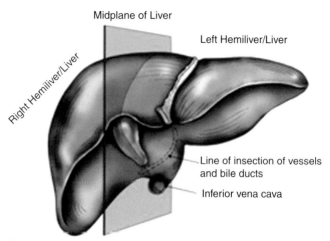

Midplane of Liver

Left Hemiliver/Liver

Right Hemiliver/Liver

Line of insection of vessels and bile ducts

Inferior vena cava

A　　First Order: The *Hemilivers or Livers*

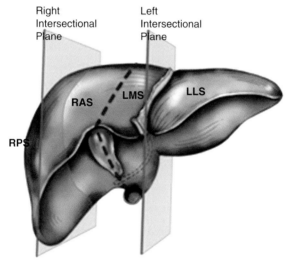

Right Intersectional Plane

Left Intersectional Plane

RAS　LMS　LLS

RPS

B　　Second Order: The *"Sections"*

FIGURE 21.2 A. First-order division of the liver into the hemilivers or livers. Midplane of the liver shown in *red.* **B.** Second-order division of the liver into sections. (RPS, right posterior section; RAS, right anterior section; LMS, left medial section; LLL, left lateral section.) The intersectional planes are shown in green.

(*Continued*)

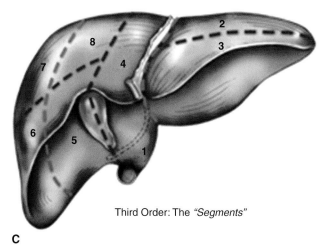

Third Order: The *"Segments"*

C

FIGURE 21.2 (Continued) C. Third-order division into numbered segments. (From Strasberg SM, Philips C. Use and dissemination of the Brisbane 2000 nomenclature of liver anatomy and resections. *Ann Surg* 2013;257(3):377–382.)

SURGICAL ANATOMY FOR LIVER RESECTIONS

Hepatic Arteries and Liver Resections

In the prevailing anatomic pattern, the celiac artery terminates by dividing into splenic and common hepatic arteries. The common hepatic artery runs anteriorly and to the right to ramify into gastroduodenal and proper hepatic arteries. The proper hepatic artery enters the hepatoduodenal ligament and normally runs for 2 to 3 cm along the left side of the common bile duct (CBD) and terminates by dividing into the right and left hepatic arteries, the right immediately passing behind the common hepatic duct (CHD). The four sectional arteries arise from the right and left arteries 1 to 2 cm from the liver. Variations from this pattern, such as replaced (aberrant) arteries, are common. "Replaced" means that the artery supplying a particular volume of the liver is in an unusual location and also that it is the

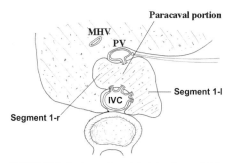

FIGURE 21.3 Anatomy of caudate lobe. Segment 1-1, caudate lobe proper; Segment 1-r, caudate process; MHV, middle hepatic vein; PV, portal vein; IVC, inferior vena cava

Anatomical Term	Couinaud Segments	Term for Surgical Resection	Diagram (pertinent area is shaded)
Right Liver OR Hemiliver	Sg 5-8	Right Hepatectomy OR Right Hemihepatectomy	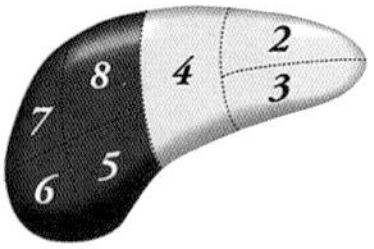
Left Liver OR Hemiliver	Sg 2-4	Left Hepatectomy OR Left Hemihepatectomy	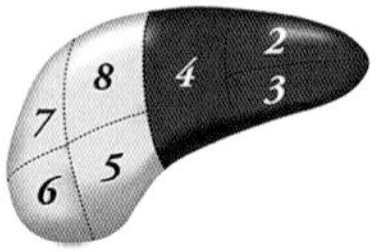

FIGURE 21.4 Resectional terminology for excision of a hemiliver or liver. (From Strasberg SM, Philips C. Use and dissemination of the Brisbane 2000 nomenclature of liver anatomy and resections. *Ann Surg* 2013;257(3):377–382.)

sole supply to that volume of the liver. This should not be confused with the term "accessory" artery. Accessory in this sense indicates that the artery is not the sole blood supply to an area (Fig. 21.8).

Part or all of the liver is supplied by a replaced artery in 25% of patients. The *replaced right hepatic artery* arises from the superior mesenteric artery

Anatomical Term	Couinaud Segments	Term for Surgical Resection Add (-ectomy) to any of the anatomical terms	Diagram (pertinent area is shaded)
Right Anterior Section	Sg 5,8	Right anterior sectionectomy	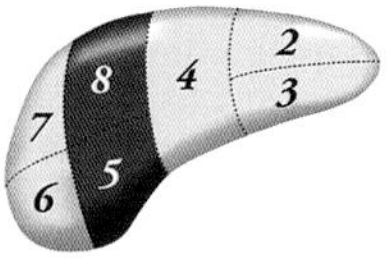
Right Posterior Section	Sg 6,7	Right posterior sectionectomy	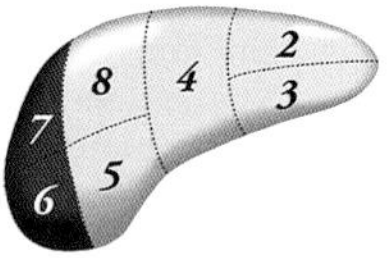
Left Medial Section	Sg 4	Left medial sectionectomy	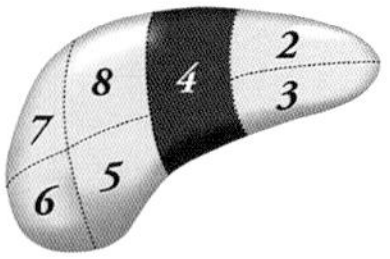
Left Lateral Section	Sg 2,3	Left lateral sectionectomy	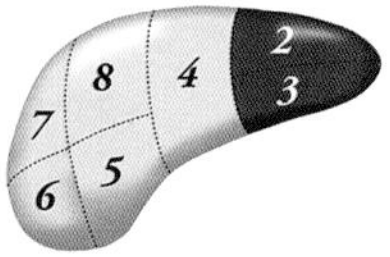

FIGURE 21.5 Resectional terminology for excision of a section. (From Strasberg SM, Philips C. Use and dissemination of the Brisbane 2000 nomenclature of liver anatomy and resections. *Ann Surg* 2013;257(3):377–382.)

Anatomical Term	Couinaud Segments	Term for Surgical Resection	Diagram (pertinent area is shaded)
Segments 1-8	Any one of Sg 1-8	Segmentectomy (e.g. segmentectomy 6)	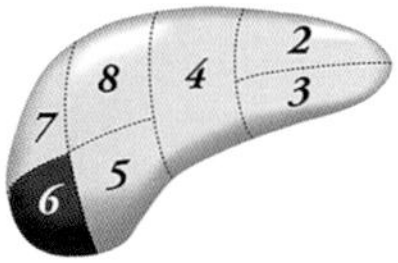
2 contiguous segments	Any two of Sg 1-8 in continuity	Bisegmentectomy (e.g. bisegmentectomy 5,6)	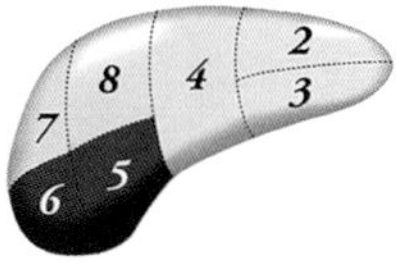

FIGURE 21.6 Resectional terminology for excision of a segment. (From Strasberg SM, Philips C. Use and dissemination of the Brisbane 2000 nomenclature of liver anatomy and resections. *Ann Surg* 2013;257(3):377–382.)

(SMA) and usually runs behind and then along the right posterior border of the CBD (Fig. 21.8), where it may often be palpated. It may supply a segment of, a section of, or the entire right hemiliver. The *replaced left hepatic artery* arises from the left gastric artery and courses in the lesser omentum to the liver. Rarely, a replaced artery supplies the entire liver, and then it is called a *replaced common hepatic artery*.

Bile Ducts and Liver Resections

The prevailing pattern of bile duct drainage from the right liver is shown in (Fig. 21.9A). There are important biliary anomalies on the right side of the liver. The right posterior sectional duct inserts into the left hepatic duct in

Extended Resections
(Trisectionectomy)

Couinaud Segments	Term for Surgical Resection	Diagram (pertinent area is shaded)
Sg 4-8	Right Trisectionectomy (preferred term) **or** Extended Right Hepatectomy **or** Extended Right Hemihepatectomy	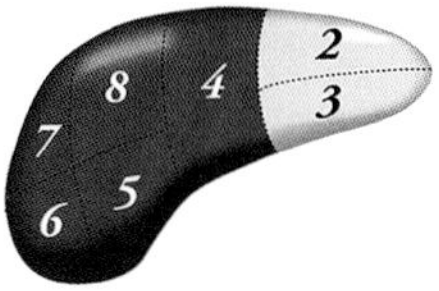
Sg 2,3,4,5,8	Left Trisectionectomy (preferred term) **or** Extended Left Hepatectomy **or** Extended Left Hemihepatectomy	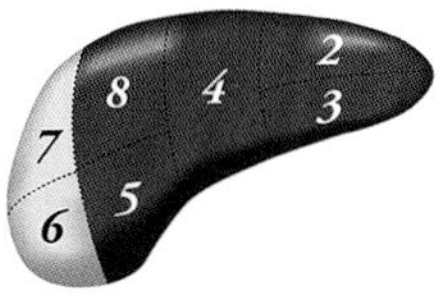

FIGURE 21.7 Terminology for extended resections (three sections). (From Strasberg SM, Philips C. Use and dissemination of the Brisbane 2000 nomenclature of liver anatomy and resections. *Ann Surg* 2013;257(3):377–382.)

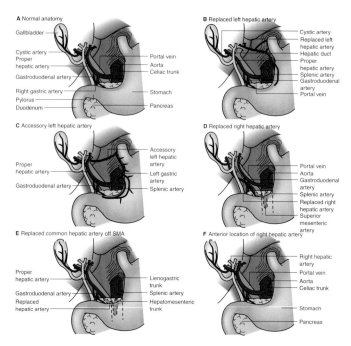

FIGURE 21.8 Prevailing pattern ("normal anatomy") and some common variations of the hepatic artery. (From Mulholland MW, Lillemoe KD, Doherty GM, et al. *Greenfield's surgery: scientific principles & practice*, 5th ed. Philadelphia, PA: Lippincott Williams & Wilkins, 2010.)

20% of persons (Fig. 21.9B), and the right anterior bile duct does so in 6% (Fig. 21.9C). A right sectional bile duct inserting into the left hepatic duct is in danger of injury during left hepatectomy. Another important anomaly is insertion of a right bile duct into the biliary tree at a lower level than the prevailing site of confluence (Fig. 21.9D). The latter anomaly places the aberrant duct at great risk for injury during laparoscopic cholecystectomy.

The prevailing pattern of bile duct drainage from the left liver and common anomalies is shown in Figure 21.10.

Portal Veins and Liver Resections

On the right side of the liver, the portal vein divisions correspond to those of the hepatic artery and bile duct, and they supply the same hepatic volumes (Fig. 21.11). It divides into two sectional and four segmental veins as do the arteries and bile ducts. The left portal vein consists of a *horizontal or transverse portion*, which is located under Sg4, and a *vertical part or umbilical portion*, which is situated in the umbilical fissure (Fig. 21.11). Unlike the right portal vein, neither portion of the left portal vein actually enters the liver, but rather, they lie directly on its surface. Often, the umbilical portion is hidden by a bridge of tissue passing between left medial and lateral sections. The junction of the transverse and umbilical portions of the left portal vein is marked by the attachment of a stout cord—the ligamentum venosum. This structure, the remnant of the fetal ductus venosus, runs in the groove between the left lateral section and the caudate lobe and attaches to the left hepatic vein/IVC junction.

VARIATIONS IN THE FORMATION OF RIGHT HEPATIC DUCTS

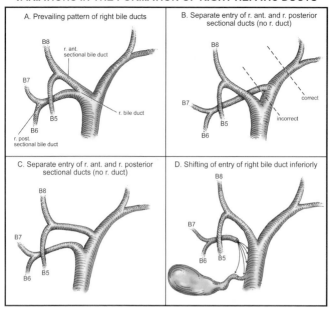

FIGURE 21.9 Prevailing pattern and important variations of bile ducts draining the right hemiliver. (From Fischer JE, Jones DB, Pomposelli FB, et al. *Fischer's mastery of surgery*, 6th ed. Philadelphia, PA: Lippincott Williams & Wilkins, 2011.)

VARIATIONS IN THE FORMATION OF LEFT HEPATIC DUCTS

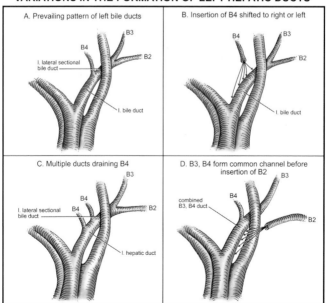

FIGURE 21.10 Prevailing pattern and important variations of bile ducts draining the left hemiliver. (From Fischer JE, Jones DB, Pomposelli FB, et al. *Fischer's mastery of surgery*, 6th ed. Philadelphia, PA: Lippincott Williams & Wilkins, 2011.)

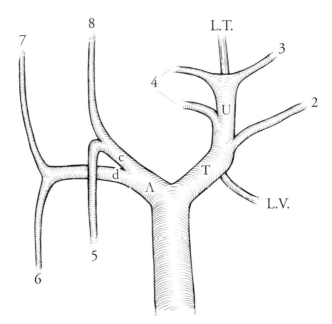

FIGURE 21.11 Ramification of the portal vein in the liver. The portal vein divides into right (*A*) and left (*T*) branches. The branches in the right liver (the sectional branches [*c*] and [*d*], and the numbered segmental branches) correspond to those of the hepatic artery and bile duct. The branching pattern on the left is unique. The left portal vein has transverse (*T*) and umbilical portions (*U*). The transition point between the two parts is marked by the attachment of the ligamentum venosum (*L.V.*). All major branches come off the umbilical portion. The vein ends blindly in the ligamentum teres (*L.T.*). (Copyright Washington University in St. Louis.)

The transverse portion of the left portal vein sends only a few small branches to Sg4. Large branches from the portal vein to the left liver arise exclusively beyond the attachment of the ligamentum venosum, that is, from the umbilical part of the vein (Fig. 21.11). Branches come off both sides of the vein—those arising from the right side pass into Sg4 and those from the left supply Sg2 and Sg3. The left portal vein terminates in the ligamentum teres at the free edge of the left liver.

The most common variation is absence of the right portal vein. In these cases, the right posterior and right anterior sectional portal veins originate independently from the main portal vein. A rare but potentially devastating anomaly is the absent extrahepatic left portal vein, an anomaly in which the main portal vein enters the right side of the liver and courses intrahepatically to supply the left liver. Division of this vein thinking that it is the right portal vein will lead to portal devascularization of the entire liver.

Hepatic Veins and Liver Resection

Three large hepatic veins run in the midplane of the liver (middle hepatic vein), the right intersectional plane (right hepatic vein), and the left intersectional plane (left hepatic vein). The left hepatic vein begins in the plane between Sg2 and Sg3 and travels in that plane for most of its length.

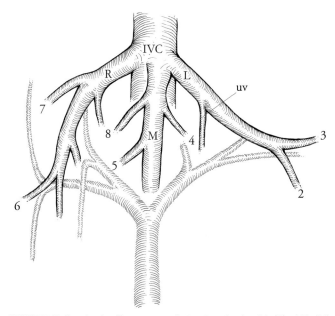

FIGURE 21.12 Hepatic veins. There are normally three hepatic veins: right (*R*), middle (*M*), and left (*L*). Note the segments drained. UV is the umbilical vein, which normally drains part of Sg4 into the left hepatic vein. The latter is proof that the terminal portion of the left vein lies in the intersectional plane of the left liver. (Copyright Washington University in St. Louis.)

In about 10% of individuals, there is more than one large right hepatic vein; in addition to the right superior hepatic vein (normally called the right hepatic vein), which enters the IVC just below the level of the diaphragm, there is a right inferior hepatic vein, which enters the IVC 5 to 6 cm below this level (Fig. 21.12).

The caudate lobe is drained by its own veins—several short veins that enter the IVC directly from the caudate lobe. When performing a classical right hepatectomy, caudate veins are divided in the preliminary portion of the dissection. As dissection moves up the anterior surface of the vena cava to isolate the right hepatic vein, one encounters a bridge of tissue lateral to the IVC referred to as the "inferior vena cava ligament." It connects the posterior portion of the right liver to the caudate lobe behind the IVC. This bridge of tissue usually consists of fibrous tissue, but occasionally is a bridge of liver parenchyma.

The Plate/Sheath System of the Liver

There is a system of fibrous plates and sheaths, which lies on the ventral surface of the liver and extends into it. Knowledge of the system is of importance in liver surgery. The fundamentals of the system can be understood by imagining a shirt with the front cut away to leave only the back and the sleeves (Fig. 21.13 inset). The back of the shirt would be a plate, and the sleeves would be sheaths. In the true plate/sheath system, there are four plates (hilar, cystic, umbilical, and arantian) and several sheaths (Fig. 21.13).

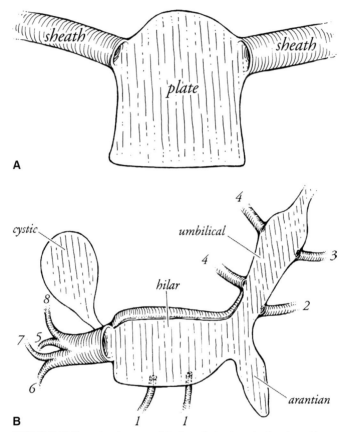

FIGURE 21.13 Plate–sheath system of the liver. **A.** A schematic of a plate with two sheaths (see text) **B.** plate sheath system. (From Strasberg SW, Linehan DC, Hawkins WG. Isolation of right main and right sectional portal pedicles for liver resection without hepatotomy or inflow occlusion. *J Am Coll Surg* 2008;206(2):390–396.)

The hilar plate, the most important plate in liver surgery, is a flat sheet, lying in the coronal plane, posterior to the main bilovascular structures in the porta hepatis. However, the upper part curves forward to enclose the right and left bile ducts, the most superior structures in the porta hepatis. It is this taut, firm, upper curved edge of the hilar plate that is dissected free from the underside of the liver when "lowering the hilar plate."

Coming off the right side of the hilar plate like a sleeve is the sheath of the right portal pedicle. It extends into the liver surrounding the portal structures that enter it on its free edge, that is, the portal vein, hepatic artery, and bile duct (Fig. 21.14). The combined structure consisting of sheath and contents is the right portal pedicle. As the right portal pedicle enters the liver, it divides into a right anterior and right posterior portal pedicle supplying the respective sections and then segmental pedicles supplying the four segments. On the left side, only the segmental structures are sheathed.

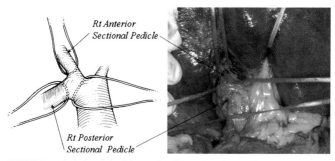

FIGURE 21.14 Isolation of the right portal pedicle and sectional pedicles by technique of dissection on surface of pedicles. No inflow occlusion or separate hepatotomies are used (see Fischer et al., 2011). The umbilical tape in the upper right of the photograph is around the bridge of the liver tissue over the umbilical fissure. (From Strasberg SW, Linehan DC, Hawkins WG. Isolation of right main and right sectional portal pedicles for liver resection without hepatotomy or inflow occlusion. *J Am Coll Surg* 2008;206(2):390–396.)

The cystic plate is the ovoid fibrous sheet on which the gallbladder lies (Fig. 21.13). In its posterior extent, the cystic plate narrows to become a stout cord that attaches to the anterior surface of the sheath of the right portal pedicle. The latter is a point of anatomical importance for the surgeon wishing to expose the anterior surface of the right portal pedicle, since this cord must be divided to do so. With severe chronic inflammation, the cystic plate may become shortened and thickened so that the distance between the top of the cystic plate and the right portal pedicle is likewise much shorter than usual. This places the structures in the right pedicle in danger during cholecystectomy in which dissection is performed "top down" as a primary strategy. The other plates are the umbilical and arantian, which underlie the umbilical portion of the left portal vein and the ligamentum venosum respectively (Fig. 21.13). The other sheaths carry segmental bilovascular pedicles of the left liver and caudate lobe.

Liver Capsule and Attachments
The liver is covered with a thin fibrous capsule that covers the entire organ except for the large "bare area" posteriorly. There, the organ is in contact with the IVC and diaphragm. The bare area stretches superiorly to include the termination of the three hepatic veins and ends in a point, which is also where the attachment of the falciform ligament ends. The limit of the bare area, where the peritoneum passes between the body wall and the liver, is called the coronary ligament. It is one of three structures, which connect the liver to the abdominal wall "dorsally," the other two being the right and left triangular ligaments. The liver also has another much smaller bare area, where the hepatoduodenal ligament and the lesser omentum attach on the "ventral" surface. It is here that the portal structures enter the liver at the hilum. The ligamentum teres ("round") is the obliterated left umbilical vein and runs in the free edge of the falciform ligament from the umbilicus to the termination of the umbilical portion of the left portal vein. The falciform (falciform = "scythe shaped") is the filmy fold that runs in between the anterior abdominal wall above the umbilicus and attaches to the anterior surface of the liver between the left medial and left lateral sections. The ligamentum venosum, the residual ductus venosus, is a filmy

cord that extends from the termination of the transverse portion of the left portal vein to the left hepatic vein along the junction of the left lateral section and the caudate lobe.

GALLBLADDER AND EXTRAHEPATIC BILE DUCTS

Gallbladder

The gallbladder lies on the cystic plate. The lower edge of the gallbladder forms one side of the hepatocystic triangle. The other two sides are the right side of the CHD and the liver. Eponyms covering this anatomy (Calot, Moosman, etc.) are confusing and should be abandoned. The hepatocystic triangle contains the cystic artery and cystic node and sometimes a portion of the right hepatic artery as well as fat and fibrous tissue. Clearance of this triangle along with the isolation of the cystic duct and elevation of the base of the gallbladder off the lower portion of the cystic plate gives the "critical view of safety," which we have described for identification of the cystic structures during laparoscopic cholecystectomy.

A large number of minor curiosities of the gallbladder, for example, phrygian cap, have been described. The following are anomalies of importance to the biliary surgeon.

Double Gallbladder

This is a rare anomaly but can be the cause of persistent symptoms after resection of one gallbladder. A gallbladder may also be bifid, which usually does not cause symptoms, or have an hourglass constriction that may cause symptoms due to obstruction of the upper segment.

Agenesis of the Gallbladder

Agenesis occurs in about 1/8,000 patients. It can be difficult to recognize. When agenesis is suspected, it may be confirmed by axial imaging. If doubt remains, laparoscopy is definitive.

Cystic Duct

A tubular structure normally 1 to 2 cm in length and 2 to 3 mm in diameter. It usually joins the CHD at an acute angle to form the CBD. The cystic duct normally joins the CHD approximately 4 cm above the duodenum. However, the cystic duct may enter at any level up to the right hepatic duct and down to the ampulla. The cystic duct may also join the right hepatic duct either when the right duct is in its normal position or in an aberrant location. The cystic duct contains a spiral valve.

There are three patterns of confluence of the cystic duct and CHD (Fig. 21.15). In 20% of patients in which there is a parallel union, injury to the CHD may occur by dissecting low on the cystic duct (Fig. 21.15). When making a choledochotomy at this level, the incision should be started slightly to the left side of the midplane of the bile duct in order to avoid entering a septum between the fused cystic duct/common hepatic duct. When performing cholecystectomy, the cystic duct should be occluded in such a way that there is a visible section of cystic duct below the clip closest to the CBD.

Although a gallbladder with two cystic ducts has been described, it is an extreme rarity. When two "cystic ducts" are identified, it is likely that cystic duct is congenitally short or has been effaced by a stone and that the two structures thought to be dual cystic ducts are, in fact, the CBD and the CHD.

Cystic Artery

The cystic artery is usually 1 to 2 mm in diameter and normally arises from the right hepatic artery in the hepatocystic triangle. The cystic artery may

Angular (75%)   **Parallel** (20%)   **Spiral** (5%)

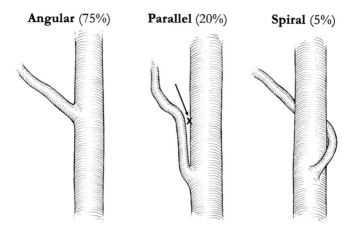

FIGURE 21.15   The three types of cystic duct/common hepatic duct confluence. The parallel union confluence is shown in the middle. Dissection of this type of cystic duct (*arrow*) may lead to injury to the side of CHD. During laparoscopic cholecystectomy, this is often a cautery injury. (Adapted from Warrren KW, McDonald WM, Kune GA. Bile duct strictures: new concepts in the management of an old problem. In: Irvine WT (ed). *Modern trends in surgery.* London, UK: Butterworth, 1966. Copyright Washington University in St. Louis.)

arise from a right hepatic artery that runs anterior to the CHD. The cystic artery may also arise from the right hepatic artery on the left side of the CHD and run anterior to this duct, while the right hepatic artery runs behind it. Such cystic arteries tend to tether the gallbladder and make dissection of the hepatocystic triangle more difficult. The cystic artery may arise from a replaced right hepatic artery arising from the SMA. In this case, the cystic artery (and not the cystic duct) tends to be in the free edge of the fold leading from the hepatoduodenal ligament to the gallbladder. This should be suspected whenever the "cystic duct" looks smaller than the "cystic artery."

Usually, the cystic artery runs for 1 to 2 cm to meet the gallbladder superior to the insertion of the cystic duct. The artery ramifies into an anterior and posterior branch at the point of contact with the gallbladder. These branches continue to divide on their respective surfaces. Sometimes, the cystic artery divides into branches before the gallbladder edge is reached. In that case, the anterior branch may be mistaken for the cystic artery proper and the posterior branch may not be discovered until later in the dissection—sometimes by inadvertent division with hemorrhage. The artery may ramify into several branches before arriving at the gallbladder giving the impression that there is no cystic artery. The anterior and posterior branches may arise independently from the right hepatic artery, giving rise to two distinct cystic arteries. There are many other variations.

Multiple small cystic veins drain into intrahepatic portal vein branches by passing into the liver around or through the cystic plate. Sometimes, there are cystic veins in the hepatocystic triangle that run parallel to the cystic artery to enter the main portal vein.

Cystic Plate

The cystic plate has been described previously. Small bile ducts may penetrate the cystic plate to enter the gallbladder. These "ducts of Luschka" are very small, usually submillimeter accessory ducts. However, when divided during a cholecystectomy, postoperative bilomas may occur. Bilomas and hemorrhage may also be caused by penetration of the cystic plate during dissection. In about 10% of patients, there is a large peripheral bile duct immediately deep to the plate, disruption of which will cause copious bile drainage. The origin of the middle hepatic vein is also in this location, and if it is injured, massive hemorrhage may ensue. There is areolar tissue between the muscularis of the gallbladder and the cystic plate. At the top of the gallbladder, the layer is very thin. As one progresses downward, the areolar layer thickens. If dissection from the top of the gallbladder downward is carried on the gallbladder leaving the areolar tissue on the cystic plate, one will arrive onto the posterior surface of the cystic artery and cystic duct. Conversely, if dissection is carried downward on the cystic plate leaving the areolar tissue on the gallbladder, one will arrive onto the surface of the right portal pedicle. If this is not anticipated, structures in the right portal pedicle may be injured. Therefore, the proper plane of dissection is between the gallbladder and the areolar tissue.

Extrahepatic Bile Ducts

The CHD is formed by the union of the right and left hepatic ducts. The union normally occurs at the right extremity of the base of Sg4 anterior and superior to the bifurcation of the portal vein. The CHD travels in the right edge of the hepatoduodenal ligament for 2 to 3 cm where it joins with the cystic duct to form the CBD. The latter has a supraduodenal course of 3 to 4 cm and then passes behind the duodenum to run in or occasionally behind the pancreas to enter the second portion of the duodenum. The external diameter of the CBD varies from 5 to 13 mm when distended to physiologic pressures. However, the duct diameter at surgery, that is, in fasting patients with low duct pressures, may be as small as 3 mm. Radiologically, the internal duct diameter is measured on fasting patients. Under these conditions, the upper limit of normal is about 8 mm. Size should never be used as a sole criterion for identifying a bile duct. Caution is required in situations in which a structure seems larger than the expected norm. Although the cystic duct may be enlarged due to passage of stones, a surgeon should take extra precautions before dividing a "cystic duct" that is greater than 2 mm in diameter because the CBD can be 3 mm in diameter and aberrant ducts may be smaller.

Anomalies of Extrahepatic Bile Ducts

As already noted, there are biliary anomalies of the right and left ductal systems, which can affect outcome of hepatic surgery. The same is true for biliary surgery. The most important clinical anomaly is low insertion of the right hepatic ducts referred to above. Because of its low location, it may be mistaken to be the cystic duct and injured during cholecystectomy. This is even more likely to occur when the cystic duct unites with an aberrant duct as opposed to joining the CHD. The anomalies of a right hepatic duct entering the gallbladder and the absent CHD have been discussed above. Left hepatic ducts can also join the CHD at a low level. They are less prone to be injured since the dissection during cholecystectomy is on the right side of the biliary tree.

Extrahepatic Arteries

The course of these arteries has been described above. Anomalies of the hepatic artery may be important in gallbladder surgery. Normally, the right hepatic artery passes posterior to the bile duct (80%) and gives off the cystic artery in the hepatocystic triangle. However, in 20% of cases, the right hepatic artery runs anterior to the bile duct. The right hepatic artery may lie very close to the gallbladder, and chronic inflammation can draw the right hepatic artery directly onto the gallbladder, where it lies in an inverse U-loop and is prone to injury. In the "classical injury" in laparoscopic chole-cystectomy in which the CBD is mistaken for the cystic duct, an associated right hepatic artery injury is very common, since that right hepatic artery is considered to be the cystic artery.

Blood Supply of Bile Ducts

Many studies, dating back to the 19th century, have examined the blood supply of the extrahepatic bile ducts in cadaveric specimens. An important observation made by Rappoport is that the bile ducts are supplied solely by the hepatic artery, unlike the liver that has a dual blood supply from the artery and the portal vein. The arterial blood supply has three anatomic elements—afferent arteries, marginal arteries, and epicholedochal plexus (Fig. 21.16).

The afferent vessels are branches of the hepatic arteries and less commonly of the SMA or other upper abdominal arteries. The most constant and important artery supplying the bile duct is the posterior superior pancreaticoduodenal artery, usually the first branch of the gastroduodenal artery. Arterial twigs are sent to the duct as the artery winds around the lower end of the duct. These branches supply the retroduodenal and intrapancreatic bile duct but also ascend the bile duct to give supply to the supraduodenal bile duct. The lowest portion of the duct near the ampulla is also supplied by the anterior superior pancreatic artery and the inferior pancreaticoduodenal artery. Other vessels, which commonly send afferents to the supraduodenal bile duct, are the proper hepatic artery, cystic artery,

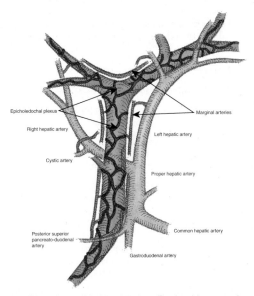

FIGURE 21.16 Blood supply to bile ducts. The three elements—the afferent arteries, marginal arteries, and epicholedochal plexus— are shown. (From Fischer JE, Jones DB, Pomposelli FB, et al. *Fischer's mastery of surgery*, 6th ed. Philadelphia, PA: Lippincott Williams & Wilkins, 2011.)

and artery to segment 4. However, virtually all extrahepatic arteries arising from the common hepatic artery can send small branches to the bile ducts. Also, body wall collaterals such as phrenic arteries can at times supply the bile ducts. The idea that the extrahepatic bile duct, that is, CHD and CBD, is supplied by the arteries that join it only at the bottom and top of its course is incorrect. Supplying arteries from the cystic artery, right and left hepatic arteries, and proper hepatic artery may join it along its length.

The afferent vessels empty into the longitudinal or "marginal" arteries, which run parallel to the long axis of the bile duct. These vessels are disposed at 3, 9, and, less commonly, 12 o'clock on the CBD/CHD or run across the top of the confluence of the right and left hepatic ducts. This hilar marginal artery is of great importance in maintaining blood supply to the liver when one hepatic artery (right or left) is occluded.

The third element, the "epicholedochal plexus," is a fine arterial plexus that lies on and surrounds the entire CBD and the left and right hepatic ducts. The part around the hepatic ducts is the hilar component of the epicholedochal plexus. The vessels of the plexus tend to run along the long axis of the ducts so that on the common duct many of the vessels are vertical while that around the confluence and the right and left ducts they are disposed horizontally. Branches of the epicholedochal plexus pierce the bile duct and supply it through the deeper and finer intracholedochal plexi within the wall of the bile duct.

Transection of the bile duct may result in ischemia of the duct. For instance, if the duct is transected at the level of the duodenum, ischemia of a portion of the bile duct above this level may occur since blood flow originating from the superior pancreaticoduodenal artery and passing up along the marginal artery is cut off. This problem is thought to be an important contributory cause to the frequent failure of choledochocholedochostomy as a form of biliary reconstruction. To avoid this problem, hepaticojejunostomy is used and the bile duct is trimmed back to within 1 cm of the confluence.

Suggested Readings

Couinaud C. *Le Foie. Etudes Anatomiqucs et Churgicales*. Paris, France: Masson & Cie, 1957.

Fischer JE, Jones DB, Pomposelli FB, et al. *Fischer's mastery of surgery*, 6th ed. Philadelphia, PA: Lippincott Williams & Wilkins, 2011.

Goldsmith NA, Woodburne RT. The surgical anatomy pertaining to liver resection. *Surg Gynecol Obstet* 1957;195:310–318.

Gunji H, Cho A, Tohma T, et al. The blood supply of the hilar bile duct and its relationship to the communicating arcade located between the right and left hepatic arteries. *Am J Surg* 2006;192:276–280.

Healey JE, Schroy PC. Anatomy of the biliary ducts within the human liver; Analysis of the prevailing pattern of branchings and the major variations of the biliary ducts. *Arch Surg* 1953;66:599–616.

Michels NA. *Blood supply and anatomy of the upper abdominal organs*. Philadelphia and Montreal: J.B. Lippincott, 1955.

Northover JMA, Terblanche J. A new look at the arterial supply of the bile duct in man and its surgical implications. *Brit J Surg* 1979;66:379–384.

Strasberg SM, Linehan DC, Hawkins WG. Isolation of right main and right sectional portal pedicles for liver resection without hepatotomy or inflow occlusion. *J Am Coll Surg* 2008;206:390–396.

Strasberg SM, Phillip C. Use and dissemination of the Brisbane 2000 nomenclature of liver anatomy and resections. *Ann Surg* 2013;257:377–382.

Terminology Committee of the IHPBA. The Brisbane 2000 terminology of liver anatomy and resections. *HPB* 2000;2:333–339.

Infections in Biliary Surgery

Massimo Arcerito and Rebecca M. Minter

INTRODUCTION

Although infection is not often the primary cause of disease in the biliary system, it is a common complication. Obstructing conditions such as gallstones, benign strictures, or endoluminal or extraluminal bile duct malignancies lead susceptible patients to develop infectious complications, which are caused by microorganisms. Gram-negative aerobic organisms (*Enterobacteriaceae* species), anaerobes, fungi, or a combination colonize the biliary system and in settings of obstruction can cause cholangitis. Biliary infections, also called infectious cholangitides, can manifest acutely or more indolently. Local infections can lead to cholangitis and subsequent liver abscesses that may spread hematogenously to cause septicemia or septic shock, requiring immediate endoscopic or surgical intervention. Bacteria predominantly cause infectious cholangitides in the Western society, while in other parts of the world parasites play a larger role in the development of biliary tract infections. In the last 30 years, immunocompromised patients (e.g., patients with AIDS or posttransplant) with viral cholangitides represent a more difficult population to treat by clinicians and surgeons.

It is well recognized that patients undergoing hepato-pancreatico-biliary surgery are at risk for infectious complications that are not limited to skin or intra-abdominal locations, but also within the biliary system and the liver parenchyma, potentially leading to the development of pyogenic liver abscesses. A very fine balance exists between the host defense mechanisms and infections of the biliary system when obstructing lesions of the biliary tree are addressed by endoscopic, percutaneous, or surgical means.

BACKGROUND

The biliary system and the liver represent a unique environment to protect the human body from hematogenous dissemination of toxins, microorganisms, and enteric pathogens delivered by the gastrointestinal system to the liver. The inferior and superior mesenteric venous systems drain into the portal vein, ultimately reaching the hepatic sinusoids where the blood is detoxified before reaching the suprahepatic veins. Typically, bile within the gallbladder and the biliary system is sterile in the absence of gallstones, obstruction, or communication with the gastrointestinal tract via either disease-driven fistula or endoscopic or surgical interventions. It is the presence of infected bile, or bacteribilia—secondary to gallstones, benign and malignant obstruction, diagnostic or therapeutic interventions—that cause infections in the hepatobiliary system.

BACTERIOLOGY

In patients with symptomatic gallstones or acute or chronic cholecystitis, the incidence of positive bile cultures ranges between 11% and 30%.

Acute cholecystitis, often characterized by fever and leukocytosis, demonstrates a higher rate of positive bile cultures as compared with chronic cholecystitis (46% vs. 22%). Cholangitis secondary to endobiliary stents, stones, or tumor presents with a positive bile culture in 100% of cases. The most common bacteria isolated are of gastrointestinal origin, specifically *Escherichia coli* (25% to 50%) followed by *Klebsiella* (15% to 20%) and *Enterobacter* species (5% to 10%) are the most common Gram-negative species. Anaerobes such as *Clostridium perfringens* and *Bacteroides* can also be present but are more commonly observed in the setting of recurrent cholangitis or following hepatobiliary surgical interventions. *Candida* species have been more often identified in the bile of critically ill patients. Achieving adequate drainage of the biliary tree by treating the underlying obstruction is critical for successful treatment, typically in conjunction with broad-spectrum antibiotic therapy covering both aerobic and anaerobic pathogens.

HOST DEFENSE MECHANISM

Physical, chemical, and immunologic properties are required to protect the liver from invasion by pathogens and toxins. Table 22.1 represents the features of the hepatobiliary host defense mechanism that function in a coordinated fashion to prevent invasion by microorganisms within the biliary system.

Division of the bile canaliculi from the bloodstream is required to protect the biliary system from pathogen invasion by the vascular system, and vice versa. This extraordinary property is provided by the hepatic tight junctions. These junctions are able to build a barrier between the biliary channels and hepatic sinusoids. The liver is the core metabolic center in humans and is responsible for fundamental physiologic functions including fatty acid, amino acid, and carbohydrate metabolism; bile secretion; and detoxification. Because of the highly vascularized nature of the liver and its hepatocytes, a microvascular network is maintained in place by the hepatic tight junctions. Deregulation of tight junction expression dismantles the parenchymal network, causing liver disease and malignant transformation. Hepatic tight junctions also represent a physical barrier within the liver preventing ascending biliary infection. Any obstruction of

TABLE 22.1	Hepatobiliary Host Defense Mechanisms
	Defense Mechanisms
Physical	Antegrade flow of bile into the duodenum
	Sphincter of Oddi preventing reflux of gastrointestinal content into biliary system
	Tight junctions between bile canaliculi and hepatic sinusoids
Chemical	Bile salts possess bacteriostatic and bacteriocidal properties
Immunologic	Kupffer cells phagocytose bacteria and bacterial products and play a critical role in bilirubin metabolism through phagocytosis of senescent erythrocytes
	IgA secreted by biliary epithelium
	Fibronectin and complement (C3, C4, and Factor B) play a critical role in opsonizing pathogens in liver

the portal vein, pre-, intra- or posthepatic, will cause portal hypertension with the development of portosystemic shunts. Those shunts will bypass the liver parenchyma and will allow the toxins and enteric pathogens to reach the systemic circulation.

Additional physical features of the hepatobiliary system serve to prevent ascending infection. Specifically, the sphincter of Oddi that prevents reflux of enteric content into the biliary tree when bile flows antegrade into the duodenum represents a dynamic physical barrier against ascending biliary infection. After cholecystectomy, there may be a decreased force of antegrade bile flow due to the loss of gallbladder contraction with retrograde reflux of enteric contents leading to colonization of the biliary tree. In addition, any surgical or endoscopic intervention on the biliopancreatic sphincter (e.g., sphincterotomy, placement of endobiliary stent, or creation of a biliary–enteric bypass) leads to loss of this physical barrier, permitting direct reflux of enteric content into the biliary tree. The mere presence of bacteria in the bile does not always lead to infection; however, in the setting of distal obstruction one must watch closely for signs and symptoms of an ascending infection.

The second protective element in the host defense mechanisms is the chemical component. Specifically, the presence of bile salts in the bile provides an excellent protection against enteric pathogens possessing both bacteriostatic and bactericidal properties. Jaundice due to mechanical obstruction of the bile duct leads to overgrowth of intestinal flora due to the absence of bile and bile salts within the gastrointestinal tract, predisposing patients to develop cholangitis when the obstruction is treated with endobiliary or surgical decompression. Fungal contamination of the bile is commonly observed in patients with biliary obstruction. This fungal colonization is secondary to the absence of bile salts that also possess antifungal properties, particularly against *Candida albicans* species.

The third protective element is the immunologic and humoral component. The liver parenchyma contains several immunologic active cells whose function is to alter and metabolize toxins coming from the gastrointestinal tract. Kupffer cells represent the largest population of tissue macrophages. Kupffer cells possess Fc, C3, and scavenger receptors that are known to phagocytize a wide variety of both opsonized and nonopsonized materials including bacteria and bacterial products. In addition, Kupffer cells play a defined role in bilirubin metabolism, controlling infections in the biliary system. Approximately 75% of bilirubin is derived from the breakdown of senescent erythrocytes by macrophages. Two isoenzymes HO-1 and HO-2 are involved in this process. HO-1, also known as heat shock protein-32, is induced by stressors and is contained in the endoplasmic reticulum and perinuclear envelope of Kupffer cells in the liver. Overall, Kupffer cells are responsible for the removal of senescent erythrocytes from the blood circulation by scavenger receptors. Depletion of Kupffer cells in the liver reduces HO-1 expression and bilirubin production, predisposing to a variety of biliary infections. Liver resections also reduce the presence of Kupffer cells and therefore reduce their immunologic effects in the liver initially following resection. Immunoglobulin A (IgA), as part of the humoral component, is produced and secreted into the hepatic system by the gallbladder and intra- and extrahepatic biliary epithelium protecting against infectious pathogens. In addition, complement C3 and C4, factor B, and fibronectin play a major role in opsonizing pathogens and helping the biliary system to defend itself from the continuous exposure to pathogens. Any alteration of these defense mechanisms predisposes to colonization and development of infection in the hepatobiliary system (Table 22.1).

BILIARY OBSTRUCTION

The etiology of biliary obstruction can be secondary to intrinsic causes like cholangiocarcinoma, choledocholithiasis, or ampullary stenosis, extrinsic causes like periampullary or pancreatic neoplasia or pancreatitis involving the distal portion of the bile duct, or functional causes such as sphincter of Oddi dysfunction. The use of endobiliary stents can often resolve the obstruction, but predisposes the patient to develop biliary infection due to the communication this creates with the gastrointestinal tract. In the presence of biliary obstruction, the lack of bile flow is considered to be a primary cause of bacterial overgrowth in the biliary system. Likewise, obstruction leads to biliary hypertension with subsequent breaking down of the hepatocyte tight junction and development of cholangiovenous reflux. This phenomenon allows the gastrointestinal endotoxins to colonize the biliary–portal system and can lead to the formation of pyogenic liver abscesses or biliary sepsis. The absence of bile salts with their bacteriostatic and bacteriocidal properties, which occurs in the setting of biliary obstruction, leads to an increase in the number of enteric pathogens in the intestinal tract.

No one clearly delineated mechanism defines how biliary obstruction specifically predisposes one to infectious complications. One theory suggests that Kupffer cell metabolism is diminished in the presence of biliary obstruction. This leads to bacterial overgrowth with inability of the existing Kupffer cells to clear the bacteria and bacterial products adequately. Bacteria can then translocate to the systemic circulation through the hepatic–sinusoid tight junctions. In addition, IgA production is limited by biliary obstruction. Clinically, the presence of bacteria in the biliary tree does not translate into cholangitis, but the combination of biliary obstruction and increased pressure in the biliary system determines a cascade of events that can often lead to acute cholangitis.

INFECTIONS IN BILIARY SURGERY

Human bile is typically sterile but may become infected in the presence of gallbladder and common bile duct stones or intrinsic or extrinsic inflammatory or neoplastic diseases leading to obstruction. The pathophysiology of infection is due either to translocation of intestinal pathogens via the portal system or more commonly due to biliary intervention with incomplete drainage. Any invasive endoscopic, radiologic, or surgical procedure on the hepatobiliary system interferes with the usual host defense mechanism, and the introduction of an indwelling biliary stent through any means constitutes a foreign body within the biliary system. Biliary–enteric anastomosis, sphincterotomy and sphincteroplasty, disruption of blood supply either locally to the liver and biliary tree or systemically (shock), blood transfusions, and the immune status of the patient are all additional important contributors to the development of an ascending biliary infection.

Hepatic resection can also predispose to the development of biliary infections. It is mandatory to analyze the hepatic reserve in patients undergoing resection of hepatic parenchyma, particularly in those who will require a bilioenteric anastomosis such as in the setting of cholangiocarcinoma. The reticuloendothelial system immunologic function is reduced after hepatic resection secondary to loss of functional liver mass. Increasingly, preoperative portal vein embolization is being utilized in preparation of planned extended hepatic resection to provide sufficient postoperative hepatic metabolic and host defense function by inducing growth of the planned hepatic remnant. A recent Cochrane review of 521 patients evaluating the use of perioperative antibiotics, duration of antibiotics, and use of probiotics did not identify any clear predictors of morbidity or mortality related to postoperative infectious complications for these variables.

ACUTE ASCENDING CHOLANGITIS

Cholangitis is caused by an acute bacterial infection of the bile duct. In 1877, Charcot first described the triad of fever, jaundice, and right upper quadrant pain. When shock and altered mental status are included in the classic clinical scenario, it is referred to as Reynolds pentad. The development of cholangitis requires biliary bacterial contamination, stagnant bile, and increased intrabiliary pressure (>20 cm H_2O). Cholangitis is a serious medical problem; mortality ranges between 3.5% and 65%. Interestingly, the severity of acute cholangitis has been shown to correlate with intrabiliary pressure. The most common cause of cholangitis is partial biliary obstruction. Complete obstruction is less likely to be associated with bacterobilia and therefore is less likely to present as cholangitis. Elevated biliary pressure increases biliary ductule permeability, allowing pathogens to enter the bloodstream. Two decades ago, the most common cause of acute cholangitis was choledocholithiasis. In more recent years, other causes of cholangitis have increased, including altered biliary anatomy due to surgical intervention and instrumentation of the biliary tree. Malignancy accounts for 10% to 30% of all cases of cholangitis. Bile cultures are polymicrobial in 30% to 80% of patients who have undergone placement of endobiliary stents or biliary–enteric anastomosis; these patients often are colonized with antibiotic-resistant organisms. The most common aerobic isolated organisms in culture from these patients are *E. coli*, *Klebsiella*, *Enterococcus* species; *Enterobacter*, *Pseudomonas*, *Serratia* and *Proteus* species, and *Bacteroides fragilis* are the most common anaerobic enteric pathogens. *C. albicans* is the most common fungus in bile cultures in patients who have undergone biliary manipulation.

The diagnosis of acute cholangitis is made based upon clinical presentation. All patients must be aggressively resuscitated and started on broad-spectrum antibiotics immediately. Blood cultures are obtained at presentation, and bile cultures are also obtained as soon as possible to guide antibiotic therapy. Initial antibiotic coverage is broad and is tailored to the severity of the clinical presentation, the patient's history of prior antibiotic usage, hepatic and renal function, allergies, and any prior culture data. Typically, community-acquired cholangitis is more commonly associated with a single biliary organism (most commonly *Klebsiella*, *E. coli*, or *Enterococcus*), and treatment with a short course (3 to 5 days) of a penicillin/β-lactamase inhibitor combination (e.g., piperacillin/tazobactam or ampicillin/sulbactam) is usually effective. Patients presenting with greater clinical severity often have anaerobic bacteria contributing to the infection, and patients in the hospital may have infection due to resistant and/or multiple organisms such as *Pseudomonas*, methicillin-resistant *Staphylococcus aureus*, and vancomycin-resistant enterococci. Antibiotic choice must be tailored to address these conditions. Patients presenting with moderate or severe cholangitis should also be treated with intravenous penicillin/β-lactamase inhibitors; however, if resistant organisms are suspected then the addition of appropriate antibiotics for methicillin-resistant bacteria like vancomycin or daptomycin for coverage of suspected vancomycin-resistant *Enterococcus* should be added. Double coverage for *Pseudomonas* should also be considered if the infection is occurring in a hospitalized patient who is not responding to first-line therapy. If the patient does not respond to the initial antibiotic choice, then addition of fluoroquinolones and carbapenems should be considered along with antifungal coverage. Antibiotics

	Antibiotic Choice for Treatment of Acute Cholangitis	
Clinical Severity	**Antibiotic Selection**	**Duration of Treatment**
Mild (Community Acquired)	Pipericillin/tazobactam or ampicillin/ sulbactam	3–5 d
Moderate/Severe[a]	Pipericillin/tazobactam and metronidazole (first-line)	Minimum 7 d[b]
	Addition of carbapenems or fluoroquinolones, and Fluconazole if fail to respond clinically	
Hospital Acquired/ Resistant Organisms Anticipated[a]	Pipericillin/tazobactam and metronidazole (first-line)	Minimum 7 d[b]
	Addition of carbapenems or fluoroquinolones, and Fluconazole if fail to respond clinically	
	Addition of Vancomycin for methicillin resistant *S. aureus*, daptomycin for vancomycin-resistant *Enterococcus*, or additional anti-*Pseudomonas* coverage should also be considered	

[a]Antibiotic regimen should be narrowed once culture data are available.
[b]Course will be determined based upon clinical context and response to therapy.

should be continued a minimum of 7 days for moderate to severe cases of cholangitis; however, the clinical context, culture data, and response of the patient will ultimately dictate the choice and length of antibiotic course required (Table 22.2).

Drainage of the biliary tree is a central tenet to the treatment of ascending cholangitis, and must occur as soon as possible in a patient with sepsis secondary to ascending cholangitis. Thus, following administration of antibiotics and initiation of resuscitation and necessary supportive care, either endoscopic retrograde cholangiopancreatography (ERCP) or percutaneous transhepatic cholangiography (PTC) is the next step in management. If the patient presents with hemodynamic instability or respiratory compromise, then appropriate supportive management must be initiated prior to transporting the patient for a planned biliary drainage procedure. Endoscopic decompression is preferred; however, PTC drainage may be necessary if endoscopic decompression of the biliary tree is not possible. If a patient presents with a clinical picture of ascending cholangitis and has an indwelling biliary stent, then this stent and the biliary tree should be interrogated to ensure that there is complete drainage of the biliary system and that the stent is functioning and is not occluded. Plastic indwelling biliary stents require replacement approximately every 8 to 12 weeks (depending on stent diameter and number of stents) to prevent occlusion. Metal biliary stents (typically only placed in patients with biliary obstruction secondary to advanced malignancy) are larger in diameter and have a lower incidence of occlusion; however, sludge and stones can develop within and above these stents leading to the development of cholangitis. Endoscopic and percutaneous intervention is then required to achieve drainage of the biliary system. If the underlying cause of the cholangitis is choledocholithiasis, then clearance of the biliary system can also typically be accomplished with either endoscopic or percutaneous interventions to clear the common bile duct, or if a stone is impacted to drain the biliary tree either internally or externally with a biliary stent. Operative intervention is rarely the first-line therapy for biliary drainage as endoscopic and percutaneous drainage have lower morbidity and mortality and can usually be achieved in a timely manner. If, however, these modalities of biliary drainage are not available for a decompensating patient with severe ascending cholangitis, then operative decompression of the biliary tree should be pursued.

ACUTE CHOLECYSTITIS

Acute cholecystitis represents sudden inflammation of the gallbladder, and is typically associated with severe right upper quadrant pain, fever, and leukocytosis. Usually, this disease is secondary to cholelithiasis with the acute development of an impacted stone at Hartmann's pouch or the cystic duct in the majority of patients (90% to 95%). Acalculous cholecystitis presents in a similar manner to acute cholecystitis without gallstone involvement and usually occurs in critically ill patients representing approximately 10% of acute cholecystitis cases. Infected bile might play a role in the development of acute cholecystitis; however, many patients with acute cholecystitis do not have infected bile. Csendes et al. analyzed 467 patients with bile samples obtained for aerobic and anaerobic culture from healthy control patients and patients with various biliary diseases including acute cholecystitis, cholelithiasis, and gallbladder hydrops. Only 22% to 46% of patients with the included biliary diseases had a bile culture that was positive for aerobic or anaeroboic organisms. Healthy control patients had sterile bile as would be expected. The most common isolated organisms in the bile were *E. coli*, *Enterococcus* species, *Klebsiella*, and *Enterobacter*. Complications of acute cholecystitis include gallbladder empyema, perforation, and emphysematous cholecystitis. Clinically, any prolonged right upper quadrant pain associated with leukocytosis with or without fever should trigger an evaluation for cholecystitis. Abdominal ultrasound and radionuclide scintigraphy represent the two primary diagnostic tests to confirm the diagnosis. Ultrasound will show the presence of gallbladder wall thickening usually in the presence of gallstones with pericholecystic fluid, while radionuclide study will demonstrate uptake of the radiotracer by the liver with excretion into the common bile duct and duodenum within 1 to 2 hours *without* filling or visualization of the gallbladder. Failure to visualize the gallbladder with radionuclide tracer simply confirms obstruction of the cystic duct but does not confirm a diagnosis of acute cholecystitis. However, it can be useful for differentiating symptomatic cholelithiasis from cholecystitis in the setting of operative decision making.

If a diagnosis of acute cholecystitis is suspected, the role of antibiotic therapy is debated. Antibiotic therapy is not recommended beyond routine perioperative antibiotics for uncomplicated acute cholecystitis. The Infectious Disease Society of America currently recommends that antibiotics should be administered for acute cholecystitis in the setting of a leukocytosis exceeding 12,500 WBC/mm^3, fever greater than 38.5 C, suggestion of emphysematous cholecystitis manifest as evidence of air in the wall of the gallbladder, and in elderly, diabetic, or immunocompromised patients. These patients should receive intravenous antibiotics with piperacillin/tazobactam or a second- or third-generation cephalosporin with duration tailored to clinical improvement.

Laparoscopic cholecystectomy is typically performed as definitive management of acute cholecystitis unless the patient is felt to have prohibitive operative risk. In these high-risk patients, percutaneous cholecystostomy can be performed in radiology under ultrasound guidance and local anesthesia for management of their cholecystitis. Patients with uncomplicated acute cholecystitis who do not undergo definitive operative management will usually see resolution of their symptoms 5 to 7 days after presentation. Cholecystectomy is typically delayed in these settings to 6 weeks or greater following their initial presentation; however, this delay in intervention is associated with an increased conversion rate to an open procedure of approximately 15% to 20% in most recent series.

Acute cholecystitis can present with severe complications including gallbladder empyema, emphysematous cholecystitis, and perforation of the gallbladder. Gallbladder perforation is a rare occurrence (5%) in the setting of acute cholecystitis and can occur within a few days or few weeks of a patient's presentation with acute cholecystitis. Presenting symptoms of these serious complications are more severe than the usual presentation of acute cholecystitis, and prompt surgical intervention is mandatory to prevent significant morbidity or mortality.

CONCLUSIONS

Physical, chemical, and immunologic properties of the liver and biliary system characterize the host defense mechanisms protecting the hepatobiliary system from infectious organisms. Although infection is not often the primary cause of biliary tract disease, it is a common complication. Many patients with gallstones obstructing the biliary tree develop infectious complications caused by normal gastrointestinal flora such as *Enterobacteriaceae, Klebsiella, E. coli,* and *B. fragilis.* Local infection can result in cholangitis and pyogenic liver abscesses or invade the bloodstream causing bacteremia, septicemia or septic shock. Removing the underlying obstruction in the biliary tree is a prerequisite to successful therapy. Broad-spectrum antibiotics, covering both aerobes and anaerobes, are almost universally utilized. Acute cholecystitis and acute cholangitis can be a primary infection due to gallstones or could be a secondary event due to endoscopic, radiologic, or surgical instrumentation to the biliary tree. Treatment of systemic infection, resuscitation, and treatment of the underlying source of infection with either cholecystectomy or gallbladder drainage in the setting of acute cholecystitis or relief of biliary obstruction in the setting of acute cholangitis are critical to the successful treatment of patients presenting with these conditions.

Suggested Readings

Csendes A, Burdiles P, Maluenda F, et al. Simultaneous bacteriologic assessment of bile from gallbladder and common bile duct in control subjects and patients with gallstones and common duct stones. *Arch Surg* 1996;131(4):389–394.

Gurusamy KS, Naik P, Davidson BR. Methods of decreasing infection to improve outcomes after liver resections. *Cochrane Database Syst Rev* 2011;(11):CD006933. doi: 10.1002/14651858.CD006933.pub2.

IDSA. ISDA Guidelines. http://www.idsociety.org/idsa_practice_guidelines. 2013.

Kinney KP. Management of ascending cholangitis. *Gastrointest Endosc Clin N Am* 2007;17(2):289–306. Accessed date: April 1, 2014.

Lillemoe KD. Surgical treatment of biliary tract infections. *Am Surg* 2000;66(2):138–144.

Mazeh H, Mizrahi I, Dior U, et al. Role of antibiotic therapy in mild acute calculus cholecystitis: a prospective randomized controlled trial. *World J Surg* 2012;36(8): 1750–1759.

23

Gallbladder Disease

Henry A. Pitt

INTRODUCTION

Gallbladder disease is a major health problem throughout the world. In the United States, approximately 12% of the population or more than 30 million Americans have gallstones. Currently, in the United States, more than 750,000 cholecystectomies are performed annually, and the cost of caring for these patients is estimated to be between 7 and 10 million dollars per year. To properly manage these patients, surgeons should understand biliary physiology; the pathogenesis, incidence, risk factors, and natural history of gallstones; cholecystitis; and biliary dyskinesia. This chapter also reviews the diagnostic imaging and management options, as well as expected outcomes.

ETIOLOGY/PATHOGENESIS

Gallstones

Gallstones represent a failure to maintain biliary solutes, primarily cholesterol and calcium salts, in a liquid state. Gallstones are classified by their cholesterol content as either cholesterol or pigment stones. Pigment stones are further classified as either black or brown. Pure cholesterol gallstones are uncommon (10%) with most cholesterol stones containing calcium salts in their center, or nidus. In most Western populations, 70% to 80% of gallstones are cholesterol, and black pigment stones account for most of the remaining 20% to 30%. An important biliary precipitate in gallstone pathogenesis is biliary "sludge," which refers to a mixture of cholesterol crystals, calcium bilirubinate granules, and mucin gel matrix. Biliary sludge has been observed clinically in prolonged fasting states and with the use of long-term total parenteral nutrition (TPN). Both of these conditions also are associated with gallstone formation. The finding of macromolecular complexes of mucin and bilirubin, similar to biliary sludge in the central core of most cholesterol gallstones, suggests that sludge may serve as the nidus for gallstone growth.

Cholesterol Gallstones

The pathogenesis of cholesterol gallstones is multifactorial but may be considered to involve four factors: (a) cholesterol supersaturation in bile, (b) crystal nucleation, (c) gallbladder dysmotility, and (d) gallbladder absorption/secretion. For many years, gallstones were thought to result primarily from a defect in the hepatic secretion of biliary lipids. More recently, gallbladder motor and mucosal functions also have been demonstrated to play key roles in gallstone formation. Cholesterol solubility depends on the relative concentration of cholesterol, bile salts, and phospholipids. Present theory suggests that in states of excess cholesterol production, large cholesterol–phospholipid vesicles also exceed their capability to transport cholesterol, and crystal precipitation occurs. These cholesterol-rich vesicles aggregate to form large multilamellar liquid vesicles that then precipitate cholesterol monohydrate crystals. Several pronucleating factors including mucin glycoproteins, immunoglobulins, and transferrin accelerate the precipitation of cholesterol in bile.

For gallstones to cause clinical symptoms, they must obtain a size sufficient to produce a mechanical injury to the gallbladder or obstruction of the biliary tree. Growth of stones may occur in two ways: (a) progressive enlargement of individual crystals or stones or (b) fusion of individual crystals or stones to form a larger conglomerate (Fig. 23.1A). In addition, defects

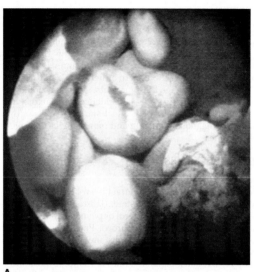

A

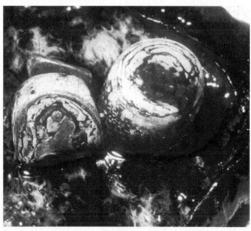

B

FIGURE 23.1 A. Pure cholesterol gallstones. **B.** Cholesterol gallstones with calcium.

(*Continued*)

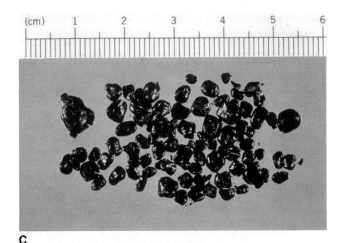

C

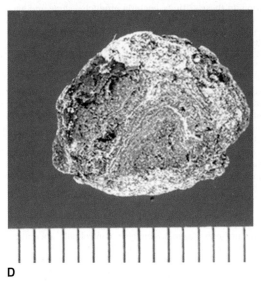

D

FIGURE 23.1 (Continued) C. Black pigment stones. **D.** Brown pigment stones.

in gallbladder motility increase the residence time of bile in the gallbladder, thereby playing a role in stone formation. Gallstone formation occurs in clinical states with gallbladder stasis, as seen with prolonged fasting, the use of long-term parenteral nutrition, after vagotomy, in diabetic patients, and in patients with somatostatin-producing tumors or in those receiving long-term somatostatin therapy.

The gallbladder is a very effective absorptive organ, and a normal function of the gallbladder is to concentrate and acidify bile. For many years, three factors have been thought to be key in cholesterol gallstone pathogenesis: cholesterol supersaturation, cholesterol crystallization, and biliary motility. However, a fourth factor, gallbladder absorption/secretion, also is key to gallstone formation. Alterations in sodium, chloride, bicarbonate, and water absorption/secretion alter the milieu for both cholesterol crystal formation and for calcium precipitation with various anions (Fig. 23.1B).

Pigment Gallstones

Precipitation of calcium with bilirubin, carbonate, phosphate, or palmitate as insoluble calcium salts serves as a nidus for cholesterol stone formation. Furthermore, calcium bilirubinate and calcium palmitate also form major components of pigment gallstones. Pigment gallstones are classified as either black or brown pigment stones. Black pigment stones are typically tarry and frequently are associated with hemolytic conditions or cirrhosis (Fig. 23.1C). In hemolytic states, the bilirubin load and concentration of unconjugated bilirubin increases. These stones usually are not associated with infected bile and are located almost exclusively in the gallbladder.

In contrast to black pigment stones, brown pigment stones are earthy in texture and are typically found in the bile ducts, especially in Asian populations (Fig. 23.1D). Brown stones often contain more cholesterol and calcium palmitate than black stones and occur as primary common duct stones in Western patients with disorders of biliary motility and associated bacterial infection. In these settings, bacteria producing slime and bacteria containing the enzyme glucuronidase cause enzymatic hydrolysis of soluble conjugated bilirubin glucuronide to form free bilirubin, which then precipitates with calcium.

Prevalence

Gallstones are uncommon in patients younger than age 20 years, but a sharp increase is noted, especially in women, with each decade to approximately 70 years. Approximately 20% of women and 10% of Western men have stones by age 60 years. In certain populations, such as Native Americans, the incidence is extremely high, especially in women. In Chileans and Bolivians of Indian ancestry, gallstones also are very common, and they are associated with a high incidence of gallbladder cancer. In the United States, the prevalence of stones is highest in Mexican American women (26%), and the prevalence in white women (17%) is higher than in black women (14%).

Risk Factors

Gallstones are more common in women, especially those who are obese, have had multiple pregnancies, are taking birth control pills, are undergoing rapid weight loss, or have elevated serum triglyceride levels. Diet plays an important role in cholesterol supersaturation, and these gallstones do not form in vegetarians. Cholesterol gallstones are common in populations consuming a Western diet, which is relatively high in overall calories as well as animal fats and carbohydrates. Diabetic patients also have an increased incidence of gallstones, which may be caused, in part, by alterations in gallbladder motor function and/or absorption/secretion. Gallstones also are known to occur more frequently in certain families. Current theory suggests that approximately 30% of the risk for gallstone formation is hereditary, whereas 70% is environmental, with diet being the primary environmental factor. As mentioned previously, prolonged fasting, TPN, ileal resection, vagotomy, hemolytic states, and cirrhosis are additional risk factors, and many of these factors lead to black pigment stone formation. Finally, bile duct stasis, as occurs with biliary strictures, congenital cysts, chronic pancreatitis, sclerosing cholangitis, and perivaterian duodenal diverticula, is the primary risk factor for brown pigment stone formation.

Degree of Symptoms	Symptoms Requiring Cholecystectomy	Complications of Gallstones
Asymptomatic	1%–2%/y	1%–2%/y
Mild symptoms	6%–8%/y	1%–3%/y
Symptomatic	5%–30%/y	7%/y

Natural History

An understanding of the natural history of gallstone disease is necessary for the appropriate management of patients with cholelithiasis. The presence or absence of symptoms remains the most important factor in the determination of the natural history of gallstones. Gallstone disease can be considered as a spectrum of clinical entities that includes asymptomatic gallstones, symptomatic gallstones, and complicated gallstone disease. The complications of gallstone disease include (a) acute cholecystitis, (b) choledocholithiasis with or without cholangitis, (c) gallstone pancreatitis, (d) gallstone ileus, and (e) gallbladder carcinoma.

Asymptomatic gallstones often are discovered at the time of laparotomy or during abdominal imaging for nonbiliary disease. The vast majority of patients with gallstones are asymptomatic. These stones remain in the gallbladder and do not obstruct the cystic duct. As a result, the gallbladder fills and empties normally, and the gallstones remain silent. However, asymptomatic gallstones can progress to symptomatic disease. Symptomatic gallstones usually present with what is termed *biliary colic*, right upper quadrant or epigastric abdominal pain that typically develops postprandially and may be associated with nausea and vomiting. The pain results from the impaction of a gallstone at the neck of the gallbladder or cystic duct.

Studies that have followed asymptomatic patients have shown that 20% to 30% of patients become symptomatic within 20 years. Approximately 1% to 2% of asymptomatic individuals with gallstones per year develop serious symptoms or complications related to their gallstones (Table 23.1). The longer stones remain silent, the less likely symptoms are to develop. In addition, almost all patients will develop symptomatic disease before developing one of the complications of gallstones. Therefore, prophylactic cholecystectomy generally is not indicated in patients with asymptomatic gallstones.

In select groups of patients, however, prophylactic cholecystectomy should be considered (Table 23.2). Children with gallstones almost always

Indications for Prophylactic Cholecystectomy

Pediatric gallstones
Congenital hemolytic anemia
Gallstones >2.5 cm in diameter
Calcified (porcelain) gallbladder
Long common channel
Bariatric surgery
Incidental gallstones found during intra-abdominal surgery
Solid organ transplantation
No access to medical care

develop symptoms and should be considered for early cholecystectomy. In patients with sickle cell disease, cholecystitis can precipitate a crisis with substantial operative risks. Therefore, these patients are best treated with elective cholecystectomy. A nonfunctioning gallbladder usually indicates advanced disease with more than 25% of these patients developing symptoms that require cholecystectomy. Large gallstones (>2.5 cm) are more frequently associated with acute cholecystitis and gallbladder carcinoma, and prophylactic cholecystectomy also may be indicated in these patients. The presence of a porcelain gallbladder (calcified gallbladder wall) is associated with a 5% to 10% risk of malignant transformation, and prophylactic cholecystectomy has been recommended for these patients. A long common channel between the bile and pancreatic ducts also is a significant risk for gallbladder cancer, and these patients should undergo prophylactic cholecystectomy. In obese patients in whom gallstones have already developed and who undergo bariatric surgery, cholecystectomy may be indicated because symptoms are likely to develop and may be difficult to distinguish from those caused by complications of the operation. Prophylactic cholecystectomy adds minimal morbidity and mortality risks to most bariatric operations and is clearly indicated in patients with gallstones. Finally, acute cholecystitis is a potentially life-threatening condition in immunosuppressed patients. For this reason, prophylactic cholecystectomy has been recommended prior to solid organ transplantation.

Patients with mild symptoms (intermittent biliary colic) are at higher risk for developing gallstone-related complications than asymptomatic patients who have gallstones (Table 23.1). Approximately 1% to 3% of mildly symptomatic patients per year will develop gallstone-related complications, and at least 6% to 8% per year will require a cholecystectomy to manage their gallbladder symptoms. The diagnosis of symptomatic gallstones requires the presence of characteristic symptoms and the documentation of gallstones on diagnostic imaging.

Cholecystitis

Chronic Cholecystitis

The term *chronic cholecystitis* implies an ongoing or recurrent inflammatory process involving the gallbladder. In more than 90% of patients, gallstones are the causative factor and lead to recurrent episodes of cystic duct obstruction manifest as biliary pain or colic. Over time, these recurrent attacks can result in scarring and a nonfunctioning gallbladder. Histopathologically, chronic cholecystitis is characterized by an increase in subepithelial and subserosal fibrosis and a mononuclear cell infiltrate. The primary symptom associated with chronic cholecystitis or symptomatic cholelithiasis is pain, often labeled *biliary colic*. The pain is usually located in the right upper quadrant and/or epigastrium and frequently radiates to the right upper back, right scapula, or between the scapulae. Other symptoms such as nausea and vomiting often accompany each episode. The physical examination is usually completely normal in patients with chronic cholecystitis, particularly if they are pain-free. During an episode of biliary colic, mild right upper quadrant tenderness may be present. Laboratory values such as serum bilirubin, transaminases, and alkaline phosphatase usually are normal in patients with uncomplicated gallstones.

Acute Cholecystitis

Acute cholecystitis is the most common complication of gallstones occurring in 15% to 20% of patients with symptomatic disease. As in biliary colic, acute cholecystitis results from a stone impaction at the gallbladder–cystic duct junction (Fig. 23.2A). The extent of inflammation and the progression of acute

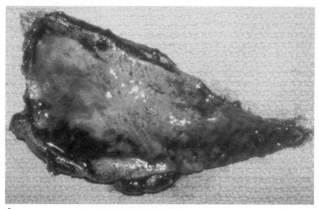

A

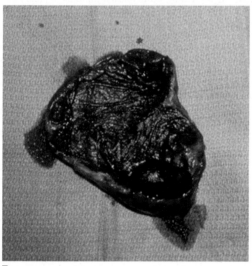

B

FIGURE 23.2 A. Acutely inflamed, edematous gallbladder with solitary pigment stone obstructing the cystic duct. **B.** Gangrenous cholecystitis with solitary black pigment stone.

cholecystitis are related to the duration and degree of obstruction. In the most severe cases (5% to 18%), this process can lead to ischemia and necrosis of the gallbladder wall (Fig. 23.2B). More frequently, the gallstone is dislodged, and the inflammation gradually subsides. Acute cholecystitis is primarily an inflammation and not an infectious process with bacterial infection appearing as a secondary event. Approximately 50% of patients with acute cholecystitis will have positive bile cultures, with *Escherichia coli* being the most common organism.

Patients with acute cholecystitis typically present with right upper quadrant pain that is similar to that of biliary colic. In acute cholecystitis, however, the pain is usually unremitting, may last several days, and is often associated with nausea, emesis, anorexia, and fever. On physical examination, patients with acute cholecystitis usually have a low-grade fever and exhibit localized right upper quadrant tenderness and guarding. The presence of Murphy sign, an inspiratory arrest during deep palpation of the right upper quadrant, is the classic physical finding of acute chole-cystitis. A palpable right upper quadrant mass is appreciated in one-third of patients and usually represents omentum that has migrated to the area around the gallbladder in response to the inflammation. Severe jaundice is rare, but mild jaundice may be present in up to 30% of patients. Severe jaun-dice suggests the presence of CBD stones, cholangitis, or Mirizzi syndrome, obstruction of the common hepatic duct by severe pericholecystic inflam-mation resulting from impaction of a large stone in the Hartmann pouch. Laboratory evaluation can show a mild leukocytosis (white blood cell [WBC] count 12,000 to 15,000 cells/mm³). However, many patients have a normal WBC. A white cell count greater than 20,000 should suggest further complications of cholecystitis, such as gangrene, perforation, or cholangitis.

Biliary Dyskinesia

A subgroup of patients presenting with typical symptoms of biliary colic (postprandial right upper quadrant pain, fatty food intolerance, and nau-sea) will not have any evidence of gallstones on ultrasound examination. The vast majority of these patients are women who frequently are over-weight or obese. Experimental work suggests that excess fat and cytokines in the gallbladder wall (steatocholecystitis) may be the underlying cause for this phenomenon. Many of these gallbladders are enlarged at rest sug-gesting that a defect in absorption/secretion may be a contributing factor.

Further investigations usually are performed in these patients to exclude any other pathology. This workup often includes an abdominal computed tomography (CT) scan, an esophagogastroduodenoscopy, or even an endoscopic retrograde cholangiogram. In these patients, the diag-nosis of biliary dyskinesia or chronic acalculous cholecystitis should be considered. The cholecystokinin-Tc-HIDA scan has been useful in identify-ing patients with this disorder. Cholecystokinin (CCK) is infused intrave-nously, and the gallbladder ejection fraction (EF) is calculated. An EF of less than 35% at 20 minutes is considered abnormal.

DIAGNOSTIC IMAGING

Abdominal X-Rays

In general, plain abdominal x-rays have a low yield in diagnosing biliary tract problems. Plain films are most useful in diagnosing other causes of acute abdominal pain such as a perforated viscus or a bowel obstruction. Only approximately 15% of gallstones contain sufficient calcium to appear radi-opaque on a plain x-ray. Rarely, abdominal films may show a calcified gall-bladder wall or pneumobilia that may aid in the diagnosis of biliary disease.

Ultrasound

Transabdominal ultrasound is the radiologic procedure of choice for identify-ing gallstones and bile duct dilation. Ultrasound is noninvasive, inexpensive, and widely available. Patients should receive nothing by mouth for several hours prior to performing an ultrasound examination so that the gallblad-der is fully distended. Gallstones create echoes that are reflected back to the ultrasound probe. The ultrasound waves cannot penetrate the stones, and therefore, acoustic shadowing is seen posterior to the stones (Fig. 23.3). In addition, gallstones that are free floating in the gallbladder will move to a dependent position when the patient is repositioned during scanning. When

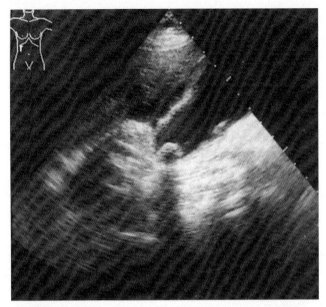

FIGURE 23.3 Gallbladder ultrasound with solitary stone with acoustic shadowing.

these two features are present, the accuracy of ultrasound at diagnosing gallstones approaches 100%. Echoes without shadows may be caused by gallbladder polyps. However, the majority of "polyps" are really small gallstones that are attached to the mucus gel.

Several features lower the diagnostic accuracy of ultrasound in detecting gallstones. Small gallstones may not demonstrate an acoustic shadow. A lack of fluid (bile) around the gallstones (stone impacted in the cystic duct, gallbladder filled with gallstones) also impairs their detection. In addition, an ileus with increased abdominal gas, as occurs with acute cholecystitis, will hamper gallbladder visualization. Overall, the false-negative rate for ultrasound in detecting gallstones is approximately 5% but may increase to 15% with acute cholecystitis.

Cholescintigraphy

Cholescintigraphy provides a noninvasive evaluation of the liver, gallbladder, bile duct, and duodenum with both anatomic and functional information. [99m]Technetium-labeled iminodiacetic acid derivatives (hepatic 2, 6-dimethyl-iminodiacetic acid [HIDA], diisopropylacetanilidoiminodiacetic acid, or p-isopropylacetanilido imidodiacetic acid) are injected intravenously, rapidly extracted from the blood, and excreted into the bile. These radionuclide scans provide functional information about the liver's ability to excrete radiolabeled substances into a nonobstructed biliary tree. Uptake by the liver, gallbladder, common bile duct (CBD), and duodenum should all be present after 1 hour. Slow uptake of the tracer by the liver suggests hepatic parenchymal disease. Filling of the gallbladder and CBD with delayed or absent filling of the intestine suggests an obstruction at the ampulla.

The primary use of cholescintigraphy is in the diagnosis of acute cholecystitis. Although used less frequently for this indication because of the

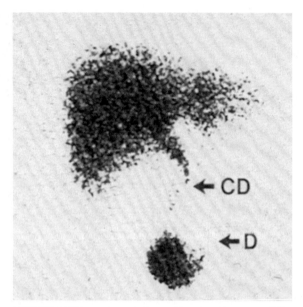

FIGURE 23.4 HIDA scan demonstrating good hepatic uptake, a patent CBD (*CD*), and visualization of the duodenum (*D*). This scan is "positive" for acute cholecystitis because the gallbladder is not visualized.

availability and accuracy of ultrasound, cholescintigraphy demonstrates the presence of cystic duct obstruction, which is invariably present in acute cholecystitis. Nonvisualization of the gallbladder 1 hour after the injection of the radioisotope with filling of the CBD and duodenum is consistent with total or partial cystic duct obstruction and acute cholecystitis (Fig. 23.4). The sensitivity and specificity of cholescintigraphy for diagnosing acute cholecystitis are each about 95%. False-positive results are increased in the setting of gallbladder stasis as in critically ill patients or in those receiving parenteral nutrition.

Computerized Tomography/Magnetic Resonance Imaging

Abdominal CT is less sensitive in diagnosing gallstones than ultrasound. Calcified gallstones are visualized in approximately 50% of patients. The role of CT scanning is primarily limited to the diagnosis of complications of gallstone disease such as acute cholecystitis (gallbladder wall thickening, pericholecystic fluid), gallbladder perforations, choledocholithiasis (intrahepatic and extrahepatic bile duct dilation), pancreatitis (pancreatic edema and inflammation), and gallbladder cancer (Fig. 23.5). Magnetic resonance imaging (MRI) also has been shown to be highly sensitive in the diagnosis of both gallstones and common duct stones when T2-weighted images are obtained. Both MRI and CT are much more expensive than ultrasound and, therefore, are not cost-effective for the initial evaluation of gallbladder disease.

MANAGEMENT

Chronic Cholecystitis

The operative management of gallstones has been the standard of care over the past 140 years. Cholecystectomy is the most common

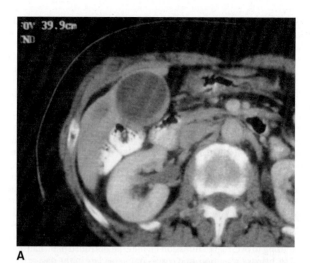

A

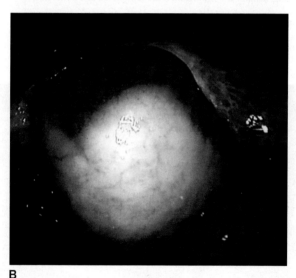

B

FIGURE 23.5 A. CT scan demonstrating a thickened gallbladder wall secondary to cancer. Note the low-density area in the adjacent liver due to metastatic disease. **B.** Laparoscopic appearance of the gallbladder in the same patient. Note that the gallbladder wall is white with neovascularization.

gastrointestinal operation performed in the United States. Since the introduction of laparoscopic cholecystectomy in the late 1980s, the number of cholecystectomies performed in the United States has increased from approximately 500,000 to 750,000 per year. Symptomatic cholelithiasis is the main indication for laparoscopic cholecystectomy. Relative contraindications to laparoscopic cholecystectomy include the inability of the patient to withstand a general anesthetic, severe bleeding disorders, and end-stage liver disease. In addition, patients with severe chronic obstructive pulmonary disease or congestive heart failure may not tolerate the pneumoperitoneum required for performing laparoscopic surgery. Morbid obesity, once thought to be a relative contraindication to the laparoscopic approach, is not associated with a higher conversion rate. Longer trocars and instruments and an increase in intra-abdominal pressure may be helpful in these patients. Prior upper abdominal surgery may increase the difficulty but rarely precludes laparoscopic cholecystectomy. Elective laparoscopic cholecystectomy also has been completed safely in patients with well-compensated cirrhosis (Child class A and B), although difficulty retracting the firm liver and increased bleeding from collaterals have been noted.

Conversion to an open cholecystectomy is required in less than 3% of patients undergoing laparoscopic cholecystectomy for chronic cholecystitis. Conversion rates are increased in male and elderly patients. Elective laparoscopic cholecystectomy can be safely performed as an outpatient procedure (Fig. 23.6). Among patients selected for outpatient management, 75% to 95% of patients can be successfully discharged the same day. Factors contributing to overnight admission include uncontrolled pain, nausea and vomiting, urinary retention, and cases completed late in the day.

Acute Cholecystitis
Once the diagnosis of acute cholecystitis is made, the patient should be given nothing by mouth, and intravenous hydration should begin. A nasogastric tube is placed if persistent nausea and vomiting or abdominal

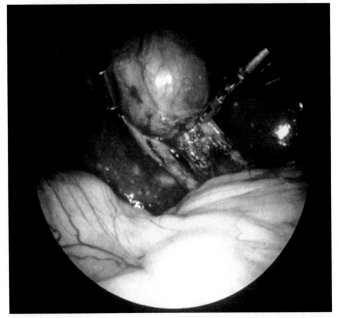

FIGURE 23.6 Laparoscopic appearance of a minimally invasive diseased gallbladder, which contained symptomatic gallstones.

distention are present. In almost all cases, broad-spectrum antibiotics, such as a broad-spectrum penicillin, should be started and maintained into the immediate postoperative period. Parenteral analgesia also should be administered. Unfortunately, narcotics increase biliary pressure, whereas nonsteroidal analgesics, which inhibit prostaglandin synthesis, reduce gallbladder mucin production and, therefore, reduce pressure and pain.

The treatment of choice for acute cholecystitis is cholecystectomy. Open cholecystectomy had been the standard treatment for acute cholecystitis for many years. Initially, acute cholecystitis was felt to be a contraindication to laparoscopic cholecystectomy. As experience has increased, however, laparoscopic cholecystectomy clearly can be performed safely in the setting of acute cholecystitis. However, the conversion rate in the setting of acute cholecystitis (10% to 20%) is higher than with chronic cholecystitis. In prospective, randomized trials, length of hospital stay and time to return to work have been lower in patients undergoing early as opposed to late laparoscopic cholecystectomy. In addition, randomized trials, population studies, and cost–utility analyses have shown that early laparoscopic cholecystectomy (within 3 days of symptom onset) can be accomplished with a similar morbidity and mortality rate and lower cost than with delayed cholecystectomy. No significant differences were observed in the conversion rate to open cholecystectomy among patients undergoing early cholecystectomy versus those managed with delayed surgery. In addition, approximately 20% of patients in whom delayed surgery is planned require an operation during the initial admission or before the end of the planned cooling off period. Moreover, a recent Canadian propensity score analysis demonstrated that patients undergoing early surgery had a lower incidence of major bile duct injuries as well as reduced mortality.

In certain high-risk patients whose medical condition precludes cholecystectomy, a cholecystostomy can be performed for acute cholecystitis. In this setting, percutaneous gallbladder drainage usually can be accomplished. In most cases, prompt improvement is seen after gallbladder drainage and appropriate antibiotics. However, patients must be observed closely, and if improvement does not occur within 24 hours, laparotomy is indicated. Failure to improve after percutaneous cholecystostomy is usually caused by gangrene of the gallbladder or perforation. After the acute episode resolves, the patient can undergo either cholecystectomy or percutaneous stone extraction and removal of the cholecystostomy tube. The latter is an option in elderly or debilitated patients for whom a general anesthetic is contraindicated.

Severe Cholecystitis

Several complications of acute cholecystitis are recognized in clinical practice. These complications include empyema of the gallbladder, emphysematous cholecystitis, gangrene, perforation, and cholecystoenteric fistula. All of these complications are associated with significant morbidity and mortality and, therefore, require prompt surgical intervention.

Empyema

Gallbladder empyema is a rare advanced stage of cholecystitis with bacterial invasion of the gallbladder and actual pus in the lumen (Fig. 23.7). Patients present with severe right upper quadrant pain, high-grade fever, rigors, and significant leukocytosis and mild elevations of bilirubin (2 to 3 mg/dL). Sepsis, including cardiovascular collapse, may be seen. Treatment consists of broad-spectrum antibiotics, including anaerobic coverage, and emergent cholecystectomy or cholecystostomy. However, cholecystostomy may not be adequate to relieve sepsis in patients with empyema of the gallbladder.

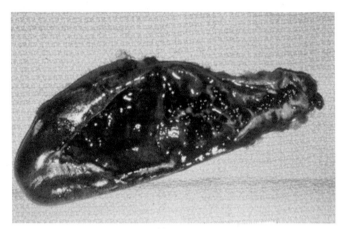

FIGURE 23.7 Empyema of the gallbladder. Note the thickened, inflamed wall and pus around the multiple pigment stones.

Emphysematous Cholecystitis

Emphysematous cholecystitis is another uncommon (1%) form of acute cholecystitis, which develops more frequently in males and in patients with diabetes mellitus. Only half of these patients have gallstones, but the majority (75%) have a gangrenous gallbladder with (20%) or without perforation (Fig. 23.8A). Severe right upper quadrant pain and generalized sepsis are frequently present. Abdominal films or CT scans may demonstrate air within the gallbladder wall or lumen (Fig. 23.8B). Prompt antibiotic therapy to cover the common biliary pathogens, including *E. coli*, *Enterococcus*, *Klebsiella*, as well as *Clostridia* species, and emergency cholecystectomy are appropriate treatments.

Gangrene/Perforation

Gangrene of the gallbladder, another rare complication, occurs when the wall becomes ischemic and leads to perforation. Again, only 50% of these patients have gallstones, and many are diabetic. Gangrene is more likely in a number of clinical situations including ruptured abdominal aortic aneurysms, following cardiac surgery, and in patients with burns, trauma, and a long intensive care unit stay as well as in patients requiring TPN. Gallbladder perforation occurs in 5% to 10% of patients with acute cholecystitis and can be categorized as either localized or free. Localized perforation generally results in the formation of a pericholecystic abscess as the omentum walls off the perforation and limits it to the right upper quadrant (Fig. 23.9A). Free perforation is less frequent (1% of cases) and occurs if the omentum is unable to wall off the inflammatory process. Free perforation results in the spilling of bile into the peritoneal cavity and a generalized peritonitis. Perforation should be suspected if the patient's clinical course deteriorates. Evidence for perforation includes an increase in pain and tenderness, fever and chills, elevation in WBC count, and hypotension. These patients require aggressive fluid resuscitation, antibiotics, and emergent operative exploration (Fig. 23.9B). Cholecystostomy usually will not be adequate therapy for patients with gangrene or perforation of the gallbladder.

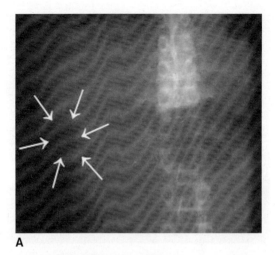

A

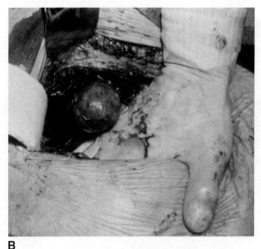

B

FIGURE 23.8 A. Plain abdominal x-ray with a round gas pattern (*arrows*) in the right upper quadrant. **B.** Open cholecystectomy in this patient demonstrating a gangrenous gallbladder fundus.

Cholecystoenteric Fistula

In 1% to 2% of patients with acute cholecystitis, the gallbladder will perforate into an adjacent hollow viscus. The duodenum (75% to 80%) and the hepatic flexure of the colon (15% to 20%) are the most common sites. Generally, after the fistula forms, the episode of acute cholecystitis resolves as the gallbladder spontaneously decompresses. If a large gallstone passes from the gallbladder into the small intestine, a mechanical bowel obstruction may result, which is termed gallstone ileus. Gallstone ileus occurs in 10% to 15% of patients with a cholecystoenteric

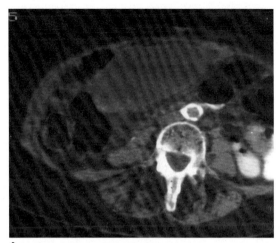

A

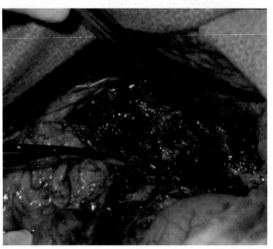

B

FIGURE 23.9 A. CT scan demonstrating a very enlarged gallbladder with a thickened wall. **B.** At surgery, this patient had a localized pericholecystic abscess. This picture demonstrates the area after gallbladder removal and abscess evacuation.

fistula. Patients with gallstone ileus present with signs and symptoms of intestinal obstruction—nausea, vomiting, and abdominal pain. The pain may be episodic and recurrent as the impacted stone temporarily impacts in the gut lumen and then dislodges and moves distally (tumbling obstruction). A history of gallstone-related symptoms (right upper quadrant pain) may only be present in 50% of these patients. Abdominal films will demonstrate small bowel distension and air–fluid levels and may give additional clues to the source of the obstruction (pneumobilia or a calcified gallstone distant from the gallbladder) (Fig. 23.10A).

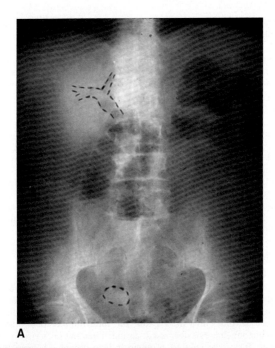

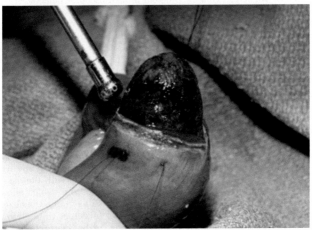

FIGURE 23.10 A. Gallstone ileus. Note air in the biliary tree (*upper right*), air–fluid levels (*middle*), and large calcified gallstone (*lower right*). **B.** At surgery, in this patient, a large gallstone was found to be obstructing the distal ileum.

The site of obstruction is most frequently in the narrowest part of the small intestine (ileum) or large intestine (sigmoid colon).

The initial management of gallstone ileus includes relieving the obstruction. Most frequently, this goal can be achieved by removing the gall-stone through an enterotomy (Fig. 23.10B). Additional gallstones should be sought as recurrent obstruction has been reported in up to 10% of patients with gallstone ileus. Takedown of the biliary–enteric fistula and cholecystectomy may be warranted as recurrent cholecystitis and cholangitis are common in patients with a biliary–enteric fistula, and gallbladder cancer has been reported in 15% of these patients. However, in patients with a significant inflammatory process in the right upper quadrant or who are unstable to withstand a prolonged operative procedure, the fistula should be addressed at a second laparotomy.

Mirizzi Syndrome

The Mirizzi syndrome is a rare form of gallbladder disease that usually presents with pain, jaundice, and/or cholangitis. Two types have been described. In type I, a large stone becomes impacted in the cystic duct on the Hartmann pouch (Fig. 23.11A). In these patients, partial cholecystectomy with "repair" of the bile duct with or without a T-tube may be possible. In type II patients, the stone erodes into the common hepatic and CBD (Fig. 23.11B). Usually, a Roux-en-Y hepaticojejunostomy is required to repair this situation.

OUTCOMES

Chronic Cholecystitis

Serious complications of laparoscopic cholecystectomy are rare, and the mortality rate is less than 0.3%. As cholecystectomy rates have risen, however, the total number of deaths has not decreased. Although the increase in cholecystectomy rates means that the total number of deaths from cholecystectomy has not decreased, an individual patient's risk for death is smaller. The single greatest problem in laparoscopic cholecystectomy is biliary injury. The incidence of major bile duct injury following laparoscopic cholecystectomy is between 0.3% and 0.6%, but if all bile leaks are considered, the injury rate in these reports ranges from 0.6% to 1.5%, which is three to four times the injury rate at open surgery. Major vascular injuries to the hepatic arteries, especially the right hepatic artery, may occur in association with biliary injuries and sometimes lead to intraoperative blood loss. Vasculobiliary injuries may complicate the management and prognosis of these patients.

Spillage of stones into the peritoneal cavity during laparoscopic cholecystectomy occurs in 10% or more of cases. Leaving stones in the peritoneal cavity may not be innocuous. Intra-abdominal abscess, subcutaneous abscess, and later discharge of stones through the abdominal wall or through the lung and trachea have all been described. Every attempt should be made to remove spilled stones by picking and irrigating them out. Clearance is usually quite successful with the use of retractors to lift the liver and the 30-degree laparoscope, which allows the depths of the recess between the liver and kidney to be visualized. Laparoscopic ultrasonography may be useful to detect these stones. Large stones or massive spills should be cleaned up by laparotomy if necessary. If concern exists that stones have been left behind, the patient should be informed.

A gallbladder containing an unsuspected cancer is excised one to three times per 1,000 laparoscopic cholecystectomies. Older patients and those requiring an open cholecystectomy (planned or converted) are at greater risk. Therefore, a good practice is to open the gallbladder and inspect it and to obtain frozen sections if a suspect lesion is observed. If cancer is suspected, the gallbladder should be extracted in an impermeable bag. If a cancer is discovered, further surgery may be indicated.

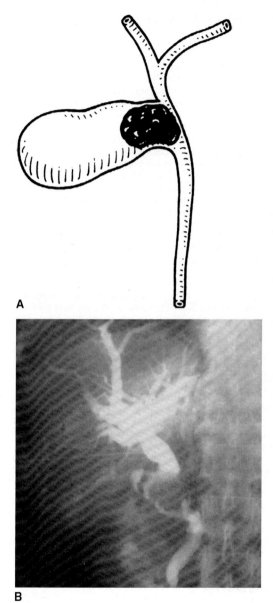

A

B

FIGURE 23.11 A. Mirizzi type II schematic. **B.** Mirizzi type II cholangiogram with a large stone eroded into the CBD.

The long-term results of laparoscopic cholecystectomy in appropriately selected patients with chronic cholecystitis are excellent. More than 90% of patients with typical biliary pain and gallstones are symptom-free following cholecystectomy. Results of open cholecystectomy are slightly worse because a small percentage of patients have persistent incisional pain. For patients with atypical symptoms or painless dyspepsia (fatty food intolerance, flatulence, belching, or bloating), the percentage of patients experiencing relief of symptoms decreases. Between 80% and 90% of patients with a low gallbladder ejection fraction and symptoms of biliary colic will be asymptomatic or improved by cholecystectomy. Most of these patients have histopathologic evidence of chronic cholecystitis. Over the past 15 years, the percentage of patients undergoing cholecystectomy for acalculous cholecystitis (biliary dyskinesia) in the United States has increased from less than 5% to more than 20% of patients having their gallbladder removed. This change parallels the obesity epidemic and may be due to abnormal gallbladder emptying as well as absorption/secretion due to fat within the gallbladder wall (cholecystosteatosis).

Acute Cholecystitis

In general, the results of patients undergoing cholecystectomy for acute cholecystitis also are quite good. As outlined above, early surgery is recommended for most patients with acute cholecystitis and is associated with fewer bile duct injuries and less mortality. On the other hand, in the small subset of patients with severe cholecystitis, the risk of hospital mortality is dramatically increased. Patients with emphysematous cholecystitis and those with gangrene or perforation of the gallbladder have a 10% to 15% mortality. Severe sepsis with associated organ failure is clearly life threatening in older, frail patients as well as those with ruptured aneurysms, recent cardiac surgery, burns, or trauma.

CONCLUSIONS

Gallbladder disease is a very common health care problem. Considerable knowledge exists regarding the etiology and pathogenesis of gallstones and biliary dyskinesia. However, strategies to prevent stones, other than diet, have not been developed. In addition, nonoperative methods to dissolve or remove gallstones have not been successful. The fact that laparoscopic cholecystectomy is quite safe and that the majority of patients undergoing this procedure can be managed as an outpatient has thwarted nonoperative challenges. In addition, with laparoscopic cholecystectomy, patients return to work quickly, and in the vast majority, the long-term quality of life is quite good. Moreover, following the introduction of laparoscopic cholecystectomy, the percentage of patients presenting with acute cholecystitis and choledocholithiasis has reduced because the threshold for patients to have their gallbladder removed has lowered. However, approximately 8% to 10% of patients still present with complex gallbladder disease that may require an open cholecystectomy and/or more complex biliary procedures.

Suggested Readings

Al-Azzawi HH, Nakeeb A, Saxena R, et al. Cholecystosteatosis: an explanation for increased cholecystectomy rates. *J Gastrointest Surg* 2007;11(7):835–843.

Doty JE, Pitt HA, Kuchenbecker SL, et al. Impaired gallbladder emptying prior to gallstone formation in the prairie dog. *Gastroenterology* 1983;85,168–174.

Friedman GD, Raviola CA, Fireman B. Prognosis of gallstones with mild or no symptoms: 25 years of follow-up in a health maintenance organization. *J Clin Epidemiol* 1989;42:127–134.

Gutt CN, Encke J, Koninger J, et al. Acute cholecystitis: early versus delayed cholecystectomy: a multicenter randomized trial. *Ann Surg* 2013;258:385–397.

de Mestral C, Rostein O, Laupacis A, et al. Comparative operative outcomes of early and delayed cholecystectomy for acute cholecystitis. *Ann Surg* 2014;259:10–15.

Nakeeb A, Comuzzie AG, Martin L, et al. Gallstones: genetics versus environment. *Ann Surg* 2002;235:842–847.

Pitt HA. Patient value is superior with early surgery for acute cholecystitis. *Ann Surg* 2014;259:16–17.

Ravikumar R, Williams JG. The operative management of gallstone ileus. *Ann R Coll Surg Engl* 2010;92:279–284.

Schmidt GH, Hausken T, Glambek I, et al. A 24-year controlled follow-up of patients with silent gallstones showed no long-term risk of symptomatic or adverse events leading to cholecystectomy. *Scan J Gastroenterol* 2001;46:949–54.

Stephen AE, McFadden DW, Cortina GR, et al. Porcelain gallbladder is not associated with gallbladder carcinoma. *Am Surgeon* 2001;67:7–11.

Stinton LM, Myers RP, Shaffer EA. Epidemiology of gallstones. *Gastroenterol Clin North Am* 2010;39:157–175.

Strasberg SM, Brunt LM. Rationale and use of the critical view in laparoscopic cholecystectomy. *Am J Surg* 1993;165:655–60.

Strasberg SM. Clinical practice. Acute calculus cholecystitis. *N Engl J Med* 2008;358: 2804–2811.

Swartz-Basile DA, Lu D, Basile DP, et al. Leptin regulates gallbladder genes related to absorption and secretion. *Am J Physiol* 2007;293:84–89.

Takada T, Strasberg SM, Solomkin JS, et al. Updated Tokyo guidelines for the management of acute cholecystitis and cholangitis. *J Hepatobiliary Pancreat Sci* 2013;20:1–7.

24

Sphincter of Oddi Dysfunction

Evan L. Fogel

INTRODUCTION

Since its original description by Ruggero Oddi in 1887, the sphincter of Oddi (SO) has been the subject of much study and controversy. Its very existence as a distinct entity has been disputed. It is therefore not surprising that the clinical syndrome of sphincter of Oddi dysfunction (SOD) and its therapy are controversial areas. Nevertheless, SOD is commonly diagnosed and treated by physicians. This chapter reviews the epidemiology and clinical presentation of SOD and currently available diagnostic and therapeutic modalities.

Postcholecystectomy pain resembling the patient's preoperative biliary colic occurs in at least 10% to 20% of patients. These patients should have appropriate noninvasive and invasive (when indicated) evaluation to rule out common bile duct stones, tumors, or strictures near the cholecystectomy site. The residual group of patients has a high frequency of SOD. SOD refers to an abnormality of SO contractility. It is a benign, noncalculous obstruction to flow of bile or pancreatic juice through the pancreaticobiliary junction (i.e., the SO) resulting from a dyskinetic or stenotic sphincter. SOD may be manifested clinically by "pancreaticobiliary" pain, pancreatitis, abnormal liver tests, or abnormal pancreatic enzymes. SO dyskinesia refers to a motor abnormality of the SO, which may result in a hypotonic sphincter but, more commonly, causes a hypertonic sphincter. In contrast, SO stenosis refers to a structural alteration of the sphincter, probably from an inflammatory process, with subsequent fibrosis. Because it is often impossible to distinguish patients with SO dyskinesia from those with SO stenosis, the term SOD has been used to incorporate both groups of patients. A clinical classification system has been developed for patients with suspected biliary or pancreatic SOD based on clinical history, laboratory results, and endoscopic retrograde cholangiopancreatography (ERCP) findings (Tables 24.1 and 24.2). A variety of less accurate terms—such as papillary stenosis, ampullary stenosis, biliary dyskinesia, and postcholecystectomy syndrome—are listed in the medical literature to describe this entity. The latter term is somewhat of a misnomer because SOD may clearly occur with an intact gallbladder.

EPIDEMIOLOGY

SOD most commonly occurs in middle-aged females, although patients of any age or sex may be affected. Although SOD typically is seen in the postcholecystectomy state, it may occur with the gallbladder in situ. The epidemiology of SOD is unclear due to a paucity of population-based data and the considerable variation that exists in currently published literature, including patient selection criteria, definition of SOD used, and whether or not one or both sphincter segments are studied by sphincter of Oddi

| **TABLE 24.1** | Modified Milwaukee Classification for Biliary Sphincter of Oddi Dysfunction, Postcholecystectomy |

Biliary Type 1
Patients with biliary-type pain, abnormal ALT or alkaline phosphatase greater than two times normal, and dilated common bile duct (CBD) >12 mm diameter
Biliary Type II
Patients with biliary-type pain and one of either abnormal ALT or alkaline phosphatase greater than two times normal OR dilated CBD >12 mm
Biliary Type III
Patients with only biliary-type pain and no other abnormalities

---

manometry (SOM). Eversman et al. performed SOM of both the biliary and pancreatic sphincter segments in 360 patients with intact sphincters. In this series, 19% had abnormal pancreatic basal sphincter pressure alone, 11% had abnormal biliary basal sphincter pressure, and 31% had abnormal basal sphincter pressure in both segments (total 61% with abnormal SOM). A more recent 14-year review of patients undergoing evaluation with SOM at our institution identified SOD in 65% of patients. These and other studies highlight the need to evaluate both the bile duct and pancreatic duct during SOM. Sphincter dysfunction may also cause recurrent pancreatitis, and manometrically documented SOD has been reported in 15% to 72% of patients previously labeled as having idiopathic pancreatitis.

PATHOGENESIS AND PATHOLOGY

The SO is a complex of smooth muscles that surrounds the terminal common bile duct, ventral pancreatic duct, and the common channel (ampulla of Vater) if present (Fig. 24.1). Its primary role is to regulate bile and pancreatic juice flow and to prevent reflux of duodenal contents into the sterile biliary and pancreatic systems. The SO has both a variable basal pressure and phasic contractile activity, which are under both neural and hormonal control. Patients with type I SOD are thought to have a stenotic sphincter rather than a sphincter in spasm, as pathologic series of sphincteroplasty resection specimens have shown significant inflammation, reactive muscular hypertrophy, and fibrosis within the papillary zone in 60% of patients. These pathophysiologic changes at the sphincter papillary orifice are likely responsible for ductal hypertension with resultant duct dilation, elevated liver enzymes, and biliary-type pain in patients with type I SOD. In patients

| **TABLE 24.2** | Modified Pancreatic Classification System for Sphincter of Oddi Dysfunction |

Pancreatic Type 1
Patients with pancreatic-type pain, abnormal amylase or lipase >1.5 times normal on any occasion, and dilated pancreatic duct (PD) >6 mm diameter in the head or 5 mm in the body
Pancreatic Type II
Patients with pancreatic-type pain and only one of abnormal amylase or lipase >1.5 times normal on any occasion OR dilated PD >6 mm diameter in the head or 5 mm in the body
Pancreatic Type III
Patients with only pancreatic-type pain and no other abnormalities

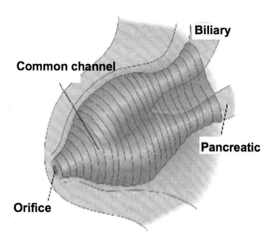

FIGURE 24.1 The sphincter of Oddi.

with type II and III SOD, the mechanism of dysfunction is not related to sphincter inflammation and scarring but is thought to be related to dysregulation of stimulatory and/or inhibitory factors.

How does SOD cause pain? From a theoretical point of view, this may be related to (a) impedance of flow of bile and pancreatic juice resulting in ductal hypertension, (b) muscular ischemia of the sphincter arising from spastic contractions, and (c) hypersensitivity of the papilla and/or duodenum. These mechanisms may potentially act alone or in concert to explain the genesis of pain.

CLINICAL PRESENTATION

The Rome III classification system has provided diagnostic criteria for SOD (Table 24.3). Abdominal pain is the most common presenting symptom. The pain is usually localized to the epigastric area or right upper quadrant, may radiate to the back or shoulder, and lasts anywhere from 30 minutes to several hours. Pain may be precipitated by food or narcotics and often is accompanied by nausea and vomiting. The pain may begin several years after cholecystectomy and is usually similar in character to the pain that initially prompted gallbladder evaluation. Alternatively, patients may have continued pain that was not relieved by cholecystectomy. Jaundice, fever, or chills are rarely observed. Physical examination typically is negative or reveals only mild abdominal tenderness. The pain is not relieved by trial medications for acid peptic disease or irritable bowel syndrome. Laboratory abnormalities consisting of transient elevations of liver tests during episodes of pain that normalize during pain-free periods may be observed. Patients with pancreatic SOD may present with typical pancreatic pain with or without pancreatic enzyme elevation or recurrent pancreatitis.

The association between SOD and chronic pancreatitis is poorly understood. It is not known whether the sphincter at times becomes dysfunctional as part of the overall scarring process or whether it has a role in the pathogenesis of chronic pancreatitis. However, a high frequency of basal sphincter pressure abnormalities in the pancreatic sphincter has been identified, with 20 of 23 (87%) chronic pancreatitis patients found to have SOD in one study. Sphincterotomy has been demonstrated to

Rome III Criteria for Functional Biliary, Gallbladder, and Sphincter of Oddi Disorders

A. Diagnostic Criteria for Functional Gallbladder and Sphincter of Oddi Disorders

Must include episodes of pain located in the epigastrium and/or right upper quadrant and *all* of the following:

1. Episodes lasting 30 min or longer
2. Recurrent symptoms occurring at different intervals (not daily)
3. The pain builds up to a steady level
4. The pain is moderate to severe enough to interrupt the patient's daily activities or lead to hospital visit
5. The pain is not relieved by bowel movements
6. The pain is not relieved by postural change
7. The pain is not relieved by antacids
8. Exclusions of other structural disease that would explain the symptoms

Supportive Criteria

The pain may present with one or more of the following:

1. Pain is associated with nausea and vomiting
2. Pain radiates to the back and/or right infrascapular region
3. Pain awakens from sleep in the middle of the night

B. Diagnostic Criteria for Functional Biliary Sphincter of Oddi Disorder

Must include BOTH of the following:

1. Criteria for functional gallbladder or sphincter of Oddi disorder met
2. Normal amylase/lipase

Supportive criteria:

Elevated serum transaminases, alkaline phosphatase, or conjugated bilirubin temporally related to at least two pain episodes

C. Diagnostic Criteria for Functional Pancreatic Sphincter of Oddi Disorder

Must include BOTH of the following:

1. Criteria for functional gallbladder or sphincter of Oddi disorder met
2. Elevated amylase and/or lipase

Adapted from Behar J, Corazziari E, Guelrud M, et al. Functional gallbladder and sphincter of Oddi disorders. *Gastroenterology* 2006;130:1498–1509.

improve pain in a subset of patients with chronic pancreatitis in uncontrolled studies.

While the diagnosis of SOD is commonly made after cholecystectomy, SOD may also exist in the presence of an intact gallbladder. However, the symptoms due to SOD may be indistinguishable from gallbladder-type pain, resulting in the diagnosis of SOD being made after cholecystectomy or less frequently after gallbladder abnormalities have been excluded. Given the potential complications of ERCP in patients with suspected SOD (see below), empiric cholecystectomy may be considered in select patients as initial therapy prior to ERCP even in the setting of normal gallbladder evaluation.

DIFFERENTIAL DIAGNOSIS

The clinical presentation of SOD may be mimicked by many organic pathologies including common bile duct stones, chronic pancreatitis, ampullary tumors, peptic ulcer disease, mesenteric ischemia, renal colic, as well as other functional disorders including irritable bowel syndrome, referred musculoskeletal pain, and functional dyspepsia. Because of the 10% to 20% complication rate seen in the evaluation and therapy of patients with suspected SOD (see below), the diagnosis should be treated as one of exclusion, with other diagnostic possibilities initially pursued with appropriate testing. As well, therapeutic trials with low-risk empirical medical therapies such as proton pump inhibitors, antispasmodics, and/or pain modulators should be made before proceeding with ERCP and SOM.

Diagnostic Methods

Initial investigations for patients with suspected SOD should include laboratory tests (liver enzymes, serum amylase and/or lipase) and abdominal imaging (ultrasound or computed tomography (CT) scan). If at all possible, the enzyme studies should be drawn during an acute attack of pain, although liver test abnormalities lack both sensitivity and specificity. Mild elevations (<2× upper limit of normal) are common in SOD, whereas greater abnormalities are more suggestive of stones, tumors, and intrinsic liver disease. Imaging of the abdomen is usually normal, but occasionally dilated bile ducts or pancreatic ducts may be found (type I or type II patients). More detailed structural evaluation may be obtained with EUS and MRI/MRCP in select patients. Several noninvasive tests have been designed in an attempt to identify those individuals with SOD. The morphine-prostigmine provocative test (Nardi test) has been shown to have an unacceptable rate of false-positive studies (>40% in patients with irritable bowel syndrome) and as such is no longer recommended. Quantitative hepatobiliary scintigraphy (HBS), with or without morphine provocation, may predict an abnormal SOM and response to biliary sphincterotomy. However, abnormal results may be found in asymptomatic controls, and HBS does not address the pancreatic sphincter, which may be the cause of the patient's symptoms. Measurement of common bile duct diameter by ultrasound after either lipid-rich meal or secretin stimulation has also been shown to have variable sensitivity (21% to 88%) and specificity (82% to 97%). Our group has prospectively compared secretin-stimulated MRCP (sMRCP) to SOM. Prediction of SOD based on sMRCP results was poor, with positive and negative predictive values of 67% and 33%, respectively. Considering the limitations of noninvasive testing, SOM demonstrating an elevated basal sphincter pressure greater than 40 mm Hg (either biliary or pancreatic) is still considered the gold standard for diagnosing SOD.

Performance of SOM

SOM is the only available method to measure SO motor activity directly and is considered by most authorities to be the most accurate evaluation for sphincter dysfunction. Although SOM can be performed intraoperatively and percutaneously, it is most commonly done in the ERCP setting. The use of manometry to detect motility disorders of the SO is similar to its use in other parts of the gastrointestinal (GI) tract. However, performance of SOM is more technically demanding and hazardous, with complication rates (in particular, pancreatitis) approaching 20% in several series. Its use, therefore, should be reserved for patients with clinically significant or disabling symptoms. One needs to appreciate, however, that SOM is not likely an independent risk factor for post-ERCP pancreatitis when the aspirating manometry catheter is used. It is the suspicion of SOD itself rather than the performance of SOM that places the patient at increased risk.

The initial step in performing SOM is to administer adequate sedation, which will result in a comfortable, cooperative, motionless patient. All drugs that relax (anticholinergics, nitrates, calcium channel blockers, glucagon) or stimulate (narcotics, cholinergic agents) the sphincter should be avoided for at least 8 to 12 hours prior to SOM and during the manometric session. SOM requires selective cannulation of the bile duct and/or pancreatic duct. It is preferable to perform cholangiography and/or pancreatography prior to performance of SOM, as certain findings (e.g., bile duct stones) may obviate the need for SOM. Once deep cannulation is achieved and the patient acceptably sedated, the catheter is withdrawn across the sphincter. Ideally, both the pancreatic and bile ducts should be studied. Current data indicate that an abnormal basal sphincter pressure may be confined to one side of the sphincter in 35% to 65% of patients with abnormal manometry, and thus, one sphincter segment may be dysfunctional and the other normal. An abnormal basal sphincter pressure is more likely to be confined to the pancreatic duct segment in patients with pancreatitis and to the bile duct segment in patients with biliary-type pain and elevated liver function tests.

Most authorities use only the basal sphincter pressure as an indicator of pathology of the sphincter of Oddi, with 40 mm Hg used as the upper limits of normal for mean basal sphincter pressure (mean value plus three standard deviations). Interobserver variability for reading SOM is minimal when the observers are experienced in reading these tracings.

It has been questioned whether the short-term pressure recording obtained during SOM reflect the "24-hour pathophysiology" of the sphincter, as patients with SOD may have intermittent, episodic symptoms. If the basal sphincter pressure does vary over time, performance of SOM on two separate occasions may lead to different results and affect therapy. Three studies have demonstrated reproducibility of biliary SOM in 34 of 36 symptomatic patients overall and 10 of 10 healthy volunteers. However, reproducibility of pancreatic SOM was found in only 58% (7/12) and 40% (12/30) of persistently symptomatic patients with previously normal SOM at two large referral centers. Other studies have also shown that SO basal pressures are not constant, perhaps due to the inherent physiologic fluctuation of SO motor activity. Newer devices capable of portable, ambulatory, prolonged SOM would be of interest.

THERAPY FOR SPHINCTER OF ODDI DYSFUNCTION

The therapeutic approach in patients with SOD is aimed at reducing the resistance to the flow of bile and/or pancreatic juice across the sphincter. Historically, emphasis has been placed on definitive intervention (i.e., surgical sphincteroplasty or endoscopic sphincterotomy). This appears appropriate for patients with high-grade obstruction (i.e., type I SOD). In patients with lesser degrees of obstruction, the clinician must carefully weigh the risks and benefits before recommending invasive therapy. Most reports indicate that SOD patients have a complication rate from ERCP, manometry, and endoscopic sphincterotomy two to five times higher than that of patients with ductal stones.

Medical Therapy

Medical therapy for documented or suspected SOD has received only limited study. Because the SO is a smooth muscle structure, it is reasonable to assume that drugs that relax smooth muscle might be an effective treatment for SOD. Vardenafil (Levitra), an inhibitor of phosphodiesterase type 5 and a smooth muscle relaxant used most commonly for male erectile dysfunction, was found to reduce basal sphincter pressure and phasic wave amplitude. However, this drug has not been investigated in clinical trials. Sublingual nifedipine and nitrates have been shown to reduce the basal sphincter pressures in asymptomatic volunteers and symptomatic patients with SOD. In a placebo-controlled crossover trial with nifedipine, 21/28 patients (75%) with manometrically documented SOD had a reduction in pain scores, emergency room visits, and use of oral analgesics during short-term follow-up. In a similar study, 9/12 (75%) type II SOD (suspected; SOM was not done) patients improved with nifedipine. Although medical therapy may be an attractive initial approach in patients with SOD, several drawbacks exist. First, medication side effects may be seen in up to one-third of patients. Second, smooth muscle relaxants are unlikely to be of any benefit in patients with the structural form of SOD (i.e., SO stenosis), and the response is incomplete in patients with a primary motor abnormality of the SO (i.e., SO dyskinesia). Finally, long-term outcome from medical therapy has not been reported. Nevertheless, because of the relative safety of medical therapy and the benign (although painful) character of SOD, this approach should be considered in all type III and less severely symptomatic type II SOD patients before considering the more aggressive sphincter ablation therapy.

Surgical Therapy

Historically, surgery was the traditional therapy of SOD. The surgical approach, most commonly, is a transduodenal biliary sphincteroplasty with a transampullary septoplasty (pancreatic septoplasty). Several series have reported that 60% to 70% of patients benefited from this therapy during a 1- to 10-year follow-up. Predictably, patients with an elevated basal sphincter pressure, determined by intraoperative SOM, were more likely to improve from surgical sphincter ablation than those with a normal basal pressure. Some reports have suggested that patients with biliary-type pain have a better outcome than patients with idiopathic pancreatitis, whereas others suggested no difference. However, most studies found that symptom improvement after surgical sphincter ablation alone was relatively uncommon in patients with established chronic pancreatitis.

The surgical approach for SOD has largely been replaced by endoscopic therapy. Patient tolerance, cost of care, morbidity, mortality, and cosmetic results are some of the factors that favor an initial endoscopic approach. At present, surgical therapy is reserved for patients with restenosis after endoscopic sphincterotomy and when endoscopic evaluation or therapy is not available or technically feasible. Among 68 surgical sphincteroplasties done at the Medical University of South Carolina over a 5-year period, 51 had prior endoscopic sphincterotomy and 17 had endoscopically inaccessible papillae because of prior gastric surgery. There was a trend toward improved outcome following surgical sphincteroplasty ($p = 0.06$) in patients who had previous gastric surgery and no prior ERCP compared to those who had endoscopic sphincterotomy prior to their surgery. In some centers, particularly where ERCP and SOM are not performed, operative therapy continues to be the standard treatment of pancreatic sphincter hypertension.

Endoscopic Therapy

Endoscopic Sphincterotomy

Endoscopic sphincterotomy is the standard therapy for patients with SOD. Most data on endoscopic sphincterotomy relate to biliary sphincter ablation alone. Clinical improvement after therapy has been reported to occur in 55% to 95% of patients. These variable outcomes are reflective of the different criteria used to document SOD, the degree of obstruction (type I biliary patients appear to have a better outcome than types II and III), the methods of data collection (retrospective vs. prospective), and the techniques used to determine benefit. In one small study of 17 type I postcholecystectomy patients undergoing ERCP and SOM,

TABLE 24.4 Response to Biliary Sphincterotomy Alone in Biliary SOD Patients

SOD Type	n Studies	n Patients (Total)	n Improved (%)	Mean Follow-up (Months)
I	5	67	57 (85)	25.2
II	10	177	122 (69)	36.8
III	7	169	62 (37)	34.7

Adapted from Sgouros SN, Pereira SP. Systematic review: sphincter of Oddi dysfunction—non-invasive diagnostic methods and long-term outcome after endoscopic sphincterotomy. *Aliment Pharmacol Ther* 2006;24:237–246.

65% had abnormal manometry. Nevertheless, during a mean follow-up interval of 2.3 years, *all* patients benefited from biliary sphincterotomy. The results of this study suggested that because type I biliary patients invariably benefit from biliary sphincterotomy, SOM in this patient group not only is unnecessary but also may be misleading. However, the results of this study have never been validated at another center. Overall, in type I biliary SOD patients evaluated in five studies, biliary sphincterotomy led to clinical improvement in 57/67 (85%) patients with a 2-year follow-up. In contrast, traditional teaching, based on results of several nonrandomized controlled trials, has emphasized that performance of SOM is highly recommended in biliary type II and is mandatory in type III patients because clinical benefit is less certain. A total of 177 type II biliary SOD patients were evaluated in 10 small studies and 122 (69%) improved following biliary sphincterotomy alone with a mean of 3-year follow-up. Of 169 type III patients culled from seven studies, only 62 (37%) improved following biliary sphincterotomy, with nearly 3-year follow-up (see Table 24.4). The addition of pancreatic sphincterotomy to biliary sphincterotomy may offer additional benefit in patients with pancreatic sphincter hypertension, regardless of the presence of biliary SOD. Eversman et al. found that 90% of patients with persistent pain or pancreatitis after biliary sphincterotomy had residual abnormal pancreatic basal pressure. Five-year follow-up data revealed that patients with untreated pancreatic sphincter hypertension were much less likely to improve after biliary sphincterotomy than patients with isolated biliary sphincter hypertension. As shown in Table 24.5, patients with pancreatic sphincter hypertension who fail to respond to biliary sphincterotomy can be "rescued" by undergoing

TABLE 24.5 Symptomatic Improvement in Pancreatic SOD Patients After Pancreatic Sphincterotomy

Author/Year	n	n (Improved %)	Mean Follow-up (Months)
Pereira, 2006	13	7 (54)	30.2
Okolo, 2000	15	11 (73)	16
Elton, 1998	43	31 (72)	36.4
Soffer, 1994	25	16 (64)	13.7
Guelrud, 1995	27	22 (81)	14.7
TOTAL	123	87 (71)	23.9

Adapted from Sgouros SN, Pereira SP. Systematic review: sphincter of Oddi dysfunction—non-invasive diagnostic methods and long-term outcome after endoscopic sphincterotomy. *Aliment Pharmacol Ther* 2006;24:237–246.

pancreatic sphincterotomy. Recent data from our unit examined the outcome of endoscopic therapy in SOD patients with initial pancreatic sphincter hypertension (with or without biliary sphincter hypertension). Patients were followed for a mean of 43.1 months (range 11 to 77 months); reintervention was offered for sustained or recurrent symptoms at a median of 8 months after initial therapy. Performance of an initial dual pancreatobiliary sphincterotomy was associated with a lower reintervention rate (70/285, 24.6%) than biliary sphincterotomy alone (31/95, 33%; $p < 0.05$). While these results appear promising, the State of the Science conference at the National Institutes of Health in 2002 called for further study in the controversial type III SOD patients, as virtually all outcome data were based on small retrospective studies. As a result, the EPISOD (Evaluating Predictors and Interventions in Sphincter of Oddi Dysfunction) study was undertaken. This sham-controlled prospective multicenter trial evaluated 214 type III SOD patients, randomized to sphincterotomy or sham therapy. Importantly, while approximately half the patients did note a reduction in pain as measured by pain disability days, those patients randomized to sham therapy did at least as well as those treated with biliary or pancreatobiliary sphincterotomy. Furthermore, results of SOM did not predict outcome. Additionally, this benefit persisted at 1-year follow-up, even in the sham group. Three-year follow-up data are currently being collected, and these results are eagerly awaited. Further study is clearly indicated in this difficult patient population, as the EPISOD study results suggest that the pain syndrome is not entirely sphincter mediated.

Some authorities argue that the current SOD classification systems might not be a good predictor of outcome. In a study of 121 patients (18 type I, 53 type II, and 50 type III) treated by biliary sphincterotomy with (49) or without (72) pancreatic sphincterotomy, Freeman et al. reported a good to excellent response in 69%. The response was not significantly different between biliary types I, II, and III. The authors found that significant predictors of a poor response to therapy were normal pancreatic manometry, delayed gastric emptying, daily opioid use, and age less than 40. Abnormal liver function tests and dilated bile duct were not significant predictors of outcome.

Taken as a whole, these results clearly indicate that the response rate and enthusiasm for sphincter ablation must be correlated with patient presentation and results of manometry (in type II patients) and balanced against the high complication rates reported for endoscopic therapy of SOD. As noted earlier, several prospective, multicenter studies examining risk factors for post-ERCP pancreatitis have identified *suspected* (i.e., not necessarily confirmed) SOD as an independent factor by multivariate analysis, with two to five times increased pancreatitis rates compared to patients with benign or malignant biliary obstruction. These studies have also shown that the risk of pancreatitis is intrinsic to the patient group ("patient-related factors") and events occurring during the procedure ("procedure-related factors") rather than the SOM when the SOM is performed with the aspirating catheter. In a multivariate analysis, SOM has not been shown to be a risk factor for pancreatitis.

Balloon Dilation and Stenting
Balloon dilation of strictures in the GI tract has become commonplace. In an attempt to be less invasive and possibly preserve sphincter function, adaptation of this technique to treat SOD has been described. Unfortunately, because of the unacceptably high complication rates, primarily pancreatitis, this technology has little role in the primary

management of SOD. Similarly, although biliary stenting might offer short-term symptom benefit in patients with SOD and predict outcome from sphincter ablation, it too has unacceptably high complication rates and cannot be advocated in this setting. Furthermore, pancreatic stent trials are strongly discouraged due to the potential for stent-induced pancreatic ductal injury.

Botulinum Toxin Injection

Botulinum toxin (Botox), a potent inhibitor of acetylcholine release from nerve endings, has been successfully applied to smooth muscle disorders of the GI tract such as achalasia. In a preliminary clinical trial, Botox injection into the SO resulted in a 50% reduction in the basal biliary sphincter pressure and improved bile flow. This reduction in pressure may be accompanied by symptom improvement in some patients. Although further study is warranted, Botox may serve as a therapeutic trial for SOD with responders undergoing permanent sphincter ablation. In a small series, 22 postcholecystectomy type III patients with manometric evidence of SOD underwent Botox injection into the intraduodenal sphincter segment. Eleven of the 12 patients who responded to botulinum toxin injection later benefited from endoscopic sphincterotomy, whereas only 2 of 10 patients who did not benefit from Botox injection later responded to sphincter ablation. However, such an approach does require two endoscopic procedures to achieve symptom relief. Moreover, patients must have relatively frequent episodes of pain to assess the benefit from Botox. Further studies are needed before recommending this technique.

Failure to Achieve Symptomatic Improvement After Biliary Sphincterotomy

There are several potential explanations as to why patients may fail to achieve symptom relief after biliary sphincterotomy is performed for well-documented SOD. First, the biliary sphincterotomy may have been inadequate, or restenosis may have occurred. Second, the importance of pancreatic sphincter ablation is being increasingly recognized, as noted previously. Third, patients may fail to respond to sphincterotomy because they have chronic pancreatitis. It has been reported that SOD patients are four times more likely to have evidence of chronic pancreatitis than those without SOD. Although SOD appears to be associated with chronic pancreatitis, a causal relationship has not been proven. These patients may or may not have abnormal pancreatograms. Intraductal pancreatic juice aspiration after secretin stimulation (with bicarbonate determination) may help make this diagnosis. EUS may show parenchymal and ductular changes of the pancreas in some of these patients suggesting chronic pancreatitis. Fourth, some patients may be having pain from altered gut motility of the stomach, small bowel, or colon (irritable bowel or pseudoobstruction variants). There is increasing evidence that upper GI motility disorders may masquerade as pancreatobiliary-type pain. Multiple preliminary studies show disordered duodenal motility in such patients. This area needs much more study to determine the frequency, significance, and/or coexistence of these motor disorders along with SOD.

Others have suggested that type III patients have duodenal-specific visceral hyperalgesia with pain reproduction by duodenal distention, as well as high levels of somatization, depression, obsessive–compulsive behavior, and anxiety compared to control subjects. Patients with SOD appear to have a higher than expected prevalence of the irritable bowel syndrome (IBS), supporting the notion that SOD may occur as part of a more generalized functional disorder of the gut. Patients with SOD not only somatize more than controls, but they may have an antecedent history of sexual or physical abuse similar to IBS. Selective SOD therapy cannot be expected to provide symptom resolution in such patients and may account for the high failure rate of sphincterotomy in many patients with type III SOD.

COMPLICATIONS AND THEIR PREVENTION

As noted earlier, patients with suspected SOD are at increased risk of post-ERCP complications. While large multicenter studies and meta-analyses have identified suspected SOD as an independent risk factor for post-ERCP pancreatitis, several approaches may be undertaken to decrease the incidence of this complication. Ensuring adequate pancreatic duct drainage post-ERCP with small diameter, temporary prophylactic pancreatic stents in all patients with suspected SOD, whether or not sphincterotomy is performed, may now be considered standard of care. As in all patients undergoing ERCP, limiting the number of pancreatic duct injections and extent of pancreatic duct opacification may further decrease pancreatitis rates. Recently, rectal indomethacin was shown to reduce post-ERCP pancreatitis by nearly 50% in high-risk (mostly SOD) patients. Despite these advances, complication rates remain significant in patients with suspected SOD. These patients should be counseled thoroughly on the risk–benefit ratio of undergoing ERCP with SOM, prior to proceeding with endoscopic intervention. Figure 24.2 illustrates a suggested algorithm for the diagnostic workup and treatment of patients with suspected type I, II, and III SOD.

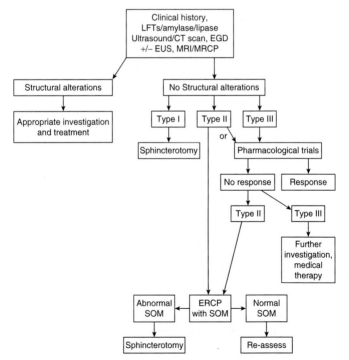

FIGURE 24.2 Suggested algorithm for the diagnostic workup and treatment of patients with suspected type I, II, or III SOD.

Suggested Readings

Behar J, Corazziari E, Guelrud M, et al. Functional gallbladder and sphincter of Oddi disorders. *Gastroenterology* 2006;130:1498–1509.

Cheng CL, Sherman S, Watkins JL, et al. Risk factors for post-ERCP pancreatitis: a prospective multicenter study. *Am J Gastroenterol* 2006;101:139–147.

Eversman D, Fogel EL, Rusche M, et al. Frequency of abnormal pancreatic and biliary sphincter manometry compared with clinical suspicion of sphincter of Oddi dysfunction. *Gastrointest Endosc* 1999;50:637–641.

Freeman ML, Guda NM. Prevention of post-ERCP pancreatitis: a comprehensive review. *Gastrointest Endosc* 2004;59:845–864.

Freeman ML, Gill M, Overby C, et al. Predictors of outcomes after biliary and pancreatic sphincterotomy for sphincter of Oddi dysfunction. *J Clin Gastroenterol* 2007;41:94–102.

Madura JA II, Madura JA. Diagnosis and management of sphincter of Oddi dysfunction and pancreas divisum. *Surg Clin North Am* 2007;87:1417–1429.

Morgan KA, Romagnuolo J, Adams DB. Transduodenal sphincteroplasty in the management of sphincter of Oddi dysfunction and pancreas divisum in the modern era. *J Am Coll Surg* 2008;206(5):908–914; discussion 914–917.

Park SH, Watkins JL, Fogel EL, et al. Long-term outcome of endoscopic dual pancreatobiliary sphincterotomy in patients with manometry-documented sphincter of Oddi dysfunction and normal pancreatogram. *Gastrointest Endosc* 2003;57:483–491.

Sgouros SN, Pereira SP. Systematic review: sphincter of Oddi dysfunction—noninvasive diagnostic methods and long-term outcome after endoscopic sphincterotomy. *Aliment Pharmacol Ther* 2006;24:237–246.

Venu RP, Geenen JE, Hogan WJ. Sphincter of Oddi stenosis and dysfunction. In: Sivak MV Jr, ed. *Gastroenterologic endoscopy*, 2nd ed. Philadelphia, PA: WB Saunders, 2000:1023.

Dr. Fogel has provided an outstanding overview of sphincter of Oddi dysfunction, pathophysiology, and treatment. This editorial side bar is focused on the technique of surgical transduodenal sphincteroplasty.

1. The patient is approached through upper midline or right subcostal incision. A wide Kocher maneuver is essential to mobilize the duodenum into the operative field. Stay sutures placed on the duodenum are useful; stay sutures placed adjacent to the papilla are helpful as well in elevating the head of the pancreas and duodenum into the operative field; however, care must be taken to avoid occluding the biliary or pancreatic sphincter. The duodenum is opened longitudinally over the major papilla, which is easily identifiable by palpation or ultrasound. In difficult cases, a probe may be passed antegrade through the cystic duct and distal common bile duct to identify the papillary orifice.

2. Once the papilla is exposed (see figures), the bile duct and pancreatic duct are intubated with small (5 French) pediatric feeding tubes. Sphincteroplasty of the biliary sphincter is performed first. The tissue may be divided sharply between fine-tipped clamps prior to suturing. Alternatively, the sphincterotomy may simply be created/extended carefully using a needle tip cautery. If the latter approach is used, my preference is to cauterize over the plastic feeding tube (not over a metal probe) to minimize chance for inadvertent tissue injury. Care must be paid at this point of the operation to avoid extending the sphincterotomy too far (both in the biliary and pancreatic sphincter)—perforation into the retroperitoneum is associated with potentially disastrous consequence. The sphincteroplasty is completed by suturing the biliary epithelium to the duodenal epithelium with long-acting absorbable sutures or nonabsorbable monofilament sutures. The pancreatic sphincteroplasty (septotomy)

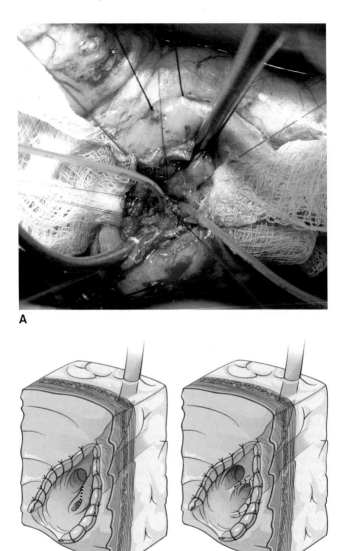

A

B

Operative **(A)** and schematic **(B)** illustration of sphincteroplasty with septoplasty.

is created between the biliary and pancreatic ductal orifice (see figures). Again, care is taken here not to extend the septotomy too deeply. It is prudent to leave a short segment (4 to 5 cm) of pediatric feeding tube in the pancreatic duct to minimize chances of postoperative pancreatitis. This tube is secured with chromic suture to ensure short-term stability but promote early passage. Should the patient have pancreas divisum, the minor papilla is addressed in a similar fashion.

3. The duodenotomy is closed transversely in two layers. Routine drainage is not necessary; however, may be considered if concern for retroperitoneal incursion is high.

4. Patients are typically counseled preoperatively to expect full liquid diet or soft mechanical diet for the first few postoperative weeks. Immediate postoperative laboratory evaluation includes liver chemistry and serum amylase or lipase. Diet advancement is delayed if the patient manifests biochemical pancreatitis. If patients have early postoperative epigastric or right upper quadrant pain, abdominal x-ray should be obtained to ensure passage of pancreatic stent.

Common Bile Duct Stones and Exploration

Attila Nakeeb

ETIOLOGY

Common bile duct (CBD) stones can be classified as either primary or secondary. Primary CBD stones develop de novo within the bile ducts, whereas secondary stones develop in the gallbladder and subsequently pass into the CBD. In the United States, more than 85% of all bile duct stones are secondary. Primary duct stones typically occur in conditions associated with biliary stasis such as benign biliary strictures, sclerosing cholangitis, choledochal cyst disease, oriental cholangiohepatitis, or sphincter of Oddi dysfunction. Bile stasis promotes the overgrowth of bacteria in bile with subsequent bilirubin deconjugation and the breakdown of biliary lipids, resulting in the formation of brown pigment stones. Secondary bile duct stones have a composition similar to gallbladder stones: approximately 75% are cholesterol stones, and 25% are black pigment stones. The classification of CBD stones into primary or secondary is of therapeutic importance because primary stones require removal of the stones and a drainage procedure (choledochoenterostomy or sphincteroplasty), whereas secondary stones can be treated by removal of the stones and cholecystectomy.

Most patients with CBD stones are asymptomatic. It is estimated that CBD stones (choledocholithiasis) are found in approximately 10% of patients with cholelithiasis. This incidence of CBD stones in patients undergoing cholecystectomy ranges between 8% and 15%. The incidence varies with age and is less than 5% in younger patients and more than 20% in older patients with gallstones. Patients with symptomatic CBD stones may present with biliary colic, extrahepatic biliary obstruction, cholangitis, or pancreatitis. Typically, the pain and jaundice associated with CBD stones are more intermittent and transient than when the biliary obstruction is caused by a malignancy. Fever and chills are present in patients with cholangitis. Gallstone pancreatitis can develop from the obstruction of the ampulla of Vater by common duct stones. In the west, CBD stones are responsible for up to 50% of all cases of pancreatitis. Most patients with gallstone pancreatitis experience a mild self-limited attack from which they recover within a few days; however, some patients will progress to develop severe pancreatitis with peripancreatic necrosis, infection, or other local complications.

DIAGNOSIS

No single clinical variable is completely accurate in predicting the presence of choledocholithiasis. Therefore, the results of a detailed history and physical examination, laboratory evaluations, and diagnostic imaging tests must be considered together when assessing the likelihood that a patient has CBD stones. Serum liver function tests (bilirubin, alkaline phosphatase, and transaminases) can be useful in predicting common duct stones.

In the setting of suspected CBD stones, if any one value of the liver profile is elevated, the risk for CBD stones approaches 20%. With two elevated values, the risk increases to nearly 40%, and with three or more elevated values, the risk for CBD stones is nearly 50%. Factors associated with a high risk of choledocholithiasis include cholangitis, CBD size greater than 6 mm, CBD stones visualized on ultrasound (US) or cross-sectional imaging, and jaundice (bilirubin >4 mg/dL).

DIAGNOSTIC STUDIES

Transabdominal Ultrasonography

US is highly sensitive for the diagnosis of gallstones within the gallbladder. Unfortunately, the sensitivity of transabdominal US for the detection of CBD stones is only 30% to 50%. US successfully identifies the presence of CBD stones in only 70% of patients because the distal bile duct is frequently obscured by duodenal or colonic gas. On the other hand, transabdominal US is very sensitive for identifying CBD dilation, which can suggest choledocholithiasis. If the extrahepatic bile duct diameter is less than 3 mm, CBD stones are exceedingly rare, whereas a CBD diameter greater than 10 mm in a jaundiced patient is associated with CBD stones in more than 90% of cases.

Magnetic Resonance Imaging

Magnetic resonance cholangiopancreatography (MRCP) has a sensitivity of 90%, a specificity of 100%, and an overall diagnostic accuracy of 97% for the diagnosis of CBD stones. MRCP (Fig. 25.1) permits direct imaging of the biliary tract without the need for contrast, radiation exposure, or an invasive

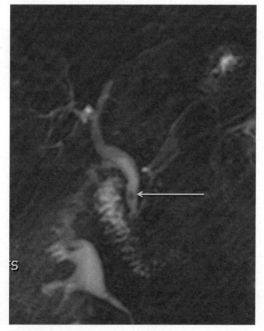

FIGURE 25.1 MRCP demonstrating CBD stones.

procedure. Disadvantages of MRCP include its relatively high cost, the need for prolonged breath holding, and a lack of therapeutic options. MRCP can be used to screen patients at low and moderate risk of having common duct stones prior to endoscopic cholangiography. A normal magnetic resonance cholangiogram can eliminate the need for an invasive endoscopic cholangiogram or intraoperative cholangiogram.

Endoscopic Ultrasound

Endoscopic ultrasound (EUS) is a semi-invasive test that can be performed with a very low rate of complications (<0.1%). The sensitivity (92% to 100%) and specificity (95% to 100%) for the diagnosis of CBD stones by EUS are excellent. The negative predictive value for EUS is more than 97%. Therefore, when EUS is negative for common duct stones, endoscopic retrograde cholangiopancreatography (ERCP) or intraoperative cholangiography (IOC) can be avoided.

Direct Cholangiography

Direct cholangiography is the gold standard for diagnosing CBD stones. Both endoscopic retrograde cholangiography (ERC) and percutaneous transhepatic cholangiography (PTC) techniques can be used to directly visualize the biliary tree. In addition to identifying CBD stones, endoscopic cholangiography (Fig. 25.2) permits safe removal of most stones and is therefore the preferred approach for patients with suspected CBD stones. Skilled endoscopists can successfully cannulate the CBD in 90% to 95% of patients. Complications of diagnostic cholangiography including pancreatitis and cholangitis occur in approximately 5% of patients; the vast majority of these complications are mild and self-limiting. ERC may be unsuccessful in patients with previous gastric surgery (Billroth II reconstruction, Roux-en-Y

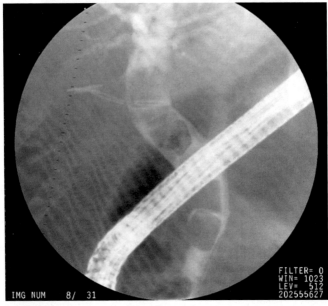

FIGURE 25.2 ERCP demonstrating CBD stones.

gastric bypass), periampullary diverticula, or tortuous bile ducts. PTC may be used to image the bile ducts if ERC is unsuccessful.

Intraoperative Cholangiography

IOC also can be successfully accomplished in more than 95% of cases. The cholangiogram should be carefully evaluated for filling defects within the ducts, presence of contrast in the duodenum, and the intrahepatic biliary anatomy (Fig. 25.3). Importantly, the surgeon must be able to interpret IOC images *in real time*, in the operating room for this study to be valuable. Debate continues over the need to perform routine IOC at the time of cholecystectomy. Advocates of routine IOC argue that asymptomatic CBD stones can be identified and biliary injuries prevented by performing routine IOC. Critics of this approach suggest that the incidence of retained stones is no greater when cholangiography is performed selectively based on clinical and laboratory criteria. The indications for performing cholangiography during cholecystectomy include (a) a dilated CBD, (b) a wide cystic duct, (c) palpable CBD stones, (d) elevated serum liver function tests or bilirubin, and (e) a history of pancreatitis. If these criteria are strictly followed, approximately 30% of patients will require IOC at the time of cholecystectomy. In addition to defining biliary anatomy, IOC can identify the size, number, and location of CBD stones. This information is critical in choosing the most appropriate treatment for CBD stones.

Intraoperative Ultrasonography

Intraoperative ultrasonography also can be used to identify CBD stones at the time of cholecystectomy. In experienced hands, intraoperative ultrasonography has been shown to be comparable to IOC for the diagnosis of CBD stones. Laparoscopic ultrasonography is performed with a high-frequency (7.5- to 10-mHz) probe, and the bile duct is imaged in the transverse and longitudinal planes. The distal bile duct can be visualized in more than 95% of cases.

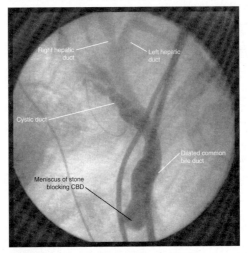

FIGURE 25.3 Intraoperative cholangiogram. (From Lillemoe K, Jarnigan W. *Master techniques in surgery: hepatobiliary and pancreatic surgery.* Philadelphia, PA: Lippincott Williams & Wilkins, 2012.)

General Diagnostic Strategy

The choice of radiologic studies used to evaluate a patient with suspected choledocholithiasis should be based on the probability of this diagnosis. A simple algorithm for the workup of patients with CBD stones is shown in Figure 25.4. Patients at highest risk for choledocholithiasis should undergo endoscopic cholangiography. Patients at intermediate risk may be screened with magnetic resonance cholangiography or EUS and proceed to laparoscopic cholecystectomy if no stones are identified. Those patients at low risk of harboring common duct stones may be evaluated with IOC at the time of laparoscopic cholecystectomy with laparoscopic CBD exploration or postoperative endoscopic stone extraction reserved for the few patients with a positive study.

MANAGEMENT

Currently, several options are available to the surgeon for the treatment of CBD stones. In choosing the most appropriate approach for an individual patient, factors such as the local endoscopic expertise, the surgeon's laparoscopic skill, and the patient's clinical condition must be considered.

ENDOSCOPIC THERAPY

ERC with endoscopic sphincterotomy permits CBD stones to be removed without the need for conventional surgery. Stones can be successfully removed from the CBD in 85% to 95% of cases. The endoscopic approach is particularly useful for patients prior to cholecystectomy in whom a high suspicion exists for CBD calculi, particularly if laparoscopic CBD exploration is not available. Endoscopic clearance of stones from the CBD precholecystectomy can obviate the need for an open operation. Furthermore, if

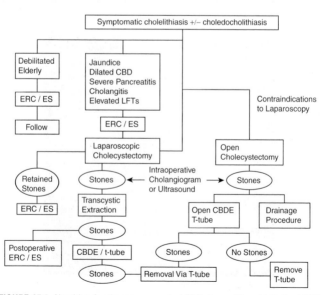

FIGURE 25.4 Algorithm for the management of CBD stones. (From Mulholland MW, Lillemoe KD, Doherty GM, et al. *Greenfield's surgery: scientific principles & practice*, 5th ed. Philadelphia, PA: Lippincott Williams & Wilkins, 2010.)

endoscopic stone extraction is not possible because of multiple gallstones, intrahepatic stones, large gallstones, impacted stones, duodenal diverticula, prior gastrectomy, or bile duct stricture, this information is known preoperatively, and an open CBD exploration or drainage procedure can be performed at the time of cholecystectomy. After sphincterotomy, most stones smaller than 1 cm in diameter pass spontaneously. A balloon catheter or stone basket also can be used to retrieve stones if needed. If endoscopic clearance is incomplete, an endoscopic stent can be placed into the CBD to maintain drainage and prevent cholangitis.

Endoscopic sphincterotomy and stone extraction is well tolerated in most patients. Complications occur in 5% to 8% of patients and include cholangitis, pancreatitis, perforation, and bleeding. The overall mortality rate is 0.2% to 0.5%. Complete clearance of all common duct stones is achieved endoscopically in 71% to 75% of patients at the first procedure and in 84% to 95% of patients after multiple endoscopic procedures.

Preoperative ERC plus endoscopic sphincterotomy is the preferred management option for CBD stones in several conditions. In the setting of acute suppurative cholangitis, morbidity and mortality are significantly decreased if preoperative biliary decompression and stone removal are accomplished before cholecystectomy. Patients with severe gallstone pancreatitis or a significant deterioration of their clinical condition also have been shown to benefit from early ERC and stone clearance. Cholecystectomy can then be performed after the pancreatitis has resolved. In patients with a dilated CBD (>8 mm) on US and jaundice, an ERC also should be performed to rule out a malignancy or biliary stricture that would alter the surgical management. In patients with a high operative risk, ERC plus endoscopic sphincterotomy can be performed or definitive treatment to remove CBD stones and the gallbladder left in place.

LAPAROSCOPIC THERAPY

Laparoscopic exploration of the CBD for choledocholithiasis enables appropriately selected patients to undergo complete management of their calculus biliary tract disease with one procedure. The laparoscopic approach is ideal for patients with CBD stones identified during IOC or US. The two approaches for laparoscopic bile duct exploration are laparoscopic transcystic duct bile duct exploration (LTCBDE) or laparoscopic choledochotomy (Table 25.1). The indications for transcystic duct exploration are

TABLE 25.1	Laparoscopic Transcystic CBD Exploration versus Laparoscopic Choledochotomy	
	Transcystic	**Choledochotomy**
Stones		
Number	<8	Any
Size	<9 mm	Any
Location	Distal to cystic duct	Entire duct
Bile duct size	Any	>6 mm
Drain	Optional cystic duct tube	T-tube
Contraindications	Friable cystic duct	Small diameter duct
	Intrahepatic stones	Inability to suture laparoscopically
Advantages	Multiple large stones	T-tube for postoperative access
	No T-tube	
	Short hospital stay	

filling defects noted on cholangiography (CBD stones), stones less than 9 mm in diameter, stones distal to the cystic duct entrance to the bile duct, and less than six stones. Contraindications to LTCBDE are a small friable cystic duct, more than eight stones in the CBD, common hepatic duct stones, and stones larger than 1 cm. Laparoscopic choledochotomy can be performed if LTCBDE fails or is contraindicated, if stones are present proximal to the cystic duct, or when multiple stones are present. The only contraindication to laparoscopic choledochotomy is a small common duct (<6 mm) that might be narrowed during its closure.

Laparoscopic Transcystic Duct Bile Duct Exploration

The technique of LTCBDE involves careful dissection of the cystic duct down to its junction with the CBD. A clip is placed on the gallbladder side of the cystic duct and a ductotomy is created sharply. After completing a cholangiogram, a guide wire should be inserted into the bile duct. A cholangiocatheter can then be advanced over the guide wire into the bile duct and saline irrigated through the catheter in an attempt to flush small stones out of the bile duct. Glucagon should be administered intravenously to encourage relaxation of the sphincter of Oddi. If the stones in the CBD are larger than the lumen of the cystic duct, the cystic duct can be dilated with a series of dilators using either the Seldinger technique or an angioplasty balloon catheter. Stone retrieval baskets can be inserted over the guide wire and stones extracted under fluoroscopic guidance. Flexible choledochoscopy via the cystic duct also can be performed and stones extracted under direct vision using baskets (Fig. 25.5). Success rates greater than 95% have been reported for bile duct clearance using choledochoscopy. To document

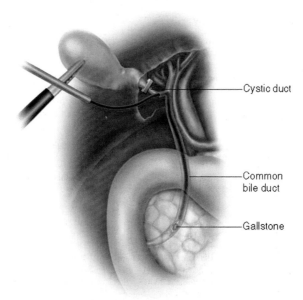

FIGURE 25.5 Laparoscopic transcystic duct CBD exploration. (From Lillemoe K, Jarnigan W. *Master techniques in surgery: hepatobiliary and pancreatic surgery.* Philadelphia, PA: Lippincott Williams & Wilkins, 2012.)

stone clearance, a completion cholangiogram should be performed. A cystic duct drainage tube can be left in place if findings on the cholangiogram are equivocal. This tube can be used postoperatively for cholangiography and radiographic treatment of retained stones if necessary. After LTCBDE, the cystic duct stump should be secured with an endoloop or a suture ligature and not be clipped.

Laparoscopic Choledochotomy

Laparoscopic choledochotomy (Fig. 25.6) is another excellent approach to CBD stones when the CBD diameter is 6 mm or greater. The anterior wall of the CBD is bluntly dissected and a longitudinal choledochotomy created in the anterior wall of the bile duct distal to the cystic duct insertion. The choledochotomy should be fashioned to accommodate the diameter of the largest stone. Two stay sutures can be placed in the common duct and used to tent up the anterior CBD wall to facilitate incision. A larger choledochoscope (3.3 mm, 2.4-mm working channel) can then be placed into the bile duct and stones extracted with baskets or balloon catheters. The choledochotomy is then closed over a T-tube with a 4-0 absorbable suture.

Advantages of laparoscopic choledochotomy relative to LTCBDE include the ability to remove larger stones (>1 cm), to remove stones from the proximal hepatic ducts, to remove multiple stones, and to use biliary lithotripsy to fragment impacted stones. The disadvantages of laparoscopic choledochotomy are that it requires a T-tube and considerable laparoscopic suturing skill to close the choledochotomy.

Clearance of all CBD stones is achieved in 75% to 95% of patients with laparoscopic CBD exploration. Results from several randomized

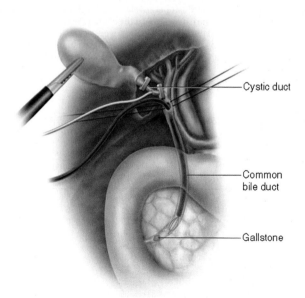

Cystic duct

Common bile duct

Gallstone

FIGURE 25.6 Laparoscopic choledochotomy. (From Lillemoe K, Jarnigan W. *Master techniques in surgery: hepatobiliary and pancreatic surgery.* Philadelphia, PA: Lippincott Williams & Wilkins, 2012.)

prospective trials comparing a single-stage approach (laparoscopic cholecystectomy + laparoscopic common bile duct exploration) versus a two-stage approach (laparoscopic cholecystectomy + either pre- or post-operative ERCP) are shown in Table 25.2. The morbidity and mortality of laparoscopic CBD exploration are similar to laparoscopic cholecystectomy alone. The overall hospital length of stay tends to be shorter for patients managed with a one-stage approach versus a two-stage approach.

Open Common Bile Duct Exploration

Open CBD exploration is performed much less frequently with the increased use of endoscopic, percutaneous, and laparoscopic techniques to remove CBD stones. The first step is to perform a full Kocher maneuver mobilizing the duodenum so that a hand can be placed behind the head of the pancreas and the distal CBD palpated. Any impacted stones may be milked proximally. The supraduodenal bile duct is then exposed, and two stay sutures are placed in the CBD just below the cystic duct. The anterior wall of the bile duct is then elevated with the stay sutures and a longitudinal choledochotomy made. The bile duct then can be explored for stones. Rigid instruments should not be used to extract stones because they can injure the delicate ductal epithelium. A soft rubber irrigating catheter can be used to gently flush out any stones or debris. Balloon-tipped catheters then can be passed proximally and distally into the ducts to retrieve stones. Adequate clearance of the duct should be confirmed visually with flexible choledochoscopy. Remaining stones can be removed by irrigation or by the use of instruments such as stone forceps, wire baskets, or balloon catheters. A T-tube should be placed in the bile duct and the choledochotomy closed with 4-0 absorbable suture. Completion cholangiography is performed before closing the abdomen to rule out the presence of retained stones or a bile leak around the T-tube. Postoperatively, a T-tube cholangiogram is performed 3 to 7 days after the exploration. If the cholangiogram is normal, the tube can be clamped and the tube pulled 3 to 6 weeks later. If retained stones are detected, the tract is allowed to mature, and percutaneous extraction can be performed by a radiologist in 4 to 6 weeks. Open CBD exploration can be accomplished with almost no mortality in patients younger than age 60 years but carries mortality of up to 4% in septic patients.

TABLE 25.2	Select Randomized Trials of One- versus Two-Stage Management of CBD Stones				
Author	Year	Treatment	N	Duct Clearance (%)	Morbidity (%)	Length of Stay (days)
Rhodes	1998	LC + ERCP	40	93	15	3.5
		LC + LCBDE	40	75	5	1
Cuschieri	1999	ERCP + LC	133	62	13	9
		LC + LCBDE	133	70	16	6
Nathanson	2005	LC + ERCP	45	96	24	7.7
		LC + LCBDE	41	97	29	6.4
Noble	2009	ERCP + LC	47	62	34	3
		LC + LCBDE	44	86	52	5
Rogers	2010	ERCP + LC	55	98	9	5
		LC + LCBDE	57	88	11	4

LC, laparoscopic cholecystectomy; ERCP, endoscopic retrograde cholangiopancreatography; LCBDE, laparoscopic common bile duct exploration.

DRAINAGE PROCEDURES

Patients with an impacted CBD stone at the ampulla that cannot be removed with a CBD exploration or those with multiple stones in a non-dilated duct may require a transduodenal sphincteroplasty. A sphincteroplasty also is indicated in the presence of an ampullary stenosis or a choledochocele. The first step in a sphincteroplasty is to perform a Kocher maneuver. A small longitudinal duodenotomy is made over the ampulla, and two stay sutures are placed on each side of the ampulla to elevate it. A small incision is made at the 11 o'clock position in the sphincter taking care to avoid the pancreatic duct, which is usually found at the 5 o'clock position. The sphincterotomy is extended through the sphincter (approximately 1.5 cm) and the impacted stone removed. The bile duct and duodenal mucosa are then approximated with interrupted 4-0 absorbable sutures. The duodenotomy should be closed transversely to prevent narrowing of the duodenal lumen.

Patients with grossly dilated bile ducts (>2 cm), multiple stones (>5), intrahepatic stones, primary CBD stones, or a distal biliary stricture should be considered for a biliary drainage procedure. The two options are a choledochoduodenostomy and a Roux-en-Y choledochojejunostomy. Choledochoduodenostomy can be performed in either a side-to-side or an end-to-side fashion. Advantages of a choledochoduodenostomy are that it can be performed rapidly, it requires only one anastomosis, and the bile duct still can be accessed endoscopically. However, a side-to-side anastomosis leaves the distal CBD in continuity and can lead to the "sump syndrome." In this situation, food debris from the duodenum can enter the distal limb of the CBD and obstruct the anastomosis or the pancreatic duct orifice leading to cholangitis or pancreatitis. Long-term complications of choledochoduodenostomy include a small but real incidence of cholangitis and liver abscess.

Roux-en-Y hepatico- or choledochojejunostomy also is an excellent option for biliary drainage. This operation is performed by dividing the hepatic or common duct and doing an end-to-side anastomosis to a 60-cm Roux limb of jejunum. Development of the sump syndrome is not a concern because a hepatico- or choledochojejunostomy completely diverts bile flow from the alimentary stream.

CONCLUSIONS

CBD stones may be approached endoscopically, laparoscopically, or by open CBDE. Choice of therapy depends on both patient considerations as well as local endoscopic and surgical expertise. Patients with primary CBD stones must be considered for a biliary drainage procedure.

Suggested Readings

Abboud BA, Malet PF, Berlin JA, et al. Predictors of common bile duct stones prior to cholecystectomy: a meta-analysis. *Gastrointest Endoscopy* 1996;44:450–459.

Alexakis N, Connor S. Meta-analysis of one vs. two-stage laparoscopic/endoscopic management of common bile duct stones. *HPB* 2012;14:254–259.

Duncan C, Riall T. Evidence-based surgical practice: calculous gallbladder disease. *J Gastrointest Surg* 2012;16:2011–2025.

Freeman M, Nelson D, Sherman S, et al. Complications of endoscopic biliary sphincterotomy. *N Eng J Med* 1996;335:909–918.

Kharbutli B, Velanovich V. Management of preoperatively suspected choledocholithiasis: a decision analysis. *J Gastrointest Surg* 2008;12:1973–1980.

Lillemoe K, Jarnigan W. *Master techniques in surgery: hepatobiliary and pancreatic surgery*. Philadelphia, PA: Lippincott Williams & Wilkins, 2012.

Liu T, Consorti E, Kawashima A, et al. Patient evaluation and management with selective use of magnetic resonance cholangiography and endoscopic retrograde cholangiopancreatography before laparoscopic cholecystectomy. *Ann Surg* 2001;234:33–40.

Mulholland MW, Lillemoe KD, Doherty GM, et al. *Greenfield's surgery: scientific principles & practice*, 5th ed. Philadelphia, PA: Lippincott Williams & Wilkins, 2010.

Rhodes M, Sussman L, Cohen L, et al. Randomized trial of laparoscopic exploration of common bile duct versus postoperative endoscopic retrograde cholangiography for common bile duct stones. *Lancet* 1998;351:159–161.

Vilgrain V, Palazzo L. Choledocholithiasis: role of US and endoscopic ultrasound. *Abdom Imaging* 2001;26:7–14.

Choledochal Cyst

Alessandro Paniccia and Barish H. Edil

EPIDEMIOLOGY

Choledochal cysts (CCs) are more appropriately defined as a cystic disorder of the biliary ducts. This rare condition is characterized by dilatation of the extrahepatic and/or intrahepatic biliary tree. It was originally described as a disease of infancy, but in recent years, an increase number of cases have been diagnosed during adulthood.

The prevalence of CCs is subject to significant geographic variation. The highest incidence, 1:1,000 births, is observed in Southeast Asian countries. The incidence of CCs in the western world is between 1:100,000 and 1:150,000 and is described within the US population as 1:13,500 live births. In general, the female-to-male ratio of CC is approximately 4:1.

The diagnosis of cystic disorder of the biliary ducts carries with it a significant lifetime risk of malignancy that appears to increase with age. The overall risk of malignant degeneration is approximately 10%.

ETIOLOGY

Different theories have been presented to describe the etiology of cystic dilatation of the biliary ducts. These theories postulate that anatomical and functional abnormalities of the biliary ducts combined with increased intraductal pressure and pancreatic enzyme activation contribute to bile duct dilatation.

Babbitt et al. in 1969 popularized the "long common channel" theory recognizing an abnormal junction of the main pancreatic and common bile ducts (APBDJ) outside the duodenal wall and proximal to the sphincter of Oddi. This anatomic anomaly may allow pancreatic secretion to reflux into the biliary tree. The subsequent enzyme activation leads to chronic inflammation of bile duct epithelium, with ductal wall injury and ultimately cystic dilation. Although APBDJ is a well-recognized anatomic anomaly and most accepted hypothesis, it is only present in 80% of all CCs.

CLASSIFICATION

The first classification system for CC was proposed by Alonso-Lej et al. in 1959 and described three different types of cystic dilation. The Todani modification of the Alonso-Lej classification was introduced in 1977 and is currently used. Todani expanded the original classification system to include intrahepatic disease resulting in a total of five types of cystic disorders based on site, shape, and extent of biliary tree involvement (Fig. 26.1).

Type I cyst is a dilation of the common hepatic duct and represents 50% to 80% of all cysts. Type 1 CC is subclassified into three types based on shape: type Ia cystic, type Ib focal, and type Ic fusiform.

Type II cyst is a supraduodenal diverticulum of the extrahepatic duct to which it is connected with a narrow stalk. It represents only 2% to 3% of all cysts.

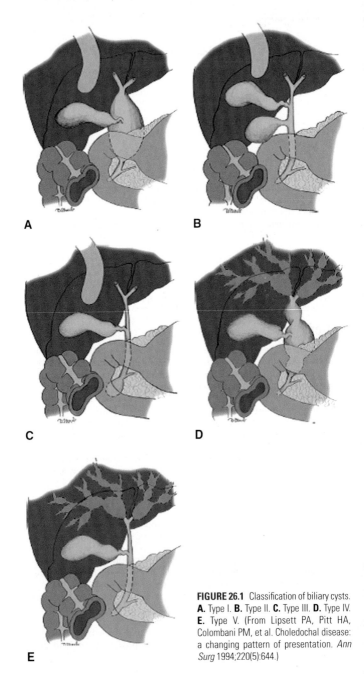

FIGURE 26.1 Classification of biliary cysts. **A.** Type I. **B.** Type II. **C.** Type III. **D.** Type IV. **E.** Type V. (From Lipsett PA, Pitt HA, Colombani PM, et al. Choledochal disease: a changing pattern of presentation. *Ann Surg* 1994;220(5):644.)

Type III cyst, also known as choledochocele, is a dilation of the common bile duct confined to the wall of the duodenum. Type III CC represents less than 10% of all cysts.

Type IV cyst refers to multiple cystic dilations of the biliary tract and is further subclassified into type IVa where multiple cysts are present in the intrahepatic and extrahepatic bile ducts and type IVb where multiple cysts only involve the extrahepatic bile duct. Type IVa cyst is the second most common type of CC representing 30% to 40%, while type IVb only accounts for less than 5% of all cysts.

Type V cyst (Caroli disease) involves only the intrahepatic biliary ducts and can be unilobar or bilobar. It represents less than 10% of all CCs.

DIAGNOSIS

Presentation

The historically described pathognomonic triad of abdominal pain, jaundice, and right upper quadrant palpable mass is only present in 10% to 17% of children. However, 85% of children present with at least two symptoms of the triad compared to only 25% of adults.

Vague right upper quadrant abdominal pain associated with nausea and emesis is often the presenting symptom in adults. Laboratory evaluation of liver function and pancreatic enzymes frequently reflects common conditions such as cholangitis or pancreatitis, where concurrent pancreatitis may be present in 30% to 70% of adult patients. Additionally, concurrent cystolithiasis and cholecystolithiasis are present in approximately 70% of patients. As a result, an interval of up to 6 years from the first presenting symptoms to the diagnosis of cystic disorder of the biliary ducts is relatively common. This delay in diagnosis often leads to additional procedures such as cholecystectomy or other surgical exploration. Most often, adults are diagnosed with CC during evaluation and treatment of complications such as cholecystitis or acute pancreatitis. Diagnosis may also be discovered incidentally during radiologic investigation for other problems. In contrast to other cyst types, patients with type III choledochal cyst (choledochocele) commonly present with acute pancreatitis.

Although rare, hepaticolithiasis and intrahepatic abscess have been described as presenting complications of type IV and V bile duct cysts. This can eventually lead to secondary biliary cirrhosis and portal hypertension with subsequent liver failure.

Cyst rupture and biliary peritonitis have been also described as presenting symptoms but usually in children. These situations are extraordinarily rare.

The most common malignancy associated with CC disease is cholangiocarcinoma, though the presence of CC also increases the risk of developing gallbladder cancer.

Imaging

Demonstration of the continuity of the cystic lesion with the biliary duct is paramount in distinguishing it from other intra-abdominal cysts such as pancreatic pseudocyst, biliary cystadenoma, or echinococcal cysts. In patients with equivocal bile duct dilation (i.e., 1 to 2 cm), the presence of APBDJ strongly suggests the diagnosis of CC.

Abdominal ultrasound (US) is often the primary and the most cost-effective imaging modality in diagnosing bile duct cyst; the sensitivity of US ranges from 71% to 97%.

Endoscopic ultrasound has been described in the literature in order to overcome the intrinsic limitations of transabdominal US such as body habitus, bowel gas, the presence of overlying intra-abdominal structures, and poor visualization of distal bile duct. It also gives you information of the pancreas and biliary duct anatomy.

Computed tomography (CT) scan is now widely available and presents several advantages in the diagnosis of CC. Some of these advantages include characterization of intrahepatic bile ducts, dilation evaluating the cysts surrounding structures, and more visualization of the distal bile duct and the pancreatic head. It also allows for evaluation of malignancy that may mimic CC or may be originating from a CC. (i.e., very thick cyst wall or portal lymphadenopathy).

Computed tomography cholangiography (CTCP) though not widely available currently has 90% sensitivity for diagnosis of CC and can correctly visualize the bile duct anatomy prior to a surgical procedure.

Magnetic resonance cholangiography (MRCP) is becoming the gold standard in diagnosis with a reported sensitivity ranging between 90% and 100%. Though MRI/MRCP is relatively more expensive than CT, MRCP offers similar excellent cross-sectional imaging evaluation as well as superior visualization of the entire biliary tree (including APBDJ).

Particularly challenging in children is proper distinction between biliary atresia and bile duct cyst. In this situation, a ^{99m}technetium IIIDA scan will demonstrate continuity of the cystic lesion with the bile duct and eventually emptying of contrast into the bowel. Retention of contrast in the biliary system is typical of biliary atresia or any condition causing distal common bile duct (CBD) obstruction. The sensitivity of a hepatobiliary iminodiacetic acid (HIDA) scan, however, is subject to wide variation ranging from 100% for type I to only 67% for type IVa. This inaccuracy is mainly due to HIDA inability to visualize the intrahepatic bile ducts.

In light of the increased accuracy of MRCP and CTCP, invasive cholangiography modalities such as percutaneous transhepatic cholangiogram (PTC) and endoscopic retrograde cholangiopancreatography are applied less frequently. However, in the scenario where biliary drainage is inadequate (type IV/V), PTC and stent placement may be required.

An exception is made for type III CC in which endoscopy is considered the principal diagnostic modality because of its potential to also provide therapeutic intervention. This modality allows cannulation of the papilla of Vater and eventually opacification of the dilated intramural common bile duct. In addition, sphincterotomy is therapeutic for these cysts.

MANAGEMENT

Surgical treatment of CCs has undergone significant changes during the last century. Several surgical techniques have been described including cyst marsupialization, choledochorrhaphy, and internal drainage via cystenterostomy to the duodenum or jejunum. The results with the above techniques have been unsatisfying due to significant associated morbidity and mortality such as ascending cholangitis, anastomosis stricture, stone formation, and a remarkable 30% incidence of postoperative malignancy occurring 15 years earlier than primary malignancy. Therefore, any treatment after complete resection is of historical interest only.

The general consensus today is that surgical management depends on cyst type and that complete cyst excision should be obtained in order to decrease the risk of associated malignancy.

Type I CC is successfully treated by complete cyst resection with a Roux-en-Y hepaticojejunostomy either in an open fashion or, when technically feasible, with a laparoscopic approach.

The technical aspects of this operation involve mobilization of the hepatic flexure and wide Kocher maneuver because the cyst extends posterior to the duodenum into the head of the pancreas. Dissection on the anterior cyst is continued caudally into the pancreatic head until the bile duct narrows, which is the inferior portion of the cyst. This area is ligated, and then, the cyst is reflected cephalad. Dividing the bile duct and displacing the cyst anteriorly allow identification of the portal vein. Posterior dissection is continued until the bile duct is transected just distal to the hepatic duct confluence. Care should be taken not to injure the right hepatic artery, which commonly passes posterior to the bile duct and anterior to the portal vein. Depending on bile duct size, some biliary surgeons prefer to reconstruct this anastomosis across soft Silastic transhepatic stents. A 60-cm limb is brought up in a retrocolic fashion for a Roux-en-Y hepaticojejunostomy. There is an associated 7% complication rate including early anastomotic leak, pancreatic leak due to injury to the pancreatic duct, and bowel obstruction. Late complications include cholangitis, pancreatitis, and anastomotic stricture. The important point is that complete cyst excision is required to prevent future degeneration of CC into cholangiocarcinoma.

Type II CC can be treated with simple cyst excision. The procedure of choice depends on cyst size and location. Commonly used surgical approaches are an extrahepatic biliary resection and Roux-en-Y reconstruction or complete excision with primary closure over a T tube. In order to prevent segmental bile duct narrowing, the defect in the wall of the common bile duct should be closed transversely or over a T tube.

Type III CCs have an extremely low risk of malignancy. These cysts more commonly present with pancreatitis or abdominal pain. They may also be diagnosed in the setting of pancreatic or biliary obstructive symptoms or much more rarely gastric outlet syndrome. Different treatments have been proposed ranging from simple endoscopic sphincterotomy to complete cyst excision through a lateral duodenostomy. If operation is undertaken, it is of primary importance to identify the pancreatic duct in order to avoid accidental injuries. Cannulation of the pancreatic duct with Silastic tubes prior to cyst resection can be used to identify the pancreatic duct and avoid injuries. Eventually the cyst can be excised and sphincteroplasty can be performed. Some authors believe that the pancreatic and biliary duct should be routinely separated and reanastomosed to the duodenum in order to avoid pancreaticobiliary mixing. Most authorities feel that endoscopic "unroofing" provides adequate therapy for type III CC.

Type IV cyst treatment is dictated by the presence or absence of intrahepatic involvement. When intrahepatic involvement is diffuse, complete cyst removal requires partial hepatectomy.

Type IVb is treated in the same fashion of type I cyst.

The treatment for type IVa cyst depends on the extent of the intrahepatic involvement and the presence of cirrhosis and/or portal hypertension. If the intrahepatic involvement is confined to a single lobe, a wide hilar hepaticojejunostomy with segmental hepatectomy can be performed. If the intrahepatic component is diffuse and bilobar involvement is encountered, extrahepatic biliary excision should still be performed, and drainage of intrahepatic biliary tree should be considered with two large-bore Silastic stents. The aim of this approach is to reduce intrahepatic biliary stasis, cholangitis, and stone formation potentially decreasing the risk of liver damage and malignant transformation. Some authors recommend having transplantation in this setting; treatment of patients with type IV CCs must be determined in the setting of an experienced multidisciplinary group.

Type V cyst (Caroli disease) treatment is dictated by extent of intrahepatic disease and the presence or absence of cirrhosis, portal hypertension, and liver failure. Early recognition of this disease is paramount in order to avoid recurrent cholangitis, biliary stasis, and intrahepatic abscess formation.

Initial nonoperative management may be warranted to treat cholangitis, intrahepatic stone formation, as well as biliary stasis in the attempt to decrease progressive liver injury.

In the absence of portal hypertension, if there is diffuse liver disease extrahepatic bile duct excision, biliary enteric anastomosis and permanent drainage of the intrahepatic cyst with large-bore Silastic stents may be considered. In cases of unilobar liver involvement, the treatment consists of extrahepatic bile duct excision and segmental hepatectomy. Orthotropic liver transplant is an option for Caroli disease with bilobar cystic involvement. Outcomes of transplantation are comparable to those for other transplant populations; however, the timing of transplant remains controversial.

OUTCOME/FOLLOW-UP

The treatment of choledocal cyst disease with complete resection is successful in preventing degeneration into cancer. Early complications include biliary anastomotic leak, pancreatic leak in case of accidental pancreatic duct injury, and bowel obstruction due to intussusception or internal hernia.

Late complications include biliary anastomotic stricture and recurrent cholangitis. These complications are seen in approximately 25% to 35% of the cases and are often associated with stone formation. Percutaneous dilation of anastomotic stricture with biliary stent placement usually provides durable treatment.

Despite excision of CCs, the risk of malignancy in the remaining bile ducts is estimated between 0.7% and 6% likely due to subclinical malignant disease not detected at the time of surgery or incomplete cyst excision. Therefore, patients diagnosed with cystic disorder of the biliary ducts require lifelong postoperative surveillance with serial imaging and monitoring of serum liver enzymes and tumor markers (CA 19–9).

CONCLUSION

Although cystic disorder of the biliary ducts remains a rare condition, in recent years, it is being recognized with increased frequency in the western population.

The importance of CCs is related to the lifetime risk of malignancy of approximately 10%. Cholangiocarcinoma remains the most common type of cancer arising from CCs, though these patients also have an increased risk for developing gallbladder cancer. Complete surgical resection of diseased bile ducts is the treatment of choice and should be pursued when technically possible in reasonable surgical candidates. When surgical excision is not possible, interventions should be considered such as transhepatic drains in order to decrease biliary stasis and improve symptomatology. Complete excision of the cyst can prevent biliary cancer. If CC disease is left behind as seen with type IV and type V, lifelong management and cancer surveillance are necessary. Even with complete CC excision, lifetime surveillance should continue, as late complications are common.

Suggested Readings

Abbas HM, Yassin NA, Ammori BJ. Laparoscopic resection of type I choledochal cyst in an adult and Roux-en-Y hepaticojejunostomy: a case report and literature review. *Surg Laparosc Endosc Percutan Tech* 2006;16(6):439–444.

Alonso-Lej F, Rever Wb, Pessagno Dj. Congenital choledochal cyst, with a report of 2, and an analysis of 94, cases. *Int Abstr Surg* 1959;108:1–30.

Ammori JB, Mulholland MW. Adult type I choledochal cyst resection. *J Gastrointest Surg* 2009;13(2):363–367.

Babbitt DP. Congenital choledochal cysts: new etiological concept based on anomalous relationships of the common bile duct and pancreatic bulb. *Ann Radiol* 1969;12:231–240.

Dhupar R, Gulack B, Geller DA, et al. The changing presentation of choledochal cyst disease: an incidental diagnosis. *HPB Surg* 2009;2009:103739.

Edil BH, Cameron JL, Reddy S, et al. Choledochal cyst disease in children and adults: a 30-year single-institution experience. *J Am Coll Surg* 2008;206(5):1000–1005; discussion 1005–1008.

Edil BH, Olino K, Cameron JL. The current management of choledochal cysts. *Adv Surg* 2009;43:221–232.

Lipsett PA, Pitt HA. Surgical treatment of choledochal cysts. *J Hepatobiliary Pancreat Surg* 2003;10(5):352–359.

Metcalfe MS, Wemyss-Holden SA, Maddern GJ. Management dilemmas with choledochal cysts. *Arch Surg* 2003, 138(3): 333–339.

Singham J, Yoshida EM, Scudamore CH. Choledochal cysts: part 1 of 3: classification and pathogenesis. *Can J Surg* 2009;52(5):434–440.

Singham J, Yoshida EM, Scudamore CH. Choledochal cysts: part 2 of 3: Diagnosis. *Can J Surg* 2009;52(6):506–511.

Singham J, Yoshida EM, Scudamore CH. Choledochal cysts. Part 3 of 3: management. *Can J Surg* 2010;53(1):51–56.

Todani T, Watanabe Y, Narusue M, et al. Congenital bile duct cysts: classification, operative procedures, and review of thirty-seven cases including cancer arising from choledochal cyst. *Am J Surg* 1977;134:263–269.

Ziegler KM, Pitt HA, Zyromski NJ et al. Choledochoceles: are they choledochal cyst? *Ann Surg* 2010, 252(4): 683–690.

27

Biliary Malignancies

Michael G. House

Cancers arising from the gallbladder and biliary tree are uncommon and often present with advanced, incurable stages. The lack of effective systemic and targeted therapies against these cancers has also added to the medical nihilism associated with biliary malignancy in general. Most histopathologic subtypes of adenocarcinoma along the biliary tract (e.g., gallbladder, extrahepatic [distal, perihilar], intrahepatic) carry infiltrative biologic behavior and long-term survival, even for individuals who undergo complete, potentially curative operative resection is exceptionally uncommon.

In the United States, approximately 10,000 new cases of biliary tract cancer are diagnosed each year, with the highest incidence among Native American and Hispanic women. Adenocarcinoma of the gallbladder stands as the most common malignancy of the biliary tree with an overall incidence of 1.5 per 100,000. Similar to all biliary tract cancers, gallbladder cancer incidence varies dramatically according to racial and geographic groups. Worldwide, high incidences of gallbladder cancer are reported in women living in India, Pakistan, Ecuador, and Chile.

Over the past three decades, the incidence of intrahepatic cholangiocarcinoma has increased worldwide while the incidence of extrahepatic bile duct cancers, excluding gallbladder cancer, has shown a downward trend. Several explanations for these observations have been hypothesized and include more accurate classification systems, improvements in diagnostic imaging, changes in etiologic factors, and greater health care access for low socioeconomic groups.

ETIOLOGY

Although most patients with gallstones do not develop cancer, the most common factor associated with gallbladder cancer is gallstones leading to chronic cholecystitis. Past studies have reported that large gallstones (i.e., 3 cm or larger) may carry a 10-fold relative risk of gallbladder cancer. Calcification of the gallbladder wall (i.e., porcelain gallbladder) reflecting chronic inflammation is also associated with malignancy. Historically, this risk was reported to be as high as 50%, but more accurately is estimated at less than 10%. Other chronic inflammatory diseases of the biliary tract, for example, anomalous pancreatobiliary junction, cholecystoenteric fistula, and typhoid bacillus, are associated with gallbladder cancer and biliary malignancy in general. While chronic inflammation is one predisposing factor for biliary malignancy, exposure to carcinogens (e.g., thorium, radon, dioxin, nitrosamines, vinyl chloride, isoniazid, and asbestos) and bile composition rich in free radicals may further potentiate malignant transformation of the biliary epithelium.

Similar to other gastrointestinal cancers, gallbladder cancer seemingly follows an adenoma to carcinoma sequence that reflects specific genetic mutation events. However, polypoid-type gallbladder cancers are extremely rare, and most patients with true multifocal polyps are not at increased risk for cancer development. Cholecystectomy is recommended for patients with true adenomatous polyps as the cancer incidence of malignancy among cholecystectomy specimens harboring polyps greater than 1 cm has been reported to be as high as 10%.

The most common risk factor associated with bile duct cancer in the United States is primary sclerosing cholangitis (PSC). The natural history of PSC varies, and the true incidence of cholangiocarcinoma within this population is difficult to calculate. An estimated 8% of PSC patients, diagnosed for at least 5 years, eventually develop cholangiocarcinoma; however, nearly 40% of liver explants at the time of transplantation contain occult bile duct cancer. The risk of developing cholangiocarcinoma in patients with ulcerative colitis-associated PSC is estimated at 30% at 20 years.

Congenital choledochal cysts are associated with an increased risk of cholangiocarcinoma especially in individuals with an anomalous pancreatobiliary junction as the risk of bile duct cancer may approach 15% in this population and appears to be time dependent. Chronic inflammation of the bile ducts as a result of pancreatic juice reflux is felt to be the etiologic factor, and similar risk has been observed in patients who undergo biliary sphincteroplasty or sphincterotomy. Outside of Caroli disease, biliary cystadenocarcinoma arising from a chronic, untreated cystadenoma is rare.

The risk of developing bile duct cancer, especially intrahepatic, is also increased in patients with underlying cirrhosis secondary to chronic hepatitis B or C infection. This finding might possibly explain the increased incidence of intrahepatic cholangiocarcinoma in Western populations over the past two decades. Recurrent pyogenic cholangiohepatitis and hepatolithiasis resulting from chronic portal phlebitis have been established as etiologies for cholangiocarcinoma, predominantly intrahepatic, in Southeast Asia. Biliary parasites, namely *Clonorchis sinensis* and *Opisthorchis viverrini*, which are endemic in various regions of Asia, increase the risk for both extra- and intrahepatic cholangiocarcinoma.

DIAGNOSIS

Three clinical situations for the diagnosis of gallbladder cancer exist: final pathology of a routine cholecystectomy specimen reveals an incidental cancer, cancer is discovered incidentally at the time of cholecystectomy, or gallbladder cancer is detected preoperatively. This latter situation is often associated with an advanced stage of disease and should be suspected in patients with right upper quadrant pain, weight loss, anorexia, and jaundice. Except for advanced stages of gallbladder cancer, laboratory testing of serum is not helpful for diagnosis. Serum CA 19-9 levels are sensitive but not specific for gallbladder cancer. Since gallbladder cancer is often asymptomatic in early stages, the majority of resected cases are diagnosed incidentally with routine cholecystectomy.

In the modern era of readily available imaging techniques, for example, ultrasound and computed tomography (CT), most patients diagnosed with gallbladder cancer have preoperative imaging available. Early stages of gallbladder cancer can be detected with dedicated ultrasound that may help to delineate echogenic mucosa associated with carcinoma compared to benign disease and the presence of modest hepatic parenchymal invasion. Cross-sectional imaging, with either CT or MRI, is crucial during the diagnostic and staging evaluation of suspected gallbladder cancer preoperatively or for complete staging when the diagnosis is established intra- or postoperatively. Both modalities provide excellent resolution for determining the local extent of disease (hepatic, vascular, and adjacent organ involvement) and the presence of local or regional lymphadenopathy. Distant sites of metastasis are best detected with CT imaging, which may be enhanced with positron emission tomography (PET) using fluorodeoxy-glucose (FDG).

The diagnosis of intrahepatic cholangiocarcinoma is typically established when a hypovascular tumor is detected on CT or MRI. Histologic confirmation is not necessary unless resection is not an option for treatment or the tumor carries atypical radiographic features. Hepatic metastasis from a primary source from the gastrointestinal tract, breast, lung, kidney, etc. can be excluded with upper and lower endoscopy and/or whole-body PET-CT functional imaging. Complete staging to evaluate for intra- and extrahepatic sites of metastasis (e.g., regional lymph nodes, peritoneum) and major vascular invasion can be accomplished with contrast-enhanced cross-sectional imaging (CT or MRI).

The diagnosis of hilar and distal cholangiocarcinoma usually follows targeted studies for the evaluation of obstructive jaundice or elevated liver enzymes. Most patients are referred after having had some initial studies done elsewhere, usually CT and some form of direct cholangiography, for example, endoscopic retrograde cholangiopancreatography (ERCP). Just as for gallbladder cancer, histologic confirmation of malignancy is not mandatory before planning operative treatment. In the absence of previous biliary tract surgery, the finding of a focal stenotic lesion along the extrahepatic biliary ducts combined with the appropriate clinical presentation (i.e., jaundice) is adequate for a presumptive diagnosis of hilar or distal cholangiocarcinoma depending on the level of stricture formation.

Distal bile duct tumors frequently are mistaken for adenocarcinoma of the pancreatic head, the most common periampullary malignancy. ERCP and (magnetic resonance cholangiopancreatography) MRCP are typically used to evaluate periampullary tumors when the diagnosis is suspected. As is true for hilar lesions, MRCP can provide images of the distal bile duct previously obtainable only with ERCP or percutaneous cholangiography. A dilated extrahepatic bile duct terminating abruptly at its distal aspect without a concomitantly dilated pancreatic duct suggests a distal bile duct cancer.

Although most patients with hilar strictures and jaundice have cholangiocarcinoma, alternative diagnoses are possible in up to 15% of patients. The most common of these are gallbladder carcinoma, Mirizzi syndrome, and benign focal strictures (e.g., lymphoplasmacytic sclerosing pancreatitis/cholangitis, granulomatous disease, and PSC). The finding of a smooth, tapered stricture on cholangiography suggests a benign stricture. Diagnostic assessments based on the cholangiographic appearance of the stricture are unreliable, and hilar cholangiocarcinoma must remain the leading diagnosis until disproved definitively. Relying on the results of percutaneous or endoscopic ultrasound needle biopsy or biliary brush cytology is not recommended because these results can be misleading. Many tumors express carcinoembryonic antigen (CEA) and carbohydrate antigen 19-9 (CA 19-9); however, serum levels of these markers, although elevated in some patients, often have little diagnostic value. Similarly, elevations of CA 19-9 or CEA levels in intraductal bile are not reliable or accurate.

The diagnosis of malignancy in patients with bile duct strictures can be challenging and depends on accurate interpretation of ERCP as well as cross-sectional imaging findings. ERCP, in particular, is a useful tool for assessing biliary tract strictures as it permits visualization of the biliary tree with the opportunity for therapeutic interventions (i.e., biliary drainage) and collection of specimens for cyto- and histopathologic evaluation. Biliary brushing cytology, although highly specific, has suffered from low to moderate sensitivity (15% to 68%). As a result, adjunctive diagnostic techniques including mutation analysis, DNA ploidy analysis, and fluorescence in situ hybridization (FISH) have been studied clinically and experimentally to improve tumor detection sensitivity. Two types of chromosomal abnormalities are frequently identified with a clinical FISH probe set, namely polysomy and trisomy 7. Polysomy has been defined as a gain of two or more of the four probes in ≥5 cells. FISH is now considered more sensitive than cytology for detecting biliary tract cancer.

In patients with a stricture of the extrahepatic bile duct and a clinical presentation consistent with cholangiocarcinoma or gallbladder carcinoma, histologic confirmation of malignancy is generally unnecessary, unless nonoperative therapy is planned. Endoscopic brushings of the bile duct have an unacceptably low sensitivity, making a negative result virtually useless. Excessive reliance on the results of endoscopic ultrasound-guided fine needle aspiration or endoscopic brush biopsies serves only to delay therapy.

The diagnosis of cancer in the setting of PSC can be difficult as a result of chronic liver disease, diffuse biliary strictures, and inflammatory changes of the biliary epithelium. New-onset jaundice, elevations of serum CA 19-9 level, clinical weight loss, dominant biliary stricture formation with or without cytologic or aneuploidic changes of dysplasia, or a detectable mass on cross-sectional imaging may signify carcinoma.

MANAGEMENT

Preoperative Staging

Radiographic studies are pivotal in selecting patients for resection of bile duct cancers. In addition to providing accurate preoperative staging information and anatomic delineation of local disease extent, cross-sectional imaging allows for careful operative planning. CT is an important study for evaluating patients with biliary obstruction. A high-quality CT scan can provide valuable information regarding the level of obstruction, vascular involvement, and liver atrophy. Advances in CT technology permits the acquisition of three distinct circulatory phases, consisting of the arterial, early, and late venous phases, in the hilar and pancreatobiliary regions.

Patients with hilar cholangiocarcinoma are difficult to stage preoperatively. The modified Bismuth-Corlette classification stratifies patients based on the extent of biliary duct involvement by tumor alone (Fig. 27.1). Although useful for operative planning, it does not predict resectability or survival. The American Joint Commission for Cancer (AJCC) TNM stage system (Table 27.1) is based largely on pathologic criteria and has little relevance for preoperative staging. A preoperative staging system should predict operative resectability and survival accurately. Preoperative assessments should include (1) the extent of tumor within the biliary tree, (2) vascular involvement, and (3) lobar atrophy (Table 27.2). This clinical staging scheme underscores the importance of considering portal vein involvement and liver atrophy in relation to the extent of ductal cancer spread. Ipsilateral involvement of vessels and bile ducts is usually amenable to resection, whereas contralateral involvement is not. Unilateral involvement of the hepatic artery is compatible with resection. Bilateral involvement of the hepatic artery usually is associated with nonresectability when the tumor is located mainly on the right. Hepatic arterial reconstruction in order to accomplish a complete resection should be reserved for highly select patients with potentially curable disease. Similarly, main portal vein invasion, while not an absolute contraindication for resection of hilar cholangiocarcinoma, will preclude a complete

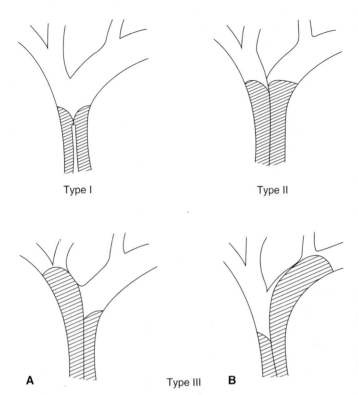

Type I   Type II

Type III

A   B

FIGURE 27.1 Bismuth-Corlette classification scheme of malignant biliary strictures.

resection with long-term benefit for the majority of patients. Unresectable hilar cholangiocarcinoma has been considered for orthotopic liver transplantation in highly selected patients with protocolized conditions and treatments.

The role of fluorodeoxyglucose positron emission tomography (FDG-PET) in the preoperative staging of patients with carcinoma of the gallbladder or biliary tract is unclear. The putative benefits of FDG-PET to identify occult metastatic disease or advanced regional lymphadenopathy have been difficult to realize in clinical practice that utilizes timely, high-resolution cross-sectional imaging routinely.

Preoperative Planning

High-resolution MRI cholangiopancreatography and direct cholangiography (e.g., ERCP or percutaneous cholangiography) provide important anatomic information, including the location of the tumor and the biliary extent of disease, both of which are crucial in operative planning. High-quality cholangiograms are essential for accurately diagnosing the extent and level of bile duct involvement. High-performance MRCP has almost replaced endoscopic and percutaneous cholangiography as the initial preoperative assessment of hilar cholangiocarcinoma. MRCP not only identifies the tumor and the level of biliary obstruction but also may reveal obstructed and isolated ducts not appreciated at endoscopic or

| TABLE 27.1 | AJCC Staging System, Seventh Edition, for Hilar Bile Duct Cancer | | |

Primary Tumor (pT)

pTX:	Cannot be assessed
pT0:	No evidence of primary tumor
pTis:	Carcinoma in situ
pT1:	Tumor confined to the bile duct, with extension up to the muscle layer or fibrous tissue
pT2a:	Tumor invades beyond the wall of the bile duct to surrounding adipose tissue
pT2b:	Tumor invades adjacent hepatic parenchyma
pT3:	Tumor invades unilateral branches of the portal vein or hepatic artery
pT4:	Tumor invades main portal vein or its branches bilaterally; or the common hepatic artery; or the second-order biliary radicals bilaterally; or unilateral second-order biliary radicals with contralateral portal vein or hepatic artery involvement

Regional Lymph Nodes (pN)

pNX	Cannot be assessed
pN0	No regional lymph node metastasis
pN1	Regional lymph node metastasis (including nodes along the cystic duct, common bile duct, hepatic artery, and portal vein)
pN2	Metastasis to periaortic, pericaval, superior mesentery artery, and/or celiac artery lymph nodes

Distant Metastasis (pM)

pMx	Cannot be assessed
pM1	Distant metastases present

Stage Groupings

Stage 0	Tis	N0	M0
Stage I	T1	N0	M0
Stage II	T2a or T2b	N0	M0
Stage IIIA	T3	N0	M0
Stage IIIB	T1, T2, or T3	N1	M0
Stage IVA	T4	N0 or N1	M0
Stage IVB	Any T	N2	M0 or M1
	Any T	Any N	M1

From Cholangiocarcinoma. In: Edge SB, Byrd DR, Compton CC (eds.). *AJCC Cancer Staging Manual*, 7th ed. New York, NY: Springer, 2010, with permission.

percutaneous study (Fig. 27.2). MRCP also provides information regarding the patency of hilar vascular structures, the presence of nodal or distant metastases, and the presence of lobar atrophy. Ultrasound, albeit operator dependent, is another useful noninvasive study during the preoperative planning process. When utilized by experienced centers, it often delineates tumor extent accurately. Ultrasound not only shows the level of biliary ductal obstruction but also can provide information regarding tumor extension within the bile duct and in the periductal tissues. Duplex ultrasound

TABLE 27.2	Preoperative Staging System for Hilar Cholangiocarcinoma

Stage	Criteria
T1	Tumor involving biliary confluence ± unilateral extension to 2 biliary radicles
T2	Tumor involving biliary confluence ± unilateral extension to 2 biliary radicles
	and ipsilateral portal vein involvement ± ipsilateral hepatic lobar atrophy
T3	Tumor involving biliary confluence + bilateral extension to 2 biliary radicles
	Or unilateral extension to 2 biliary radicles with contralateral portal vein involvement
	Or unilateral extension to 2 biliary radicles with contralateral hepatic lobar atrophy
	Or main or bilateral portal venous involvement

From Jarnagin WR, Fong Y, DeMatteo RP, et al. Staging, resectability, and outcome in 225 patients with hilar cholangiocarcinoma. *Ann Surg* 2001;234:507–519, with permission.

is firmly established as a highly accurate predictor of vascular involvement and technical resectability.

ERCP, when performed skillfully, provides useful ductal detail and can effectively drain functional liver segments prior to operative planning. Percutaneous cholangiography, while invasive, outlines the extent of intrahepatic bile duct involvement and has been the preferred study in the past for patients with hilar cholangiocarcinoma. Compared to endobiliary drainage, PTC may provide more reliable biliary drainage of the functional liver remnant when major hepatectomy is planned along with biliary resection. The benefits of preoperative biliary drainage have been difficult to prove, but most centers currently advocate for such intervention prior to resection of the extrahepatic bile ducts along with major hepatectomy.

The absolute indications for preoperative biliary drainage for jaundiced patients prior to pancreatoduodenectomy are not clear. Randomized controlled trials fail to demonstrate an improvement in postoperative outcomes for patients with periampullary cancers; however, most experts continue to advocate for preoperative endobiliary drainage for patients with deep jaundice, that is, serum total bilirubin greater than 15 mg/dL. Preoperative ERC with endobiliary drainage is the preferred approach in this situation.

For patients with hilar and intrahepatic cholangiocarcinoma who will require major hepatectomy, three-dimensional CT offers the capacity to generate volumetric models of the total liver, planned hepatic resection, and functional remnant liver volume. Since patients subjected to resection of more than 70% of functional liver parenchyma have substantially a higher risk of postoperative liver failure regardless of existing cholestatic liver disease, routine preoperative volumetry may help to identify patients who may be at considerable risk for postoperative hepatic failure and select candidates for preoperative portal vein embolization. The purpose of portal vein embolization is to increase the functional liver mass by inducing compensatory hypertrophy in the future liver remnant with the ultimate goal to minimize postoperative liver dysfunction that contributes to mortality substantially.

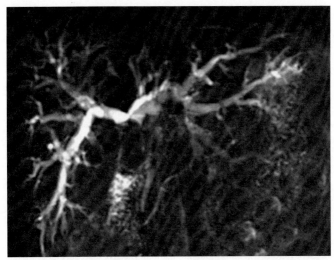

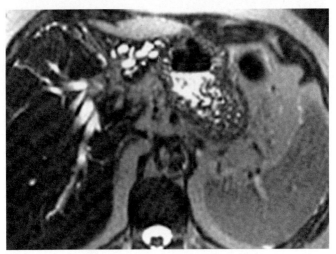

FIGURE 27.2 Coronal **(A)** and axial **(B)** MRCP images of a patient with hilar cholangio-carcinoma. The tumor involves the right and left hepatic ducts. The bile ducts in this study appear white. Extreme atrophy of the left hemiliver is apparent.

In right portal vein embolization, the volume of the left lobe increases by 130 cm^3 on average within 2 weeks after embolization, and the estimated resection volume decreases by an average of approximately 10%. In the absence of randomized controlled trials, the indications for portal vein embolization remain somewhat arbitrary, but many centers utilize this technique preoperatively for patients undergoing extended right hepatectomy in the presence of underlying liver disease. In recent years, some centers have experimented with associating liver partition and portal vein ligation for staged hepatectomy (ALPPS) as a perioperative technique to induce rapid hypertrophy of the future liver remnant and avoid postoperative liver dysfunction.

OPERATIVE INDICATIONS AND THERAPY

Staging laparoscopy for biliary tract malignancy should be considered for all patients with suspicious clinicopathologic findings for metastatic disease (e.g., remarkable elevations of serum CA 19-9 level, extreme weight loss, rapidly declining performance status, indeterminant nodules involving the liver or peritoneum). With an overall yield of 30%, staging laparoscopy should be utilized for all patients with gallbladder cancer and intrahepatic cholangiocarcinoma involving the liver capsule. Since the detection rate for occult metastases is stage dependent, most surgeons apply staging laparoscopy selectively for patients with extrahepatic bile duct cancer.

For gallbladder cancer in general, operative resection is indicated for patients with localized disease, that is, tumors limited to the gallbladder, liver bed, and regional lymph nodes. Peritoneal dissemination, extensive liver or bile duct (especially left hepatic duct) involvement, nodal metastases beyond the hepatoduodenal ligament (i.e., N2 disease, Fig. 27.3), left hepatic artery or portal vein encasement, or pancreatoduodenal infiltration

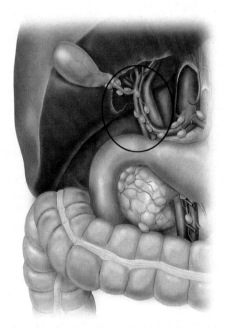

FIGURE 27.3 Regional lymph nodes associated with gallbladder cancer. The subhilar N1 level lymph nodes within the hepatoduodenal ligament are encircled. Lymph nodes outside of the circle (e.g., celiac, aortocaval, and mesenteric nodes) are considered N2 level. (Figure borrowed from Lillemoe K, Jarnagin WR (eds.). *Hepatobiliary and pancreatic surgery.* Philadelphia, PA: Lippincott Williams & Wilkins, 2013.)

should serve as contraindications for reasonable attempts at curative resection. Intraoperative ultrasound is a useful tool to further delineate spatial relationships between the tumor, liver, and surrounding hilar structures.

Tumors limited to the mucosa (T1a) can be treated sufficiently with cholecystectomy alone. Patients with deeper invasion require en bloc partial hepatectomy (wedge resection of adjacent liver for T1b tumors; segment IVb + V resection for T2-3 tumors) with regional subhilar periportal lymphadenectomy. Resection of the extrahepatic bile ducts followed by reconstruction with hepaticojejunostomy should be reserved for tumors that extend into the hepatic or common bile duct. Tumor invasion of the right hepatic duct and/or right hepatic artery is not a contraindication to operative resection, which requires an extended right hepatectomy in this circumstance.

Appreciating the extent (size, multifocality, major vascular involvement) of intrahepatic bile duct cancer on preoperative imaging and intraoperative ultrasound is crucial for planning hepatic resections for this disease. These tumors frequently arise from the segment IV ducts and involve the central liver inflow anatomy. Three phenotypes of intrahepatic cholangiocarcinoma have been described: periductal infiltrating, mass-forming, and intraductal/papillary. Usually large, these tumors often require a major hepatectomy that warrants serious preoperative consideration for the size and status of the future liver remnant (described above under preoperative planning). Proper incision and exposure are essential elements of a safe hepatectomy. Hemostatic hepatic parenchymal transection has been aided by several energy devices, including the ultrasonic aspirator, saline-linked cautery, bipolar electrocoagulation, and ultrasonic scalpel. A solitary tumor located peripherally, especially within an anterior segment, is often amenable to a safe laparoscopic technique that focuses on segmental anatomy for optimal tumor clearance. The spatial relationship of the tumor to the sectoral bile ducts and hepatic ducts needs to considered in all cases. A periductal infiltrating phenotype of a tumor with involvement of the left, right, or common hepatic ducts will require extrahepatic biliary resection often with the need for biliary reconstruction.

The Bismuth-Corlette classification scheme provides a rudimentary guide for planning operative resection for hilar cholangiocarcinoma. Type I tumors without involvement of the right hepatic artery can be treated with resection of the entire extrahepatic biliary tree (without hepatectomy), subhilar lymphadenectomy, and bilateral cholangiojejunostomy. Since biliary branches of the hepatic caudate are involved in most cases of type II-III hilar cholangiocarcinoma, caudate resection en bloc with a major hepatectomy and extrahepatic bile duct resection is indicated for these tumors. Type IIIa tumors, which may encase the right hepatic artery, are approached with an extended right hepatectomy or formal right trisectionectomy with caudate resection. In the absence of right hepatic artery involvement, type IIIb tumors are resected with extrahepatic bile duct excision, left hepatectomy, and caudate resection. The final bile duct margin status, both proximally and distally, should be assessed intraoperatively with frozen section histopathology. Sub- and perihilar lymphadenectomy should be considered routine for all operations. Kocherization of the duodenum and head of the pancreas during early exploration permits examination of the retropancreatic and aortocaval spaces to exclude advanced levels of lymph node metastases and limited opportunity for long-term benefit following operative resection.

Pancreatoduodenectomy for periampullary carcinoma has been described extensively throughout this text. Understanding the longitudinally spreading nature of cholangiocarcinoma, most surgeons recommend a high transection of the common hepatic duct in patients with distal bile duct cancer. The proximal hepatic duct margin should be analyzed intraoperatively to ensure tumor clearance.

PREVENTION AND TREATMENT OF POSTOPERATIVE COMPLICATIONS

Postoperative fluid collections after hepatectomy are usually related to either bleeding or bile leaks from the transected liver surface. Intraoperative transcystic leak tests after hepatectomy can be performed, but have not been shown to affect the incidence of postoperative bile leaks. Leaks from small biliary radicals rarely require intervention; however, 8% of all hepatectomies result in bile leaks from segmental ducts requiring percutaneous drainage. Percutaneous drainage alone will treat the majority of perihepatic fluid collections. Persistent bile leaks after percutaneous drainage should raise suspicion for a stricture of the native distal bile ducts or biliary–enteric anastomosis. In these situations, endoscopic or percutaneous biliary stenting may be necessary for resolution.

The reported association between deep organ space infection after hepatectomy and biliary–enteric anastomosis encourages judicious operative drain placement. Decompression of the biliary–enteric anastomosis with transhepatic stenting has been utilized by some surgeons to decrease the incidence of infectious complications after hepatectomy.

The risk of postoperative hepatic failure after major hepatectomy is related to the volume and quality of the functional liver remnant. Factors that predispose patients to postoperative hepatic failure include age, gender, diabetes mellitus, fatty liver disease, operative blood loss, small liver remnant (<20% normal liver volume, <40% cirrhotic liver volume), cholestasis, and postoperative infection. Preoperative factors can be addressed with techniques to improve the functional liver remnant, for example, biliary drainage and portal vein embolization. Postoperative liver failure must be addressed promptly in the postoperative period with drainage of perihepatic fluid collections and appropriate treatment of infection.

OUTCOMES

Stage-dependent survival after resection for gallbladder adenocarcinoma is summarized in Figure 27.4. Median survival for stage IV gallbladder cancer is less than 6 months; thus, operative intervention, even with palliative intent, for this stage of disease is never advocated. Simple cholecystectomy for pathologically staged T1a cancer results in cure in most cases, whereas more advanced stages of disease requiring extensive operations for tumor clearance lend themselves to long-term survival infrequently. The role of adjuvant therapy for gallbladder adenocarcinoma remains unclear. Past studies of 5-fluorouracil or gemcitabine with or without external beam radiotherapy failed to show a benefit in long-term survival; however, the addition of cisplatin to gemcitabine has improved treatment response rates for unresectable biliary tract cancers considerably. Future collaborative trials are necessary to study the benefits of adjuvant platinum-based chemotherapy for bile duct cancer.

Aggressive operations for hilar cholangiocarcinoma have been associated with major postoperative complications and mortality. But, improvements in operative technique along with better patient selection and avoidance of postoperative hepatic failure have decreased postoperative morbidity and mortality substantially over the past two decades. Long-term survival is realized only for patients who undergo

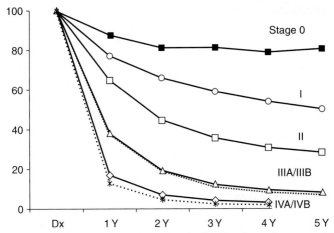

FIGURE 27.4 Overall 5-year survival for resected gallbladder adenocarcinoma, according to AJCC seventh edition cancer stage. (Figure borrowed from Lillemoe K, Jarnagin WR (eds.). *Hepatobiliary and pancreatic surgery.* Philadelphia, PA: Lippincott Williams & Wilkins, 2013.)

an R0 resection and do not carry lymph node metastases. Orthotopic liver transplantation for hilar cholangiocarcinoma can achieve excellent long-term outcomes for highly selected patients (i.e., no lymph node or distant metastases) who demonstrate no evidence of disease progression with neoadjuvant chemoradiotherapy. Liver transplant for cholangiocarcinoma is only performed in select centers with extremely close clinical selection criteria.

Patients with unresectable, locally advanced hilar tumors but without evidence of widespread disease may be candidates for palliative radiation therapy. A combination of stereotactic external beam radiation (5,000 to 6,000 cGy) with or without intraductal iridium-192 (2,000 cGy) delivered percutaneously or endoscopically can be applied. Intraluminal (either endoscopic or transhepatic) photodynamic therapy has been utilized for unresectable hilar cholangiocarcinoma. This two-step procedure involves systemic administration of a photosensitizer followed by direct illumination via cholangioscopy, which activates the compound causing local tumor cell death. Two randomized studies in patients with unresectable cholangiocarcinoma suggested improved survival with biliary stenting combined with photodynamic therapy compared with biliary stenting alone, but the improved survival observed with photodynamic therapy is likely related to better biliary decompression and avoidance of early segmental duct isolation and subsequent cholangitis, rather than any significant reduction in tumor burden.

Several pathologic features of intrahepatic cholangiocarcinoma have adverse effects on prognosis even after complete resection. Lymph node metastases, multifocality, and major vascular invasion all have negative impact on survival. Liver transplantation has been utilized for highly selected patients with technically unresectable tumors confined to the liver. Transarterial chemoembolization and radioembolization can be offered to patients with unresectable disease in an attempt to slow disease progression and possibly improve survival.

CONCLUSION

Enhanced radiologic imaging and greater understanding of malignancies of the biliary tract have permitted improved operative outcomes over the past few decades. Progress in these two areas has allowed better patient selection, preoperative preparation of the future liver remnant, and techniques to treat bile duct cancer from a surgical standpoint. Even in the modern era, highly effective systemic agents for cholangiocarcinoma are lacking, which leaves a large therapeutic gap for patients with advanced stages of disease. One of the main goals of treating patients with bile duct cancer is palliation from biliary obstruction, which can be accomplished endoscopically, percutaneously, or operatively. With recent improvements in chemotherapy, endoluminal therapy, and brachyradiotherapy, a multidisciplinary approach toward treating bile duct cancer should be advocated in order to achieve optimal individualized treatments for patients.

Suggested Readings

D'Angelica M, Fong Y, Weber S, et al. The role of staging laparoscopy in hepatobiliary malignancy: prospective analysis of 401 cases. *Ann Surg Oncol* 2003;10:183–189.

Endo I, House MG, Klimstra D, et al. Clinical significance of intraoperative bile duct margin assessment for hilar cholangiocarcinoma. *Ann Surg Oncol* 2008, 15(8):2104–2112.

Farges O, Belghiti J, Kianmanesh R, et al. Portal vein embolization before right hepatectomy: prospective clinical trial. *Ann Surg* 2003; 237:208–217.

Jarnagin WR, Fong Y, DeMatteo RP, et al. Staging, resectability, and outcome in 225 patients with hilar cholangiocarcinoma. *Ann Surg* 2001;234:507–519.

Kawasaki S, Imamura H, Kobayashi A. Results of surgical resection for patients with hilar bile duct cancer: application of extended hepatectomy after biliary drainage and hemihepatic portal vein embolization. *Ann Surg* 2003;238:84–92.

Kennedy TJ, Yopp A, Qin Y, et al. Role of preoperative biliary drainage of liver remnant prior to extended liver resection for hilar cholangiocarcinoma. *HPB* 2009;11(5):445–451.

Loehrer AP, House MG, Nakeeb A, et al. Cholangiocarcinoma: Are North American outcomes optimal? *J Am Coll Surg* 2013;216(2):192–200.

Nagino M, Kamiya J, Arai T, et al. Two hundred forty consecutive portal vein embolizations before extended hepatectomy for biliary cancer: surgical outcome and long-term follow-up. *Ann Surg* 2006;243:364–372.

Quyn AJ, Ziyaie D, Polignano FM, Tait IS. Photodynamic therapy is associated with an improvement in survival for patients with irresectable hilar cholangiocarcinoma. *HPB* 2009;11(7):570–577.

Rea DJ, Heimbach JK, Rosen CB, et al. Liver transplantation with neoadjuvant chemoradiation is more effective than resection for hilar cholangiocarcinoma. *Ann Surg* 2005; 242:451–458.

Schnitzbauer AA, Lang SA, Goessmann H, et al. Right portal vein ligation combined with in situ splitting induces rapid left lateral liver lobe hypertrophy enabling 2-staged extended right hepatic resection in small-for-size settings. *Ann Surg* 2012;255(3):405–414.

Valle J, Wasan H, Palmer DH, et al. Cisplatin plus gemcitabine versus gemcitabine for biliary tract cancer. *NEJM* 2010;362(14):1273–1281.

Van der Gaag, NA, Rauws EA, van Eijck CH, et al. Preoperative biliary drainage for cancer of the head of the pancreas. *NEJM* 2010;362(2):129–137.

28

Minimally Invasive Biliary Surgery

Eugene P. Ceppa

Minimally invasive biliary surgery is indicated in only a few isolated complex biliary disease processes when technical expertise is available. Historically and currently, the vast majority of biliary surgery is performed through an open approach. However, the benefits of laparoscopic surgery have been established in numerous other areas of general surgery including cholecystectomy, gastric bypass, and colectomy. Currently, a paucity of data exists regarding the role of minimally invasive biliary surgery. Through the improvement of surgical skill (experience and fellowship training) and technology (optics, robotics, surgical staplers, and tissue-sealing devices), surgeons have begun to challenge the standard of care in biliary surgery. In order to avoid overlap, this chapter focuses primarily on laparoscopic Roux-en-Y hepaticojejunostomy as the preferred biliary–enteric reconstruction for the treatment of biliary disease.

PREOPERATIVE CONSIDERATIONS

Preoperative considerations focus primarily on patient variables that affect minimally invasive surgery and preparation of the patient for surgery. Patient variables to consider include comorbid conditions, past surgical history (especially abdominal surgery), body habitus, and hepatoduodenal ligament anatomy. Comorbid conditions play a role in laparoscopic approach primarily as a function of length of anesthetic time and ability to clear carbon dioxide from the pneumoperitoneum. Patients with advanced cardiopulmonary disease are particularly fragile if the length of anesthetic time is excessive. This may negate the typical benefits of the laparoscopic approach. As a surgeon gains experience, operative times typically decrease dramatically, yet the learning curve in complex biliary surgery is unknown. Airway pathology (obstructive sleep apnea) and pulmonary disease (chronic obstructive pulmonary disease) can be exacerbated as a result of prolonged anesthetic and subsequent insufflation with carbon dioxide. Nearly 100% of patients who possess a body mass index (BMI) of greater than 45 have obstructive sleep apnea (with or without documented sleep studies), and patients with home oxygen requirements or room air arterial CO_2 concentration of greater than 44 mmHg should be identified as high risk prior to entering the operative theater. A history of portal hypertension or cirrhosis can be a major deterrent regardless of approach.

Past surgical history is a major component for surgeon decision making in terms of peritoneal access, port placement, the ability to perform the jejunojejunostomy, and whether the Roux limb will reach the porta hepatis for bile duct reconstruction. History taking and examination are critical to determine previous abdominal operations and location of concurrent cicatrices. Ventral hernia repair with mesh should also be specifically determined as peritoneal access and contamination of synthetic mesh with bile can create new infectious problems. More extensive open abdominal operations tend to have more robust adhesions around the small bowel, which can either prevent formation of an adequate Roux limb or increase operative times for the required enterolysis.

Body habitus is not a contraindication to laparoscopy but deters some surgeons for multiple reasons. Larger patients (BMI > 35) require longer instruments; thus, reach to the porta hepatis can be difficult. Abdominal wall tension on laparoscopic instruments can place undue stress to long, thin instruments and can either limit the ability to use some necessary instruments or damage them beyond functional use. Mobilization of the hepatic flexure and a Kocher maneuver are made more difficult when the transverse mesocolon and omentum contain more fat and organs are larger in size overall; once mobilized, the hepatic flexure and the retroperitoneum lateral to the duodenum can be more difficult to retract for exposure purposes when fatty or large. Finally, super morbidly obese (BMI > 50) patients typically have engorged livers as a result of fatty liver disease and are prone to lacerations (hemorrhage within the operative field significantly impairs image brightness) and fractures leading to further surgery to correct the problem. These patients should be considered for a preoperative liquid diet with protein supplementation (7 days prior) to diminish the water weight of the liver resulting in a temporary reduction in liver size to optimize the intraoperative exposure and minimize surrounding tissue injury.

Mastering the patient's preoperative diagnostic imaging can make intraoperative decision making clearer. Cholangiography provides an intra-luminal roadmap of the biliary tree. Identification of cystic duct or cystic duct clips can be performed safely and provide intraoperative details about the location of the bile duct. Also, knowledge of bile duct anomalies helps avoid injury when they are expected prior to surgery. Cross-sectional imaging with arterial and venous phases assists in determining the location of the hepatic arterial branches (specifically if the right hepatic artery traverses anterior to or passes posterior to the common hepatic duct to avoid inadvertent injury or ligation). Replaced right or completely replaced common hepatic artery branches should be identified with imaging to avoid injury during mobilization of the bile duct. Portal vein, superior mesenteric vein, and splenic vein thrombosis should be sought out prior to surgery as collateral veins can make the hepatoduodenal ligament dissection treacherous. Finally, a large, pathologically dilated bile duct can be easily seen on diagnostic imaging, and some surgeons will only attempt a laparoscopic hepaticojejunostomy on dilated bile ducts as a tenet of patient selection.

Patients with complex biliary disease commonly have other medical issues that require treatment prior to surgery. Preoperative biliary obstruction exposes the patient to the effects of jaundice, bactibilia, and external manipulation of the biliary tree (endoscopic or transhepatic). When infection is present in the form of cholangitis or biloma, antibiotics are indicated, and treatment of the obstruction with biliary endoprosthesis or percutaneous biliary drains and/or percutaneous peritoneal drains is required for source control. Patients with infection or biliary insensible losses may be malnourished, may be dehydrated, possess electrolyte abnormalities, and are deficient in vitamin K altering coagulation parameters. All of these factors should be corrected prior to surgery to minimize postoperative complications.

OPERATIVE INDICATIONS AND TECHNICAL TIPS

Indications for hepaticojejunostomy are listed in Table 28.1. Biliary obstruction secondary to benign and malignant strictures is the primary indication for hepaticojejunostomy. Benign complex biliary disease includes iatrogenic biliary stricture, choledochal cysts, chronic pancreatitis, Mirizzi

TABLE 28.1	Indications for Biliary–Enteric Reconstruction

Benign
    Iatrogenic bile duct injury
    Chronic pancreatitis
    Choledochal cysts
    Mirizzi syndrome
    Traumatic bile duct injury
Malignant
    Cholangiocarcinoma (mid–bile duct)
    Pancreatic adenocarcinoma—palliative
    Cholangiocarcinoma (distal)—palliative
    Duodenal adenocarcinoma—palliative
    Ampullary adenocarcinoma—palliative
    Portal lymphadenopathy—palliative

syndrome, and traumatic bile duct injuries. Choledocholithiasis and mini-mally invasive treatment thereof can be found in Chapter 25 (common bile duct exploration). Indications for treatment of malignant biliary strictures include extrahepatic bile duct resection and reconstruction of cholangio-carcinoma (Bismuth II) or palliation of periampullary tumors (pancreatic adenocarcinoma, distal cholangiocarcinoma, duodenal adenocarcinoma, and ampullary adenocarcinoma) and portal lymphadenopathy resulting from metastasis of secondary malignant tumors. Periampullary tumor treatment with curative intent via a laparoscopic pancreaticoduodenec-tomy can be found in Chapter 8 (laparoscopic pancreatic surgery).

Most studies indicate that a Roux-en-Y hepaticojejunostomy is the saf-est and most reproducible method of biliary–enteric reconstruction possess-ing the best long-term patency rate. The critical skill set for this procedure is intracorporeal suturing using laparoscopic needle drivers and graspers. The following are the critical steps toward biliary–enteric reconstruction:

1. Patient position with both arms out is suitable.
2. Port placement can vary among surgeons, but Figure 28.1 demonstrates an accepted configuration. The ports consist of a 5 mm port in both the right and left subcostal margins, a 12-mm right upper quadrant port (surgeon's primary port), and a 5- or 12-mm port in both the left upper quadrant and umbilicus (primarily for the camera). A subxiphoid incision can be made without a port for placement of a liver retractor.
3. To create the Roux limb, starting in the supine position is best. The liga-ment of Treitz is identified at the base of the transverse mesocolon.
4. A window is created between the vasa recta of the small bowel, and the small bowel is divided using a laparoscopic stapler with a 3.5-mm staple load approximately 50 cm distal to the ligament of Treitz.
5. Use the tissue-sealing device to divide the mesentery evenly in order not to encroach on the arterial arcade on either side of the divided bowel (optional). This maneuver provides a slightly longer reach to the bile duct and avoids undue tension on the anastomosis. The bowel proximal to the staple line is the alimentary limb; an additional 50 cm of small bowel distal to the staple line is measured and referred to as the Roux limb.
6. A side-to-side jejunojejunostomy is fashioned:
    a. Two 3-0 absorbable stay sutures are placed 6 to 10 cm apart.
    b. Enterotomies are created with the cautery.

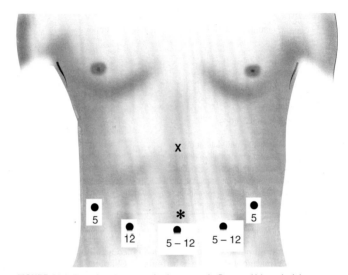

FIGURE 28.1 Port site placement for laparoscopic Roux-en-Y hepaticojejunostomy. *, Camera port; X, optional liver retractor.

    c. An articulating 60-mm cartridge of a 2.5-mm staple load is introduced into the bowel via the enterotomies. This load is generally more hemostatic than is the typical 3.5-mm load used commonly for bowel cases.

    d. The bowel is manipulated so that the mesentery is outside the staple load.

    e. The anastomosis between the alimentary and Roux limbs is created with the stapler.

    f. The common enterostomy is oversewed with a 3-0 absorbable running suture.

    g. The jejunojejunostomy mesenteric defect is closed with a running 2-0 nonabsorbable suture to prevent future internal hernias. Avoid full-thickness bites across the bowel mesenteric edge that was previously sealed with an energy device, which can lead to unnecessary hemorrhage, ischemia, or hematoma near the anastomosis. The subsequent complications include bleeding, perforation, and obstruction postoperatively. Solely suture the peritoneum superficially together.

    h. Visualize the Roux limb mesenteric edge, and travel down toward the root of the mesentery to ensure the mesentery is not twisted (this is worth double or triple checking as peripheral visualization is limited during laparoscopic surgery).

    i. Create a defect in the transverse mesocolon with the tissue-sealing device to the right of the middle colic artery. Preserve the left space in case a future pancreatic Roux limb is needed.

    j. Mark the Roux limb staple line with a stitch or a Penrose drain/colored tourniquet to make passing the bowel through the transverse mesocolon defect easier (optional).

7. Mobilization of the common bile duct within the hepatoduodenal ligament—mobilizing the hepatic flexure of the colon and performing wide Kocher maneuver should be used liberally to expose the porta hepatis:

a. If no cholecystectomy has been performed previously, use the gall-bladder to identify the cystic duct, and travel proximally toward the common hepatic–bile duct junction. The gallbladder also provides a useful "handle" (Fig. 28.2) for a lateral to medial approach when dissecting the soft tissues of the hepatoduodenal ligament. Typically, there is a station 12 lymph node just cephalad to the duodenum along the lateral border of the ligament to mark the location of the distal common bile duct.

b. Incise the peritoneum anteriorly to expose the bile duct and hepatic arterial supply. The bile duct will be lateral to the proper hepatic artery. Be mindful that the right hepatic artery travels anterior to the common hepatic duct in 10% of patients.

c. Mobilize the ligament further by incising the peritoneum laterally toward the inferior vena cava to open near the shared border of the common bile duct and portal vein. This maneuver will allow for less resistance when dissecting medially to laterally posterior to the bile duct.

d. Encircle the bile duct with a vessel loop or Penrose drain; use metallic clips to secure both tails together for retraction purposes.

e. Pass a right-angled instrument posterior to the bile duct, and use the cautery to divide the bile duct. The cautery can be used to obtain hemostasis at the 3 and 9 o'clock arterial supple at the cut edge of the bile duct. The bile duct should bleed briskly; if it does not, then consider dissecting the bile duct proximally to better perfused tissue.

f. If a biliary endoprosthesis or percutaneous biliary drain is across the bile duct, either can be used to stent your anastomosis. Otherwise, if it is cumbersome, stents can be removed as it may make the anastomosis more difficult. If stenting the biliary–enteric anastomosis is desired, the ideal situation is to place your own 12-Fr biliary stent across the anastomosis after the posterior row has been completed.

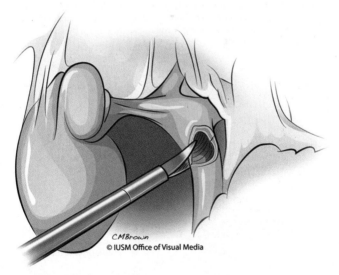

CMBrown
© IUSM Office of Visual Media

FIGURE 28.2 The gallbladder (if in situ) provides a useful landmark and "handle" to distract the bile duct laterally.

g. A laparoscopic bulldog clamp is commercially available and can be used to clamp the proximal cut edge of the bile duct; in some cases, this may allow for a slight dilatation of a smaller bile duct and minimize biliary soilage of the peritoneum.

h. The distal bile duct should be oversewn or may be closed with a staple (or clips if small).

8. Biliary–enteric anastomosis:

a. Some surgeons prefer the Trendelenburg position (head down) at the time of an intracorporeal hand-sewn hepaticojejunostomy to take tension off of the anastomosis by way of the small bowel mesentery using gravity to bring the Roux limb closer. Reverse Trendelenburg position is useful in obese patients by using gravity to retract the hepatic flexure away from the porta hepatis. The Roux limb is usually supported with a grasper from one of the assistant port sites in either scenario.

b. For larger bile ducts, tie two separate 4-0 absorbable sutures together leaving it double armed. Each suture is cut to a shorter length typically 15 to 20 cm each in length but can be adjusted based on the size of the bile duct. For small bile ducts, interrupted 4-0 absorbable sutures are used for the posterior and anterior rows (Fig. 28.3).

c. An enterotomy is created on the anterior aspect (i.e., bowel side closest to the camera) of the antimesenteric border of the Roux limb.

d. A stay suture is placed at 12 o'clock on the bile duct for retraction of the anterior wall during creation of the posterior row.

e. The suture is introduced into the peritoneum; one arm is passed outside-in on the bowel and the other on the bile duct (starting at 3 o'clock).

f. The posterior row is created first by suturing inside out on the bowel then outside-in on the bile duct. Special attention is necessary during the first bite with the suture as most leaks will occur posteriorly on the bile duct side after the initial anchoring of the double-armed suture.

g. Upon completion of the posterior row, a bulldog clamp is placed on the remainder of the posterior row stitch to maintain tension preventing unraveling of the posterior row.

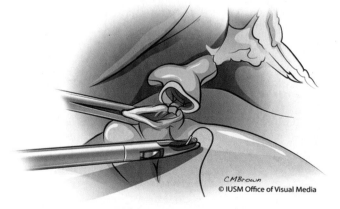

CMBrown
© IUSM Office of Visual Media

FIGURE 28.3 The posterior row of absorbable sutures is placed with knots on the inside of the anastomosis to facilitate visualization of the knots being tied.

h. The 12 o'clock stay suture should be removed now to prevent confusion.

i. Stenting the biliary–enteric anastomosis would occur either now or midway through completing the anterior row.

j. The anterior row is completed by suturing outside-in on the bowel then inside out on the bile duct.

k. The anastomosis is completed by tying the two sutures on the outside at the 9 o'clock position.

l. After completion of the anastomosis, the redundant Roux limb is pulled back through the mesocolon defect toward the jejunojejunostomy. Furthermore, the limb is secured directly to the peritoneum at the mesenteric defect with 3-0 nonabsorbable suture to prevent herniation.

m. Surgical drainage of the anastomosis is by surgeon preference.

POSTOPERATIVE MANAGEMENT, INCLUDING COMPLICATIONS

The majority of the postoperative management centers on bowel function and the advancement of the patient's diet. The previously established overall complication rate for open hepaticojejunostomy is 10% to 20% and mortality of 1% (Table 28.2). The principal complication for hepaticojejunostomy is the development of a biliary fistula (early) or stricture (late). The number of laparoscopic hepaticojejunostomy reports is so low that a true incidence of these complications is undetermined. A recent systematic review reported 19 studies to date describing a collective experience with true laparoscopic choledochoduodenostomy, cholecystojejunostomy, or hepaticojejunostomy for benign or malignant biliary disease (Table 28.2); the authors reported a biliary fistula or early stricture rate that appears to be greater than that of the open approach. The corresponding question that presently has no answer is whether a biliary fistula in the laparoscopic approach has worse outcomes as compared to the open approach. When comparing laparoscopic and open reconstruction, it is important to note that many surgeons with open biliary reconstruction currently do not internally stent or externally drain this anastomosis. Routine drainage of laparoscopic biliary–enteric anastomosis may be prudent as the incidence of early biliary fistula may be slightly higher using the laparoscopic approach. Although not common, it is possible to see bile in the surgical drain on postoperative day 1. Nevertheless, in limited experience with these biliary fistulas, they resolve in 2 to 3 days later and the majority prior to the date of discharge.

TABLE 28.2	Comparison of Laparoscopic and Open Biliary–Enteric Reconstruction	
	Laparoscopic	**Open**
Patients	Review[a] (N = 89)	Historical Comparison
Conversion to open	2 (2%)	N/A
Early patency rate (90 d)	85 (96%)	>90%
Mortality	5 (6 %)	1%
Morbidity	11 (12%)	15%
Biliary fistula	2 (2%)	1%
Early biliary stricture (1 y)	2 (2%)	1%
Long-term patency rate (>20 y)	N/A	70%–90%

[a]Toumi Z, Aljarabah M, Ammori B. Role of laparoscopic approach to biliary bypass for benign and malignant disease: a systematic review. *Surg Endosc* 2011;25:2105–2116.

If a prolonged fistula is seen, then the surgical drain is left in place at the time of discharge, and the suction bulb is changed to a gravity drainage bile bag. Prolonged fistulas are managed as an outpatient as long as the patient is asymptomatic, and at each clinic visit, the drain is retracted a short distance (2 to 3 cm) away from the fistula and secured to the skin. As long as the surgical drain is in place, rarely does a biliary fistula require intervention or lead to biliary sepsis. A high-volume (i.e., >100 to 200 mL) biliary fistula demands more thorough interrogation and more aggressive treatment.

Further complications include a jejunojejunostomy leak (<1%), which is exceedingly rare and does not typically require external drainage. The likely cause of this complication is due to ischemia of the bowel by inattentive division of the arterial supply with the tissue-sealing device within the mesentery while creating the Roux limb. If the bowel appears dusky or blue, it is best to repeat the anastomosis instead of hoping it improves. Some surgeons routinely create BP and Roux limbs 50 cm each, which gives extra length of bowel in case one needs to repeat anastomosis either at the time of the index procedure or during a take-back/revision. Internal hernia is more likely in larger patients and those where the mesocolon and jejunojejunostomy mesenteric defects were not closed. In spite of suture closure of defects, patients still likely have a 5% to 10% lifetime risk of developing a symptomatic internal hernia. These hernias present as a bowel obstruction, and any patient with a Roux limb should have an increased suspicion for internal hernia and a low threshold for operative exploration especially considering nonoperative management rarely resolves this type of bowel obstruction. The development of port site hernia is rare for 5-mm port sites and less than 1% for 12-mm port sites. Port sites do not require fascial closure if they are 5 mm; some surgeons do not close 12-mm port sites above the umbilicus since they are "protected" by the liver and stomach. A prudent approach is to close all fascial defects at 12-mm port sites either conventionally in thin patients or laparoscopically with the suture passer in obese patients.

OUTCOMES/FOLLOW-UP

The primary long-term outcome of interest following biliary–enteric reconstruction is patency rate. Open series report a 70% to 90% patency rate two decades following Roux-en-Y hepaticojejunostomy (Table 28.2). Data for laparoscopic biliary reconstruction are scant; no long-term data exist documenting true patency rates.

Follow-up varies widely, yet most surgeons see their patients 3 to 4 weeks postoperatively with a history and physical exam and laboratory studies (CBC, CMP) to determine if the patient has any signs of biliary fistula or stricture and to ensure adequate biliary drainage. A more thorough approach is to obtain a right upper quadrant ultrasound at 12 weeks to determine the presence of any dilated intrahepatic ducts or postoperative fluid collection in the gallbladder fossa, followed by a 99mTc choletech scan in nuclear medicine at 24 weeks to document filling of the Roux limb with radiotracer from the liver. In cases where a biliary fistula or stricture is identified in the postoperative period, cholangiography is indicated; the percutaneous approach is favored over double-balloon enteroscopy via the Roux limb since intervention is more accessible via the percutaneous approach.

CONCLUSION

Minimally invasive biliary surgery has not progressed as rapidly as minimally invasive liver or pancreatic surgery. The principal hurdle is the technical challenge and paramount reliance of intracorporeal suture at difficult angles in the "faraway" porta hepatis where retraction and exposure are technically challenging. Optimal outcomes are achieved by proper patient selection as well as surgeon experience both with biliary pathology and with complex laparoscopic skills.

Suggested Readings

Bismuth H. Postoperative strictures of the bile duct. In: Blumgard LH, ed. *The biliary tract*. Edinburgh, UK: Churchill Livingstone, 1982:209–218.

Branum G, Schmitt C, Baillie J, et al. Management of major biliary complications after laparoscopic cholecystectomy. *Ann Surg* 1993;217:532–540.

Chowbey PK, Katrak MP, Sharma A, et al. Complete laparoscopic management of choledochal cyst: report of 2 cases. *J Laparoendosc Adv Surg Tech A* 2002;12:219–223.

Chowbey PK, Soni V, Sharma A, et al. Laparoscopic hepaticojejunostomy for biliary strictures. The experience of 10 patients. *Surg Endosc* 2005;19:273–279.

Lillemoe KD, Melton GB, Cameron JL, et al. Postoperative bile duct strictures: management and outcome in the 1990s, *Ann Surg* 2000;232:430–441.

Shimura H, Tanaka M, Shimizu S, et al. Laparoscopic treatment of congenital choledochal cysts. *Surg Endosc* 1998;12:1268–1271.

Stewart L, Way LW. Bile duct injuries during laparoscopic cholecystectomy, *Arch Surg* 1995;130:1123–1128.

Strasberg SM, Hertl M, Soper NJ. An analysis of the problem of biliary injury during laparoscopic cholecystectomy, *J Am Coll Surg* 1995;180:101–125.

Toumi Z, Aljarabah M, Ammori B. Role of laparoscopic approach to biliary bypass for benign and malignant disease: a systematic review. *Surg Endosc* 2011; 25:2105–2116.

Bile Leak and Bile Duct Injury

Jordan P. Bloom and Keith D. Lillemoe

INTRODUCTION

A biliary leak is defined as leakage of bile from any site in the biliary tree including the bile duct, cystic duct, liver, or gallbladder. In the United States, a bile duct injury (BDI) is most commonly the result of iatrogenic injury during cholecystectomy. Cholecystectomy is one of the most commonly performed abdominal operations with over 750,000 performed yearly in the United States. Over 90% of these operations are being performed laparoscopically. The overall incidence of bile duct injuries during laparoscopic cholecystectomy is reported to range from 0.2% to 0.5%. This incidence is higher than the reported incidence in the "open cholecystectomy" era (0.1% to 0.2%). However, concerns currently exist that surgeons trained almost exclusively in laparoscopic cholecystectomy may lack adequate training and experience in the difficult open cholecystectomy. Therefore, the incidence of BDIs during open or converted cholecystectomy may increase in both frequency and severity.

A major challenge associated with biliary injuries is that such injuries are recognized at the time of laparoscopic cholecystectomy less than 40% of the time. Thus, most injuries present in the early postoperative period often with a biliary leak or jaundice. The therapeutic options, as well as the condition of the patient varies greatly based on the timing and mode of presentation, but in most cases, there should be no rush to return the patient to the operating room without proper evaluation and often nonsurgical intervention. Timely diagnosis and appropriate therapy are, however, necessary to promote optimal clinical outcome. The diagnosis and management of biliary leaks have been greatly facilitated by recent advances in imaging as well as percutaneous and endoscopic interventional techniques. The optimal management of such patients is best provided in centers that offer a multidisciplinary team approach. The basic principles of management of almost all biliary leaks includes control of the biliary leak by drainage of the biliary tree, control of the intra-abdominal sepsis, definition of biliary anatomy, and, when appropriate, definitive repair. This chapter reviews the etiology, clinical presentation and diagnosis, management, and outcomes with respect to BDI and biliary leak.

ETIOLOGY OF BILIARY LEAK

A bile leak is almost always the result of iatrogenic injury or a complication of surgical, percutaneous, or endoscopic procedures (Table 29.1).

There are a number of classifications of biliary leaks and injuries. In the United States, the Strasberg classifications have become the most commonly employed classification (Fig. 29.1). The majority of bile leaks are a result of Strasberg type A injuries.

	Etiology of Bile Leak

Abdominal operations
- Cholecystectomy
  - Major BDI
  - Minor bile leak (cystic duct, duct of Luschka)
- Pancreaticobiliary resection
- Biliary reconstruction
- Hepatic resection
- Hepatic transplantation
- Gastroduodenal surgery

Percutaneous interventions
- Transhepatic cholangiography/drainage (PTC)
- Stricture dilation
- Radiofrequency tumor ablation
- Embolization
- Liver biopsy

Endoscopic retrograde cholangiography perforation
Trauma (blunt and penetrating)

Biliary leaks can also be classified as either a minor bile leak or a major biliary ductal injury. Minor bile leaks are typically a result of cystic duct stump leak (60% to 75%) or duct of Luschka injuries (10% to 20%). Ducts of Luschka are accessory bile ducts located in the gallbladder bed that do not communicate with the lumen of the gallbladder. While they do not drain any liver parenchyma, they are a common source of minor bile leak after cholecystectomy. Major biliary ductal injury is most often an injury to the common bile duct (CBD) or common hepatic duct and includes avulsion, ligation, and transection. A bile leak can also be classified based on the volume of drainage. Low-output drainage is considered less than 300 mL of bile per day with high-output drainage being greater than 300 mL/day.

While cholecystectomy is the commonest cause of bile leak, it is important to remember that bile leakage can complicate any procedure that has a bilioenteric anastomosis. The exact incidence of biliary leak after these procedures is difficult to determine due to the wide variety of possible procedures; however, it is likely in the range of 2% to 5%. One of the greatest challenges in the diagnosis of leak after a bilioenteric reconstruction is that typically a jejunal Roux-en-Y limb is involved, which creates an access problem for traditional endoscopic diagnostic techniques.

In the last 15 years, there has been a marked increase in the complexity of liver surgery with a concomitant increase in the bile leak rate. The incidence of bile leak after hepatic resection is between 2% and 10% with most of the leaks being minor. A recent prospective analysis of 2,628 hepatic resections found that while liver-related complication rates remained stable since 1997, bile leak rates increased (5.9% from 3.7%). These authors reported that independent predictors of bile leak included bile duct resection, extended hepatectomy, repeat hepatectomy, en bloc diaphragmatic resection, and intraoperative transfusion. Since it is known that bile leak is associated with both increased hospital stay and mortality, novel techniques to minimize leak after hepatic resection have been introduced with numerous ongoing trials of new methodologies to accomplish this goal.

Bile leaks continue to be an uncommon complication of liver transplantation. Despite great improvements in surgical technique, biliary

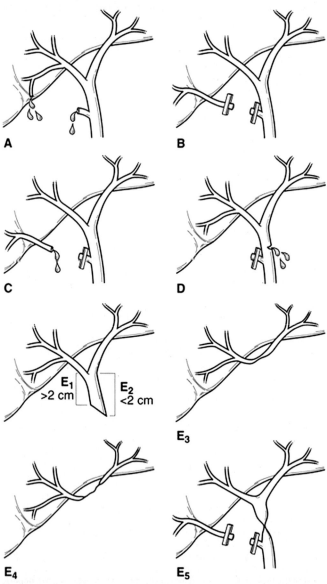

FIGURE 29.1 Strasberg classification. Type A: Injury to the cystic duct or from minor hepatic ducts draining the liver bed. Type B: Occlusion of biliary tree, commonly aberrant right hepatic duct(s). Type C: Transection without ligation of aberrant right hepatic duct(s). Type D: Lateral injury to a major bile duct. Type E (1–5): Injury to the main hepatic duct; classified according to level of injury (i.e., below). E1 (Bismuth type 1): Injury more than 2 cm from confluence; E2 (Bismuth type 2): Injury less than 2 cm from confluence; E3 (Bismuth type 3): Injury at the confluence; confluence intact; E4 (Bismuth type 4): Destruction of the biliary confluence; E5 (Bismuth type 5): Injury to aberrant right hepatic duct. (Reproduced from Winslow ER, Fialkowski EA, Linehan DC, et al. "Sideways": results of repair of biliary injuries using a policy of side-to-side hepatico-jejunostomy. *Ann Surg* 2009;249(3):426–434, with permission.)

complications are a common source of morbidity, which result in the need for intervention including percutaneous, endoscopic, or even surgical procedures. The incidence of biliary complications currently ranges from 5% to 25% with biliary strictures (9% to 12%) and leaks (5% to 10%) being the most common complications. Bile leak after liver transplant is almost always related to the biliary reconstruction and is complicated by the need for immunosuppression in the patient population.

A bile leak after blunt and penetrating abdominal trauma involving the liver is seen in 5% to 10% of reported cases and can occur after either operative or nonoperative management.

ETIOLOGY OF BILE DUCT INJURY

In the United States, BDIs are most commonly the result of injury during laparoscopic cholecystectomy. CBD injury during cholecystectomy can occur due to either a technical error or more commonly misidentification of the ductal anatomy. The Stewart-Way classification is a clear and concise method of classifying for the type of CBD injury based on the specific mechanism of injury (Table 29.2). The most common mechanism is a class III injury where the CBD is mistaken for the cystic duct with the error being unrecognized at the time of injury (Fig. 29.2). The duct is then transected and a segment usually resected. In the case series used to generate the Stewart-Way classification scheme, class III injuries were observed in 60% of the cases.

Contributing factors to BDI include acute or chronic inflammation in the triangle of Calot, a short cystic duct, excessive cephalad retraction on the gallbladder fundus, and insufficient or excessive lateral retraction of the gallbladder infundibulum. Other factors that can increase the likelihood of injury include use of an end-viewing scope, excessive use of cautery, physician inexperience, and aberrant biliary anatomy.

The "critical view of safety" (CVS) was first described in 1995 by Strasberg et al. This method has been adopted increasingly by surgeons around the world for performance of laparoscopic cholecystectomy (Fig. 29.3). The CVS has three requirements. First, the triangle of Calot must be cleared of fat and fibrous tissue. The second requirement is that the lowest part of the gallbladder be separated from the cystic plate, the flat fibrous surface to which the nonperitonealized side of the gallbladder is attached. The third requirement is that two structures, and only two, should be seen entering the gallbladder. Once these three criteria have been fulfilled, CVS

TABLE 29.2	Mechanism of Common Bile Duct Injury (Stewart-Way Classification)
Class I	CBD mistaken for cystic duct but recognized
	Cholangiogram incision in cystic duct extended into CBD
Class II	Lateral damage to the CHD from cautery or clips placed on duct
	Associated bleeding, poor visibility
Class III	CBD mistaken for cystic duct, not recognized
	CBD, CHD, R, L. hepatic ducts transected and/or resected
Class IV	RHD mistaken for cystic duct, RHA mistaken for cystic artery, RHD and RHA transected
	Lateral damage to the RHD from cautery or clips placed on duct

CBD, common bile duct; CHD, common hepatic duct; L, left; R, right; RHA, right hepatic artery; RHD, right hepatic duct.
Reprinted from Way LW, et al. Causes and prevention of laparoscopic bile duct injuries. *Ann Surg* 2003;237(4):460, with permission.

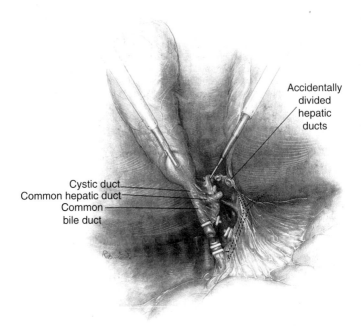

FIGURE 29.2 Classic laparoscopic BDI. The CBD is mistaken for the cystic duct and transected. A variable extent of the extrahepatic biliary tree is resected with the gallbladder. The right hepatic artery, in background, is also often injured. (Adapted from Branum G, Schmidt C, Baillie J, et al. Management of major biliary complications after laparoscopic cholecystectomy. *Ann Surg* 1993;217:532.)

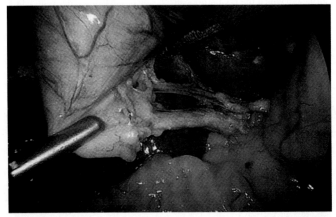

FIGURE 29.3 Operative photo demonstrating the CVS with extensive separation of the lower gallbladder from the cystic plate. The cystic duct and cystic artery are clearly defined.

has been attained. There is no level I evidence that CVS reduces BDI, and there likely never will be as the incidence of injury is so low that it would be difficult to adequately power a prospective randomized trial. There are numerous case series, however, which show a reduction in the incidence of BDI when the CVS is attained, such that it is widely considered to be the "safest" technique for performing laparoscopic cholecystectomy.

The role of intraoperative cholangiography (IOC) in preventing BDI during laparoscopic cholecystectomy is controversial. Individual institutional series have failed to demonstrate that either routine or selective cholangiography affects the incidence of BDI. Furthermore, large databases have provided mixed results as to whether IOC is an effective strategy to reduce the incidence of BDI.

CLINICAL PRESENTATION

The clinical presentation of postoperative bile leak is variable. If surgical drains are in place, a leak is obvious and easily detectable. Assuming there are not drains in place or the drains do not communicate with the area of leakage, bile can leak freely into the peritoneal cavity or it can loculate as a collection. The presentation can be subtle ranging from nonspecific complaints such as abdominal discomfort, nausea, and low-grade temperate to severe abdominal pain and/or a "septic" appearance due to bile peritonitis. Therefore, clinicians should have a high index of suspicion for bile leak in patients who have undergone right upper quadrant surgical procedures and who have any postoperative deviation from the projected clinical course.

DIAGNOSIS

There are numerous diagnostic modalities to consider in the evaluation of a potential bile leak. After history and physical exam, the first step in the workup of suspected bile leak should be basic laboratory studies. While laboratory values may be totally normal, a mild elevation in the serum total bilirubin, often due to bile absorption from the peritoneum, may be seen. Other liver function tests are often normal. Leukocytosis representing inflammation or infection is common.

Following laboratory evaluation, there are numerous imaging modalities to consider.

Ultrasonography is an inexpensive and noninvasive imaging technique that may be a useful first step in identifying an intra-abdominal fluid collection; however, numerous studies have concluded that the sensitivity of ultrasound for detection of bile leak is significantly inferior to other modalities. Abdominal axial imaging with CT provides a more detailed view of the pertinent structures as well as fluid collections or bile ascites (Fig. 29.4). Although the exact nature of the fluid as being bile may be unconfirmed, such collections certainly warrant suspicion and further workup.

The gold standard for diagnosis of biliary leakage is cholangiography. There are numerous ways that a cholangiogram can be achieved in the postoperative patient. If the patient has operative drains in place, contrast can be injected in a retrograde fashion that may demonstrate the point of leakage and biliary anatomy. Operatively placed T tubes or transhepatic stents also provide direct access to the biliary tree. In patients who have no access to the biliary tree, cholangiography can be performed either antegrade via percutaneous transhepatic puncture (PTC) or, more commonly, retrograde via endoscopic retrograde cholangiopancreatography (ERCP). Both of these techniques require skilled operators and confer some degree of risk. Assuming the patient has native anatomy, the first option would be ERCP. Although ERCP is generally well tolerated by patients and

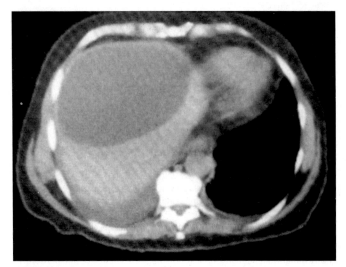

FIGURE 29.4 Large bile duct collection (biloma) occurring after BDI.

allows therapeutic intervention (stent placement and/or sphincterotomy) at the time of diagnosis, a recent large European study reported an overall complication rate of 10%. Post-ERCP pancreatitis occurred in 4.2%, bleeding in 3.6% (0.4% clinically relevant), cholangitis in 1.4%, cardiopulmonary complications in 1.2%, perforation in 0.6%, and procedure-related deaths in 0.1% of procedures. The limitation of ERCP is that in cases with disruption of the normal biliary anatomy, either through biliary transection or anastomosis, an ERCP will not demonstrate the proximal biliary tree and therefore not define the location of the leak or the anatomy necessary for reconstruction (Fig. 29.5). PTC may therefore be the only access to the biliary tree in certain situations (Fig. 29.6). PTC is another safe technique with a major complication rate of 2% to 10% (sepsis, cholangitis, bile leak, hemorrhage, or pneumothorax). After gaining access to the biliary tree, PTC also offers the potential for therapeutic intervention.

A noninvasive modality for imaging the biliary tree that might be useful in patients who are clinically stable is magnetic resonance cholangiopancreatography (MRCP). Recent developments in imaging technology have enabled MRCP to replace invasive alternatives for the pre- and postoperative assessment of biliary disease. MRCP enables rapid, noninvasive evaluation of both the biliary tree and pancreatic duct without the use of intravenous contrast media. Attention has recently focused on the utility in evaluation of the biliary system in suspected biliary injuries to help select the most appropriate next step if any (Fig. 29.7). The major limitation to MR-based biliary imaging is that there is no potential for therapeutic intervention. Other limitations include high cost, patient size restrictions, and the requirement of lying still for a prolonged period of time, which might be difficult in the acutely ill patient.

Finally, technetium-99m–labeled hydroxy iminodiacetic acid (HIDA) is commonly used as initial, noninvasive imaging modality for a suspected biliary leak. HIDA scintigraphy is a dynamic study in which an ongoing bile leak may be detected. However, it provides suboptimal anatomic detail. A biliary leak will be demonstrated by extravasation

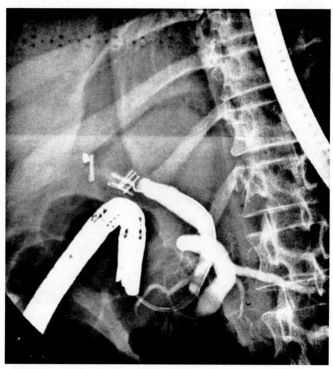

FIGURE 29.5 An ERCP performed in a patient with a major BDI. Contrast does not fill the proximal biliary tree due to operatively placed clips.

of radionuclide from the biliary system; however, these studies always require further investigation to define the true nature of the leak and to perform biliary drainage.

MANAGEMENT OF BILE LEAKS AND INJURIES

Management of Minor Bile Leaks after Cholecystectomy

Minor bile leakage following laparoscopic cholecystectomy is most commonly due to cystic duct stump leak (60% to 75%) or from a duct of Luschka (10% to 20%). The same basic management strategy applies to any minor bile leak, which includes decompression of the biliary tree, usually via endoscopic means, and drainage of the intra-abdominal collections to control sepsis. The most effective method of decompressing the biliary tree is lowering the pressure gradient across the sphincter of Oddi. This may be accomplished endoscopically via sphincterotomy with or without transampullary stenting. These techniques decompress the biliary tree and allow bile to take the path of least resistance into the duodenum, which usually allows healing of the upstream pathology. The endoscopic route with or without stenting is preferred as the endoscopic approach is easier, particularly as the intrahepatic bile ducts are often not dilated, and it is better tolerated by patients. Percutaneous transhepatic drainage is another option although is seldom necessary

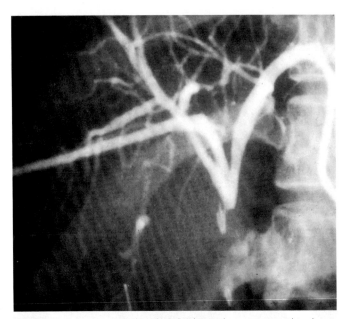

FIGURE 29.6 Percutaneous transhepatic cholangiogram demonstrates complete obstruction of the biliary tree at the site of bile duct transection.

since most minor bile leaks following cholecystectomy involve intact biliary anatomy. An increasingly common indication for PTC is a bile leak or injury following cholecystectomy after gastric bypass procedures. While the success in healing minor bile leaks using various methods have not been compared to each other using randomized studies, most series quote success rates of nonoperative decompression greater than 90%. A recent study by Pitt et al. analyzed 528 patients with biliary leak or duct injury managed by endoscopists, interventional radiologists, and surgeons. They concluded that bile leaks from the cystic duct or a duct of Luschka were managed almost exclusively by endoscopists with excellent results.

Management of Bile Leak after Liver Resection

Bile leak after liver resection continues to be a fairly common problem complicating 5% to 10% of cases. The majority of cases are minor leaks from the transected liver parenchymal surface that do not cause significant morbidity. However, major biliary complications may occur and cause significant morbidity and even mortality. Such injuries include injury to the common bile or hepatic duct, from the stump of a ligated main biliary trunk or from a biliary–enteric anastomosis. Bile may also leak from an immature T tube or transhepatic stent tract. Many investigators have tried to determine risk factors for bile leak after liver surgery. There does not seem to be a significant correlation with the preoperative condition of the patient, liver pathology, or technique used to divide the hepatic parenchyma. Some studies have suggested that longer operative times and the removal of Couinaud segment 4 may be independent risk factors for bile leak.

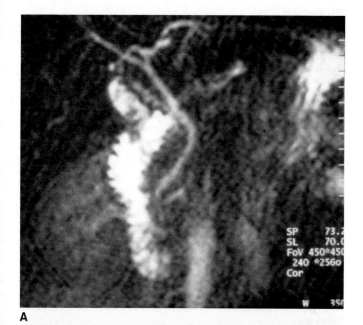

A

B

FIGURE 29.7 A: MRCP demonstrates intact biliary anatomy with a small leak from the cystic duct. In such a case, a therapeutic ERCP would be indicated. **B:** MRCP demonstrates complete transection of the common hepatic duct. In this case, ERCP would be of no value, and a percutaneous approach would be necessary to access the biliary tree should drainage be necessary. Alternatively, if appropriate, the patient could be taken directly to the operating room for reconstruction as the anatomy is nicely defined.

Bile leaks after hepatectomy may present in the early postoperative period (days 2 to 4) with bile detectable in surgically placed drains. However, since drains are not routinely used by many liver surgeons, there may be significant delay in recognition of bile leak in patients who do not have drains in place. These patients often present 6 to 8 days postoperatively with one or more of the following: abdominal pain, low-grade fever, leukocytosis, hyperbilirubinemia, ileus, or protracted hiccups. Rarely, a biliary leak may present as a severe septic or hemorrhagic event.

The workup of bile leak after hepatic resection is similar to that for postcholecystectomy bile leak. The most likely source of bile leak after hepatic resection is leakage from the parenchyma, which tends to be low volume and will often resolve with external drainage of the collection and antibiotics. If the bile leak persists, decompression of the biliary tree usually via endoscopic techniques is appropriate if native anatomy is present.

Management of Bile Leak after Liver Transplantation

Biliary complications continue to be a major source of morbidity in hepatic transplantation. The major biliary complications are bile leak and stricture, occurring in 5% to 25% of transplants. While there are exceptions, most bile leakage after transplant occurs at the biliary anastomosis. Currently, the most common anastomotic techniques are direct choledochocholedochostomy (end-to-end or side-to-side) with or without T-tube stenting or Roux-en-Y choledochojejunostomy with no clear difference in the incidence of biliary leak.

Bile leakage in transplant patients presents similar to other patient populations discussed earlier. However, due to a suppressed immune response, these patients may not mount the same magnitude of response mostly with respect to fever, leukocytosis, and abdominal pain. As such, a high awareness of the potential for bile leak in the early postoperative period is important.

Treatment strategies for bile leak after liver transplant are essentially the same as discussed for other types of bile leaks. The use of nonoperative strategies has nearly obviated the need to return to the operating room for anastomotic revision except in the most drastic situations. In patients with direct choledochocholedochostomy, ERCP with sphincterotomy and stenting is the treatment of choice with a frequency of success approaching 90%. However, in patients with Roux-en-Y choledochojejunostomy, ERCP is more difficult and requires a highly skilled interventional biliary endoscopist. Percutaneous transhepatic stenting of the biliary anastomosis may also be technically difficult in patients who do not have intrahepatic biliary ductal dilation and often the transplant surgeon wishes to avoid this route.

Management of Bile Leak after Trauma

The liver is the most frequently injured abdominal organ in both penetrating and blunt trauma. Nonoperative management has become well established as the standard of care for treatment of patients who have blunt liver injury. This development has resulted, in large part, from the widespread use of abdominal CT, which allows more precise definition of the extent of injury, and from the increased availability and application of angiography/embolization to control hemorrhage in these patients. Currently, 60% to 85% of all patients who have blunt hepatic trauma are managed successfully without operation. As a result of this paradigm change, it is difficult to estimate accurately the true incidence of bile leak after hepatic trauma. Biloma or bile ascites has been reported in as few as 0.5% to as many as 20% of all patients suffering blunt liver injury. In the most comprehensive study of bile leak after blunt liver trauma, Wahl et al. reported 24 bile leaks in 258 patients for an overall incidence of 9%. Several reviews have found an increased incidence of bile leak in patients who have more complex injuries and in those undergoing angiographic embolization, with an overall incidence of 30% to 40% in these populations.

The diagnosis of bile leak may prove particularly difficult in patients who have blunt trauma managed nonoperatively. Associated injuries may mask the typical symptoms and physical signs of bile peritonitis. Conversely, nonspecific symptoms or abnormal laboratory values may be attributed to other known or suspected injuries. Routine imaging studies (CT and ultrasound) can demonstrate intra-abdominal and perihepatic fluid collections. Such screening of patients managed nonoperatively at high risk for bile leak (those who have complex injuries or are undergoing angiographic embolization) may prove particularly useful in the trauma population.

As may be expected, with the paucity of data in the literature, no clear treatment strategy has evolved for managing bile leaks after liver injury. Several authors have reported success with simply percutaneous drainage of bile collections. Like with other causes of bile leak, draining the biliary tree using ERCP +/– sphincterotomy, or endoscopic stent placement, are options for persistent leaks. In some cases with major ductal injuries, operative management including reconstruction or even resection may be necessary.

Recently, laparoscopy with peritoneal lavage and operative drain placement has been suggested as a useful modality for treating patients who have hepatic trauma. Wahl noted that patients who were diagnosed as having a bile leak and were treated early by laparoscopic peritoneal lavage made more rapid recovery and had earlier hospital discharge than those diagnosed and treated later in the postinjury course. This finding prompted them to recommend early (postinjury day 3 or 4) screening for bile leak with HIDA scan in patients at high risk for bile leak, with laparoscopic peritoneal lavage applied to patients who had positive scans. Although early laparoscopic peritoneal lavage has not been studied in a randomized fashion, it may hold promise for this specific group of patients.

Most penetrating liver injuries continue to be managed operatively. Furthermore, a small percentage of patients who have blunt liver injury still require operative intervention. Diagnosis and management of bile leaks in these cases is similar to the management of bile leaks following other operative procedures on the liver or biliary tree. Biliary leak in these cases generally is suggested by the presence of bile in an operatively placed drain. Clinical findings of low-grade fevers, tachycardia, ileus, increased serum bilirubin, or leukocytosis may prompt abdominal CT and reveal an undrained fluid collection. External drainage of bile collections (by CT-guided percutaneous drainage), control of sepsis with tailored antibiotic treatment, and subsequent endoscopic or percutaneous transhepatic decompression of the biliary tree generally leads to resolution of bile leak in these situations.

Management of Major Bile Duct Injury

Most major bile duct injuries in the United States occur during laparoscopic cholecystectomy. Optimal management depends on timing of recognition of the injury. Most of these injuries (60% to 70%) go unrecognized at the time of laparoscopic cholecystectomy. Figure 29.8 shows the suggested management of injuries associated with laparoscopic cholecystectomy.

If the injury is recognized at the time of cholecystectomy, the first step is to determine if the operating surgeon is technically capable of performing the necessary repair. If he or she is not, we suggest consulting another surgeon at the original hospital who is experienced in biliary tract

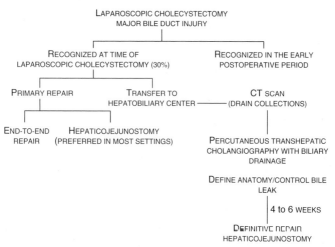

LAPAROSCOPIC CHOLECYSTECTOMY
MAJOR BILE DUCT INJURY

RECOGNIZED AT TIME OF
LAPAROSCOPIC CHOLECYSTECTOMY (30%)

RECOGNIZED IN THE EARLY
POSTOPERATIVE PERIOD

PRIMARY REPAIR

TRANSFER TO
HEPATOBILIARY CENTER

CT SCAN
(DRAIN COLLECTIONS)

END-TO-END
REPAIR

HEPATICOJEJUNOSTOMY
(PREFERRED IN MOST SETTINGS)

PERCUTANEOUS TRANSHEPATIC
CHOLANGIOGRAPHY WITH BILIARY
DRAINAGE

DEFINE ANATOMY/CONTROL BILE
LEAK

4 to 6 WEEKS

DEFINITIVE REPAIR
HEPATICOJEJUNOSTOMY

FIGURE 29.8 Algorithm for diagnosis and management of BDI associated with laparoscopic cholecystectomy.

reconstruction. If there is no one available who can perform such a repair, the patient should be transferred to a tertiary care center for further management. Once an injury is recognized, it is usually best to avoid further dissection or clipping of the proximal ducts. It is, however, mandatory to create a controlled biliary fistula prior to closing. This can be easily accomplished by placing a small drainage catheter retrograde into the biliary ductal system as well as placing a closed suction drain into the gallbladder bed. At this point, the patient should be closed and transferred to a center with skilled multidisciplinary teams to manage the injury.

A few specific scenarios deserve further discussion. One such situation is the placement of a clip across the CBD without cutting or dividing the duct (Fig. 29.9). In such cases, the clip can be removed, the gallbladder is removed, and no further treatment is necessary. If a small choledochotomy has been made to perform a cholangiogram, it should be closed with simple fine absorbable sutures and a drain should be placed in the gallbladder bed. The procedures can be performed laparoscopically; however, conversion to open operation is advisable for most surgeons. The patient is at risk to develop a late stricture, but in most cases, endoscopic balloon dilation and stenting will result in successful management.

The other situation in which minimal intervention is appropriate is when a minor bile duct is transected. In such cases, if the duct is less than 4 mm in diameter and cholangiography demonstrates only subsegmental liver drainage with the remainder of biliary anatomy intact, simple ligation is preferable than an attempt at reconstruction.

If a major duct injury is suspected and the surgeon is capable of repairing the injured duct, the first step is to convert to an open procedure and use gross anatomic identification combined with cholangiography to better define the nature of the injury. As discussed above, if the combination of exploration and cholangiography reveal an injured duct less than 4 mm, which drains subsegmental hepatic parenchyma, simple ligation is acceptable. If the injured duct is larger than 4 mm, it likely drains a larger area of hepatic parenchyma and will typically require operative repair.

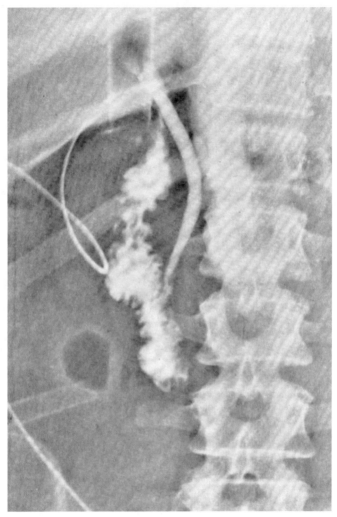

FIGURE 29.9 Intraoperative cholangiogram demonstrating a normal distal bile duct with drainage into the duodenum. The proximal biliary tree cannot be visualized due to a clip placed across the duct. Such a cholangiogram should alert the surgeon that a major BDI will occur unless steps are taken to redefine anatomy before transecting the duct.

If the injury is to the common hepatic or CBD, it should be repaired immediately. The two most common methods of repair are primary end-to-end repair or a bilioenteric anastomosis, typically a Roux-en-Y hepaticoje-junostomy. If a primary end-to-end repair is to be undertaken, the injured segment of the bile duct should be less than 1 cm and the ends must be able to be approximated without tension. This is usually accomplished by per-forming a generous Kocher maneuver (mobilizing the duodenum by taking down the lateral attachments from the retroperitoneum). After the Kocher

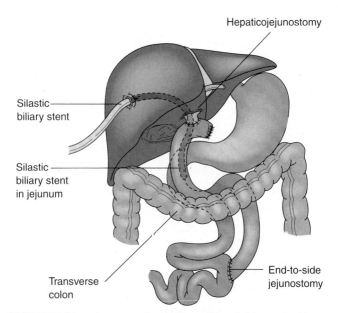

FIGURE 29.10 Schematic representation of a Roux-en-Y hepaticojejunostomy with trans-anastomotic stent to repair a BDI. (From Mulholland MW, Lillemoe KD, Doherty GM, et al., eds. *Greenfield's surgery: scientific principles and practice*, 4th ed. Philadelphia, PA: Lippincott Williams & Wilkins, 2006.)

maneuver, there is typically enough length to facilitate approximation of the injured ends. The anastomosis should be decompressed with a T tube placed either above or below the suture line. If the end-to-end repair is contraindicated, the distal bile duct should be oversewn and repair undertaken with a bilioenteric anastomosis.

The long-term results of end-to-end repair have often been criticized for having a high failure rate with late stricture occurring in over half of reported cases. However, by keeping normal biliary anatomy intact, endoscopic balloon dilatation with stenting is an option for treatment of such strictures. The results for such treatment are excellent and spare the patient the need for percutaneous procedures that are often painful and associated with the need for long-term external stents, which are unpopular with patients.

Most major bile duct injuries, however, will require a bilioenteric anastomosis with a Roux-en-Y limb of jejunum. The jejunum is divided about 25 cm from the ligament of Treitz. A 60-cm tension-free Roux limb is prepared in standard fashion with a stapled functional end-to-side enteroenterostomy. The stapled end of the jejunum is then pulled up through a rent made in the transverse mesocolon to the right of the middle colic vessels. Reconstruction is performed using a hand-sewn end-to-side anastomosis ensuring that the mucosa of the bile duct is brought into contact with the mucosa of the jejunum (Fig. 29.10). Many hepatobiliary surgeons believe that external biliary drainage preferably by an operatively placed transhepatic stent is necessary in all cases of biliary reconstruction after BDI. This catheter provides decompression of the biliary tree as well as allows recognition of and protection against the consequences of an anastomotic

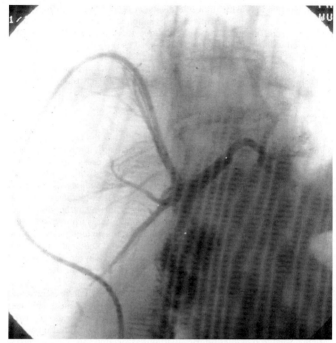

FIGURE 29.11 Postoperative cholangiogram after immediate reconstruction of a major BDI.

leak. This can be easily accomplished intraoperatively by placing a silastic stent retrograde through the hepatic parenchyma and externalized prior to completing the anastomosis. Another benefit of the catheter is the ability to easily study the repair and biliary anatomy postoperatively with cholangiography (Fig. 29.11).

Unfortunately, most patients who sustain a major BDI are not recognized during cholecystectomy. These patients usually present with pain, nausea, vomiting, bloating, and fever early in their postoperative course (days 2 to 5). These symptoms necessitate further diagnostic evaluation as described previously. A CT should be performed to evaluate for bile ascites or a bile collection. Such studies should also include arterial phase contrast, as up to 20% of major BDI may have an associated hepatic arterial injury. Assuming there is evidence of bile leak, decompression and external drainage of the biliary system is mandated. In cases in which there is evidence of a bile duct transection, the only reliable route for biliary drainage is using a percutaneous transhepatic approach. If there are drainable collections, these should also be drained by interventional radiology (IR). Although most patients with a bile leak do not have "infected bile," broad-spectrum antibiotics to cover typical biliary pathogens should be started as well as used to provide prophylaxis for various procedures. Once the leak is controlled via external drainage (often allowing operatively placed or IR-placed drains to be removed), and the biliary system is decompressed, there is no immediate rush to repair. It is clearly beneficial to allow resolution of the inflammatory process prior to performing definitive repair. An adequately controlled bile leak with total bile diversion is well tolerated for several weeks; however, both electrolytes and volume status must be monitored and optimized. The temptation to reexplore patients early with a major BDI associated with a bile leak should be avoided as the associated inflammation makes dissection and anastomosis quite difficult. Usually 4 to 6 weeks is a suitable time to plan definitive reconstruction. In those patients with a major bile duct transection presenting with obstruction without a bile leak, repair can be completed early after defining the anatomy.

OUTCOMES/FOLLOW-UP

Management of both postoperative bile leaks and bile duct injuries requires a multidisciplinary team. Minor bile leaks that are appropriately managed have excellent outcomes with nonoperative success rates over 90%. Bile duct injuries even when treated at major centers still are associated with significant morbidity and even mortality. Delay in diagnosis, failure to control the bile leak, and uncontrolled sepsis can lead to a fatal outcome particularly in elderly patients. Multiple series reporting outcomes following repair have reported postoperative morbidity rates from 25% to 40% and mortality rates of less than 2%. Complications include postoperative wound infections, cholangitis, septicemia, intra-abdominal abscess, anastomotic leak, biliary fistula, and hepatic insufficiency. In most patients, IR plays an important role in managing complications without the need for reoperation.

Fortunately, the long-term results for BDI following biliary reconstruction at major referral centers are generally excellent with successful outcomes reported in 85% to 95% of cases with follow-up in excess of 5 years. The development of liver failure or the need for liver transplantation is very rare for isolated bile duct injuries (without associated vascular injuries) if timely and appropriate treatment is provided. Finally, for most patients, quality of life following BDI with successful repair eventually returns to levels of healthy controls, which is particularly important as the majority of patients in most series are middle-aged women.

CONCLUSION

Biliary leakage is a complication that usually occurs after interventions on the gallbladder, bile ducts, and liver as well as after abdominal trauma. The overwhelming majority of biliary leaks are minor and will resolve with minimal intervention and morbidity. Advances in imaging and minimally invasive techniques permit nonoperative treatment in most cases. A BDI is a major complication with significant deleterious effects to the patient with respect to morbidity, cost of medical care, and disruption of short-term quality of life. Prompt recognition, appropriate management, and definitive repair are necessary to ensure the best possible outcome.

Suggested Readings

Branum G, Schmitt C, Baillie J, et al. Management of major biliary complications after laparoscopic cholecystectomy. *Ann Surg* 1993;217:532.

Flum DR, Cheadle A, Prela C, et al. Bile duct injury during cholecystectomy and survival in Medicare beneficiaries. *JAMA* 2003;290:2168–2173.

Flum DR, Dellinger EP, Dheadle A, et al. Intraoperative cholangiography and risk of common bile duct injury during cholecystectomy. *JAMA* 2003;289:1639–1644.

Lillemoe KD, Melton GB, Cameron JL, et al. Postoperative bile duct strictures: management and outcome in the 1990s. *Ann Surg* 2000;232:430.

Massarweh NN, Flum DR. Role of intraoperative cholangiography in avoiding bile duct injury. *J Am Coll Surg* 2007;204:656.

Melton GB, Lillemoe KD, Cameron JL, et al. Major bile duct injuries associated with laparoscopic cholecystectomy: effect of surgical repair on quality of life. *Ann Surg* 2002;235:888.

Pitt HA, Sherman S, Johnson MS, et al. Improved outcomes of bile duct injuries in the 21st century. *Ann Surg* 2013;258:490.

Sheffield KM, Riall TS, Han Y, et al. Association between cholecystectomy with vs without intraoperative cholangiography and risk of common duct injury. *JAMA* 2013;310:812–820.

Sicklick JK, Camp MS, Lillemoe KD, et al. Surgical management of bile duct injuries sustained during laparoscopic cholecystectomy: perioperative results in 200 patients. *Ann Surg* 2005;241:786.

Stewart L, Way LW. Bile duct injuries during laparoscopic cholecystectomy: factors that influence the results of treatment. *Arch Surg* 1995;130:1123–1129.

Strasberg SM, Hertl M, Soper NJ. An analysis of the problem of biliary injury during laparoscopic cholecystectomy. *J Am Coll Surg* 1995;180:101.

Strasberg SM. Biliary injury in laparoscopic surgery: Part 2. Changing the culture of cholecystectomy. *J Am Coll Surg* 2005;201:604.

Walsh RM, Henderson JM, Vogt DP, et al. Long-term outcome of biliary reconstruction for bile duct injuries from laparoscopic cholecystectomies. *Surgery* 2007;142:450.

Way LW, Stewart L, Gantert W, et al. Causes and prevention of laparoscopic bile duct injuries. *Ann Surg* 2003;237:460–469.

Wohl W, Brandt MM, Hammila M, et al. Diagnosis and management of bile leaks after blunt liver injury. *Surgery* 2005;138:742–748.

Multidisciplinary HPB Care

Liver and Pancreas Transplantation

Richard S. Mangus and Jonathan A. Fridell

BRIEF HISTORY OF LIVER TRANSPLANTATION

Though orthotopic liver transplantation (LT) first became a reality in the early 1960s, outcomes were inadequate to make it the standard of care for end-stage liver disease until the 1980s. Two primary factors drove the ultimate success of this procedure: (1) the introduction of calcineurin inhibitors (cyclosporine) to provide adequate, stable, long-term immunosuppression and (2) the passage of brain death laws that drastically improved the quality of deceased donor organs. Subsequent improvements in organ preservation, surgical technique, and intensive care unit management have now led to survival approaching 90% at 1 year and 60% to 70% at 10 years. This success has resulted in an unprecedented demand for LT and has driven the field of LT in search of more organs. The primary expansion of donors for LT has come from (1) the use of nonideal (extended criteria) deceased donors and (2) the use of partial grafts from both deceased and living donors.

INDICATIONS AND CONTRAINDICATIONS FOR LIVER TRANSPLANTATION

The primary indications for LT are separated into two disease mechanisms: cholestatic and noncholestatic liver disease. Additionally, LT may be indicated for certain tumors that meet specific criteria (Table 30.1). Simultaneous transplantation of the liver with other solid organs has been well described, including the kidney, pancreas, lung, heart, and intestine. Unlike kidney and pancreas grafts that are allocated according to time on the transplant wait list, liver allografts are allocated solely based upon severity of illness. The model for end-stage liver disease score (MELD) was developed to predict the risk of death while awaiting LT. The MELD score is calculated from three commonly measured laboratory values (international normalized ratio [INR], serum total bilirubin, and serum creatinine) and serves to assess synthetic (INR) and excretory (bilirubin) function of the liver as well as systemic decompensation (creatinine). The MELD score ranges from 6 (low) to 40 (maximum), and patients are generally not transplanted until their score is greater than 15. MELD exception points may be granted for the presence of malignant tumor (hepatocellular carcinoma) or quality of life issues.

Most contraindications to LT are relative but may include active substance abuse, systemic infection, cancer, HIV infection, poorly managed psychiatric disorders, lack of social support, and significant disease of the cardiopulmonary or neurologic systems. Surveillance for hepatocellular carcinoma (HCC) is mandatory for all patients with cirrhosis; 70% to 90% of all HCC cases arise in the cirrhotic liver. Scoring systems have been developed to determine acceptable HCC tumor volume that still permits

	Common Diseases for Which Liver Transplantation May Be Indicated

TABLE 30.1

Cholestatic Liver Disease	Noncholestatic Liver Disease	Other
Primary sclerosing cholangitis (PSC)	Viral hepatitis	Hepatocellular carcinoma
Primary and secondary biliary cirrhosis (PBC)	Alcoholic liver disease (ALD)	Cholangiocarcinoma
Biliary atresia	Nonalcoholic fatty liver disease (NAFLD)	Acute liver failure
Cystic fibrosis	Autoimmune hepatitis	
	Hepatic toxicity from chronic drug or toxin exposure	
	Metabolic or genetic disorders	

LT, the two most common of which are the Milan and the University of California, San Francisco (UCSF) criteria (Table 30.2). Liver-directed therapies for HCC such as transarterial embolization and radiofrequency ablation are useful and serve to control disease burden while awaiting LT; these therapies may also be used to downstage HCC volume to meet transplant criteria.

End-stage liver disease is frequently accompanied by a host of comorbidities that may impact the outcome of the transplant. Hepatorenal syndrome (HRS) is a condition in which chronic liver disease is associated with renal insufficiency. Though some of the effects of severe HRS may be reversed with LT, patients do not generally return to completely normal renal function. Hepatopulmonary syndrome (HPS) results from differences in vascular pressures related to the primary liver disease. The vasodilation resulting from liver failure leads to a direct vasodilatory effect in the lungs, which results in increased blood flow in relation to ventilation and a ventilation–perfusion mismatch. This is seen clinically as a right-to-left shunt, and the patient experiences dyspnea. As with HRS, HPS is an important marker of disease severity, and prognosis is poor without a timely LT. Symptoms of HPS improve markedly with LT.

TABLE 30.2

	Criteria for Liver Transplantation in Patients with Hepatocellular Carcinoma	
	Milan Criteria	**UCSF Criteria**
Number and size of tumors	Solitary tumor with maximum diameter of 5 cm	Solitary tumor with maximum diameter of 6.5 cm
	Up to three tumor nodules, each of which is <3 cm, with no vascular invasion or extrahepatic metastases	Up to three tumor nodules, with largest nodule <4.5 cm, or a total tumor diameter <8 cm, with no vascular invasion or extrahepatic metastases

PROCEDURE/TECHNIQUE

Organ Procurement from Deceased Donors

The organ procurement operation from a deceased donor is standardized with little variation among surgeons. Safe preservation of the organs is dependent upon two primary principles: (1) rapid organ exsanguination and vascular flushing with an appropriate preservation solution and (2) rapid organ cooling. After the organs have been prepared in the donor, an aortic cannula is placed that is used to flush the arterial system. Some surgeons choose to place a second cannula in the portal vein (through the inferior mesenteric vein) to flush the portomesenteric system. The abdominal aorta is clamped superior to the celiac trunk and also near the iliac bifurcation to isolate the abdominal organs. The outflow for the blood and preservation solution is generally through the suprahepatic vena cava at its junction with the right atrium. As the clamps are placed and the preservation solution is infused, iced normal saline is placed throughout the abdominal cavity to topically cool the organs. The heart arrests during this process, and the organs are then removed. For living donor partial liver procurement, the liver resection is performed in the donor with dissection completed while vascular inflow and outflow remains intact. Clamps are applied simultaneously, and the donor graft is removed, followed by rapid flushing and cooling (Fig. 30.1A and B). Donation after cardiac death (DCD) is currently used in 4% of deceased donors and requires complete cessation of cardiopulmonary function prior to organ procurement. This necessarily results in several minutes of graft warm ischemia time, which results in inferior outcomes. In all cases, once procured, the liver allograft must be transplanted and reperfused within 12 hours, after which there is an increased risk of complications.

Liver Transplant Operation

There are three components to the liver transplant operation: (1) preparation of the transplant organ, (2) recipient hepatectomy, and (3) implantation of the graft. Preparation of the graft involves removal of residual tissue from the donor operation including residual diaphragm and pericardium around the vena cava and hepatic veins. The gallbladder is always removed from the donor liver, and the cystic duct is ligated. Accessory hepatic arteries are carefully dissected and preserved. An accessory right hepatic artery requires reconstruction prior to transplantation. Frequently, an accessory left hepatic artery cannot be safely reconstructed, because of small size, and is dissected and preserved in situ.

The recipient hepatectomy is performed in one of two ways: (1) conventional (standard bicaval) or (2) the piggyback or "cava-preserving" technique (Fig. 30.2A and B). Both approaches to the hepatectomy require initial takedown of the falciform and gastrohepatic ligaments, followed by dissection of the hilum of the liver with transection of the hepatic artery, common bile duct, and portal vein. The conventional approach then proceeds with clamping of the vena cava above and below the liver with transection of the vena cava between the clamps and removal of the liver. This technique necessarily requires complete clamping of the vena cava for a prolonged period of time. The piggyback technique varies from this approach with no clamping of the vena cava required. For the piggyback hepatectomy, the liver is carefully retracted away from the vena cava with perforating branches between the vena cava and the liver individually ligated and transected. Eventually, the liver remains attached only by the hepatic veins. The veins are clamped and transected, and the liver is removed. The piggyback technique is technically more difficult than the conventional approach, but

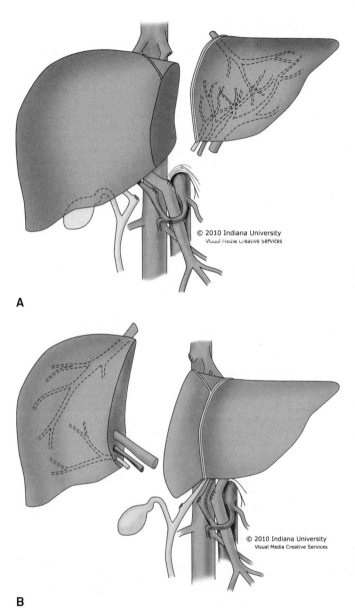

A

B

FIGURE 30.1 A. Living donor left lateral segment graft for a pediatric recipient. **B.** Living donor right lobe graft for an adult recipient.

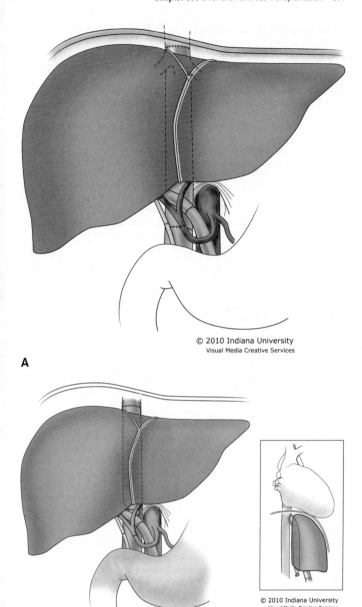

© 2010 Indiana University
Visual Media Creative Services

A

© 2010 Indiana University
Visual Media Creative Services

B

FIGURE 30.2 A. Conventional or standard bicaval anastomosis of the vena cava.
B. Piggyback or "cava-preserving" technique for LT.

the recipient tends to remain more hemodynamically stable as the preload to the heart from the lower body is never interrupted. Some surgeons who use the piggyback approach construct a temporary portacaval shunt to decompress the portomesenteric system until the time of liver allograft reperfusion. The piggyback approach may be the preferred method in high-risk patients such as the elderly, those with poor physiologic reserve, or patients who are hemodynamically unstable. The piggyback technique tends to preserve hemodynamic and physiologic stability throughout the transplant, which may then be associated with less perioperative morbidity and mortality.

Finally, the transplant is performed. For the conventional approach, the vena cava must be reanastomosed both above and below the liver. For the piggyback technique, the liver outflow is through the clamped hepatic veins so that a single anastomosis is required. This reduction from two to one vena cava anastomosis can decrease critical warm ischemia time by as much as 5 to 10 minutes. Next, the portal vein and hepatic artery are anastomosed. Finally, the common bile duct can be anastomosed, after the liver has been fully reperfused, either to the recipient common bile duct or to a Roux-en-Y limb of the small intestine. At our center, 90% of our transplants employ a primary duct-to-duct reconstruction, and we never use a T tube.

In countries with limited access to deceased donors, partial liver allografts from living donors may be the only option available for patients in need of transplantation. Also, splitting of a whole deceased donor liver can result in two viable grafts, though each split portion carries an increased risk of complications when compared to a whole organ allograft. The living donor partial liver transplant requires use of the piggyback hepatectomy because there is no vena cava available from the living donor. Therefore, the donor hepatic vein is anastomosed to the recipient hepatic veins, with portal and arterial inflow constructed directly to the native portal vein and hepatic artery (Fig. 30.3). The bile duct is transected close to the liver graft and is generally reconstructed with a Roux-en-Y limb of jejunum.

COMPLICATIONS

Immediate posttransplant complications may result from technical issues related to the transplant procedure, poor function of the graft, or recipient health issues. The most critical early posttransplant complication is thrombosis of the hepatic artery or the portal vein. Thrombosis of the hepatic vein anastomosis is very uncommon. The liver requires both hepatic artery and portal vein inflow for survival, and thrombosis of either anastomosis places the graft at imminent risk of failure. Doppler ultrasound is utilized post-LT to assure that vascular flow remains adequate. A loss of flow in either vessel generally necessitates emergent return to the operating room to reestablish flow. Posttransplant bleeding in the first 24 to 48 hours is not uncommon and requires reexploration to identify and control the source. Primary nonfunction (PNF) is a definition of exclusion in which there is graft failure within 7 days of the transplant with no other identifiable cause. PNF occurs in 1% to 5% of liver transplants and may be related to prolonged ischemia time, old donor age, and severe steatosis. Small for size graft is a syndrome seen almost exclusively in partial LT. The small size of the transplant graft in relation to the recipient blood flow results in persistent portal hypertension and liver congestion as the portomesenteric flow is too great for the partial liver graft segment. This syndrome is a major cause of early graft loss in living donor transplantation.

Biliary complications may be seen within the first week posttransplant but may also occur several weeks or months later. There are three

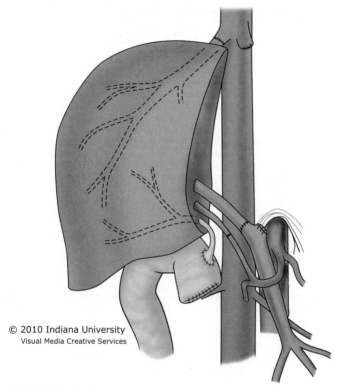

© 2010 Indiana University
Visual Media Creative Services

FIGURE 30.3 Implantation of the right lobe graft into an adult.

primary complications of the bile duct: (1) biliary leak, (2) anastomotic stricture, and (3) intrahepatic strictures. Biliary leak is encountered in the perioperative period and may be technical in nature or may result from bile duct necrosis. Biliary complications are particularly problematic in living donor LT and are a major cause of graft loss and patient death in this population. Most anastomotic strictures, and many anastomotic leaks, can be treated nonoperatively with endoscopic retrograde cholangiopancreatography or percutaneous transhepatic cholangiography. Through these techniques, stents can be placed across the anastomosis to facilitate drainage, and these can be increased in size over time to dilate the duct. Intrahepatic strictures appear as multiple diffuse strictures within a region of the liver or across the entire liver. Diffuse intrahepatic structuring points to a systemic problem usually related to arterial blood flow. Liver allografts procured from deceased donors using a DCD protocol are at increased risk of diffuse intrahepatic strictures. Patients who develop diffuse intrahepatic biliary strictures have a high rate of graft loss and frequently require retransplantation within 1 year.

An important impediment to success in the field of LT is the side effects of immunosuppressive drugs. These powerful agents, though effective at preventing rejection, continue to have major side effects that impact on long-term patient morbidity and mortality. Many centers now use antibody-based immunosuppression induction at the time of transplant, followed by one, two, or three drug maintenance regimens. Rejection of the liver allograft is less common than that seen for other solid organs. In fact, the liver appears to lessen the rejection risk of other organs when they are transplanted simultaneously. The reason for this finding is unclear. Because the liver transplant procedure itself is clean, intraabdominal infections post-LT are rare. Bacterial wound infections, however, are common for a variety of reasons. The liver transplant incision is quite large, and patients with liver failure are malnourished and have poor healing capacity. Many liver transplant recipients receive perioperative steroids, which impacts wound healing directly. Finally, clinical comorbidities such as diabetes and obesity contribute to poor wound healing and infection. The most common opportunistic viral infection in the liver transplant patient is cytomegalovirus (CMV) infection with a 1-year risk of 5% to 20%. Anti-CMV prophylaxis with valganciclovir and minimization of immune suppression lower the rate of this infection. Fungal infections can occur in up to 20% of patients and are most commonly seen in the mouth, esophagus, and urine. These infections almost always result from Candida species and respond to standard treatments.

Nearly all post-LT immunosuppression protocols utilize calcineurin inhibitors as the primary immunosuppressant drug. Use of these agents has resulted in nephrotoxicity being one of the primary long-term major complications associated with solid organ transplantation. Finally, the immune system plays a critical role in neoplasm surveillance in the human body. The chronic immune suppression required by all transplant patients places them at increased risk for the development of cancer, and this is well documented. The cancers found in transplant patients tend to mirror those seen in the general population, but with increased frequency. Therefore, the cancer most commonly seen in transplant patients is skin cancer (squamous and basal cell). Patients with HCC at the time of transplant have a risk of HCC recurrence posttransplant, but their survival is similar to that for non-HCC patients if they are within the Milan criteria at the time of transplant. Posttransplant lymphoproliferative disorder (PTLD) is well described and appears to have increasing risk with increasing levels of immune suppression.

PANCREAS TRANSPLANTATION

Introduction
Pancreas transplantation can restore normal insulin secretion and euglycemia in insulinopenic diabetic recipients. Since the first pancreas transplant performed by Lillehei and Kelly at the University of Minnesota in 1966, pancreas transplantation has evolved to the point where there are more than 1,500 procedures performed annually in the United States and it is routinely offered at most abdominal organ transplant centers. Outcomes have improved steadily over the decades, owing to improvements in organ preservation, surgical technique, postoperative care, and immunosuppression. Nonetheless, the need for a major operation and the requirement for lifelong immunosuppression have limited the application of pancreas transplantation to very select diabetic populations.

INDICATIONS

The majority of pancreas transplants are performed in association with another organ transplant in recipients with type 1 diabetes mellitus. The other organ transplanted is almost always a kidney transplant for end-stage diabetic nephropathy. These patients are already committed to lifelong immunosuppression for the renal allograft and therefore only have the added surgical risk of implanting the pancreas. Simultaneous liver–pancreas and lung–pancreas transplants have also been reported applying the same philosophy. The kidney and pancreas transplants can be performed either simultaneously (simultaneous pancreas and kidney [SPK]) from a single cadaveric donor or sequentially if a potential living donor can be identified for the kidney allograft (pancreas after kidney [PAK]). A few select centers offer simultaneous cadaveric pancreas and living donor kidney transplantation (SPLK).

Less frequently, a pancreas transplant alone (PTA) is offered for difficult to control and potentially life-threatening diabetes mellitus, usually with documented episodes of hypoglycemia unawareness. In these instances, the constant risk of untreated hypoglycemia that can result in hypoxic brain injury, accidents, and mortality outweighs the risk of the procedure and the immunosuppression. PTA is also offered for recipients who had previously undergone total pancreatectomy and exhibit poor glycemic control. In these cases, enteric exocrine drainage has the additional advantage in this recipient population of restoring exocrine function and improving nutrition.

CONTRAINDICATIONS

Absolute contraindications to pancreas transplantation include substance or alcohol abuse, uncorrectable cardiac disease, and active malignancy or infection. Prior to listing, all patients undergo cardiac evaluation, including a cardiac stress test with coronary angiography investigation of all abnormal studies. Only candidates with normal or corrected cardiac status are considered eligible. There is no specific upper limit for age or body mass index that contraindicates pancreas transplantation, although these are both features that may increase the risk of the procedure. Similarly, although not considered a contraindication, candidates who have undergone extensive prior abdominal operations or with advanced atherosclerotic arterial disease certainly present technical challenges that increase the risk of surgery.

SURGICAL TECHNIQUE

Pancreas allografts are procured following an aortic flush with preservation solution. The spleen is usually retained with the pancreas until implantation to avoid direct handling of the pancreas. The duodenum is also included with the allograft in order to facilitate creation of exocrine drainage. The backbench preparation of the pancreas includes a donor splenectomy and reconstruction of the donor superior mesenteric and splenic arteries with a donor iliac artery Y graft. Ultimately, when ready for implantation, the iliac artery Y graft will serve as the arterial inflow and the portal vein the venous outflow.

Pancreas transplantation is usually performed through a midline incision. SPK transplants are routinely performed with the kidney on the left and the pancreas on the right, although ipsilateral placement with both organs on the right side has also been described. Surgical techniques for pancreas allograft implantation have evolved with time. The original pancreas allograft was implanted with a ligated pancreatic duct. The subsequent series of transplants were performed with enteric exocrine drainage and were plagued with early allograft failures because the surgical techniques, organ preservation, and immunosuppression were still in their infancy. The introduction of bladder drainage of the exocrine secretions in the 1980s had several advantages over enteric drainage, particularly the ability to monitor exocrine function by measuring urinary amylase excretion. Furthermore, anastomotic leak from a bladder-drained pancreas is much easier to manage compared to an enteric leak. Unfortunately, bladder drainage has its own separate list of complications, particularly metabolic complications related to the loss of bicarbonate in the urine, cystitis, urethritis, and reflux pancreatitis in recipients with neuropathic bladders. Recently, as graft survival outcomes following pancreas transplantation have improved, enteric drainage has become the exocrine drainage procedure of choice at most centers. In fact, it has also become fairly common for the pancreas to be implanted with the head oriented toward the upper abdomen in order to facilitate a tension-free enteric anastomosis (Fig. 30.4).

Endocrine graft drainage through the portal vein is most commonly performed to the systemic venous circulation, usually to the right external or common iliac veins or vena cava. An alternative technique is mesenteric drainage through the recipient superior mesenteric vein. Regardless of the venous outflow, the donor iliac artery Y graft is still most commonly anastomosed to the right external or common iliac artery or, less often, the aorta. The theoretical advantage of mesenteric drainage is that it more closely imitates the normal endocrine physiology as the insulin is drained directly into the portal vein, as it is in the native setting. This allows for the first-pass

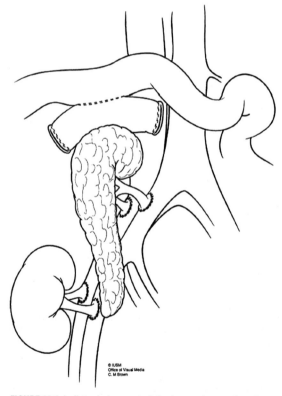

© IUSM
Office of Visual Media
C. M Brown

FIGURE 30.4 Ipsilateral placement of simultaneously transplanted pancreas and kidney allografts. The iliac artery extension Y graft and portal vein from the pancreas are anastomosed to the recipient common iliac artery and vein, respectively.

effect through the liver, where approximately half of the insulin is removed resulting in relatively lower systemic insulin levels. Both endocrine drainage techniques establish normoglycemia, although with different systemic insulin levels, and similar graft and patient survival.

Immunosuppression

A detailed discussion of immunosuppression is beyond the scope of this chapter, but some highlights are provided. The most common protocols include induction immunosuppression with depleting antibodies such as alemtuzumab (Campath), a monoclonal antibody to CD52, or rabbit antithymocyte globulin (Thymoglobulin). Maintenance immunosuppression most commonly includes a combination of tacrolimus and mycophenolate mofetil or sirolimus. It has also become a relatively common practice to avoid steroids as maintenance immunosuppression. In addition to the toxicities of the various immunosuppression agents, there is also an associated risk for opportunistic infections, particularly CMV and BK virus in kidney and pancreas transplant recipients, and opportunistic malignancies such as skin cancers and lymphoma (including PTLD). Prophylaxis against CMV and *Pneumocystis jiroveci* is routinely required following induction immunosuppression.

COMPLICATIONS

Technical failure, defined by the International Pancreas Transplant Registry as graft loss secondary to vascular thrombosis, bleeding, anastomotic leaks, or infection/pancreatitis, is responsible for more than half of all pancreas grafts lost in the first 6 months following transplantation, representing approximately 8% to 10% of transplants. Thrombosis accounts for more than half of these technical failures and may be influenced by donor and recipient factors, preservation and ischemic injury, immunologic issues, and surgical technique. Timely re-exploration is critical because, if there is indeed vascular thrombosis, the resulting allograft inflammation may initiate a systemic response with consequent recipient hemodynamic compromise or segments of the clot may form pulmonary emboli if the portal vein is systemically drained. Additionally, if explored early enough, vascular thrombectomy with graft salvage is occasionally possible. In cases where allograft pancreatectomy is required, immediate retransplantation is an option that offers the motivated patient an opportunity to regain the benefits of a functional allograft.

Postoperative hemorrhage can present with intraperitoneal bleeding from the pancreas allograft or retroperitoneum or with gastrointestinal bleeding at the site of an enteric anastomosis. If the enteric anastomosis is created at the level of the proximal jejunum, this is approachable endoscopically and can often be treated without returning to the operating room. It is a good practice to intubate the recipient prior to push enteroscopy in order to protect the airway. In the event of severe gastrointestinal bleeding for which angiography is considered, it is essential that it be communicated to the interventional radiologist that the iliac arteries be interrogated in addition to the mesenteric vessels as the donor duodenum or an arterioenteric fistula may be the source of bleeding. An option to manage severe bleeding from the pancreas allograft endovascularly is placement of a covered stent in the recipient iliac artery to totally bypass the takeoff of the donor artery prior to emergency laparotomy and accept the loss of the pancreas allograft in the event of life-threatening bleeding.

As with other pancreatic operations and enteric anastomoses, enteric or pancreatic leaks may develop and usually present with an abscess or fistula. Options for management include operative and percutaneous drainage. A drained abscess or fistula with low output will usually heal with time, although if the fluid collects around the area of the vascular anastomoses, it may predispose to the formation of arterial pseudoaneurysm. A high index of suspicion is required to diagnose and treat this life-threatening complication; *any bleeding into an abscess drain should be presumed to represent a herald bleed until pseudoaneurysm is ruled out radiologically.* Pseudoaneurysms can be managed endovascularly, and graft salvage, although uncommon in this setting, has been described.

Small bowel obstruction (SBO) can complicate any laparotomy. In addition to adhesions, two etiologies of SBO are specific to pancreas transplantation. First of all, the enteric anastomosis, particularly when the pancreas is oriented with the head upward, creates an internal hernia defect that is prone to incarceration and intestinal volvulus if not specifically closed at the time of transplantation (Fig. 30.5). Second, the anterior surface of the pancreas in the retroperitoneum presents a raw surface that is prone to adhesion formation. It is our own practice to cover the pancreas with a sheet of adhesion barrier at the end of the operation. Similarly, the

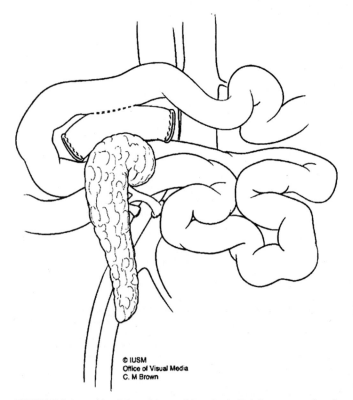

© IUSM
Office of Visual Media
C. M Brown

FIGURE 30.5 Internal herniation of the small intestine behind the pancreas allograft through a defect created at the time of transplantation. The opening is defined by the aorta and iliac artery posteriorly, the small bowel mesentery superiorly, the pancreas and enteric anastomosis anteriorly, and the pancreatic vascular anastomoses inferiorly.

intraperitoneal renal allograft should be covered with colon in order to prevent contact with the small intestine.

OUTCOMES

In the United States, approximately 1,200 to 1,500 pancreas transplants are performed annually. SPK makes up the majority of the pancreas transplants performed, accounting for approximately two-thirds of the total. Patient survival is currently similar for all three categories of pancreas transplantation, approximately 96% at 1 year (Fig. 30.6). Pancreas allograft survival has historically been superior for SPK compared to isolated pancreas transplantation (85% vs. 78% at 1 year) (Fig. 30.7). The difference in graft survival is often attributed to increased immunologic pancreas graft loss in isolated pancreas allograft recipients (PAK and PTA) compared to SPK recipients (5% vs. 2% at 1 year). This increased pancreas graft loss to rejection has been attributed to delayed detection and initiation of treatment for rejection because these recipients lack the early warning of a deterioration in renal function, which may be considered a harbinger of pancreas rejection in SPK recipients. Recent data from large centers using depleting antibody induction and steroid-free maintenance immunosuppression protocols suggest that we have entered a new era of immunosuppression where immunologic graft loss is becoming an infrequent occurrence. With this cause of graft failure practically eliminated, it is likely that pancreas allograft survival in isolated pancreas transplantation will begin to approach that of SPK. In fact, in the most recent update of the International Pancreas Transplant Registry, the 1-year graft survival for all three categories of pancreas transplantation was similar at 89% to 90% for programs using anti–T-cell antibody induction and maintenance with tacrolimus and sirolimus.

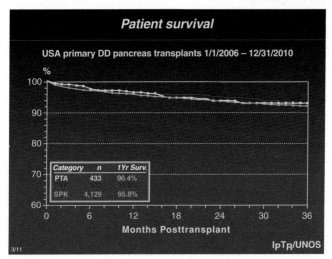

FIGURE 30.6 Patient survival following primary deceased donor pancreas transplantation in the United States between 1/1/2006 and 12/31/2010. Pancreas transplants are categorized by type as pancreas transplant alone (PTA), pancreas after kidney (PAK), and simultaneous pancreas and kidney (SPK). (Reprinted with permission from the International Pancreas Transplant Registry.)

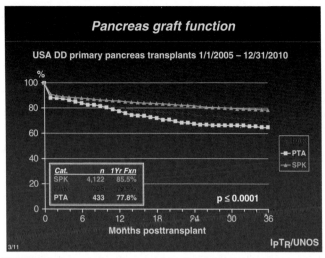

FIGURE 30.7 Pancreas allograft survival following primary deceased donor pancreas transplantation in the United States between 1/1/2005 and 12/31/2010. Pancreas transplants are categorized by type as simultaneous pancreas and kidney (SPK), pancreas after kidney (PAK), and pancreas transplant alone (PTA). (Reprinted with permission from the International Pancreas Transplant Registry.)

Suggested Readings

Liver Transplantation

Abu-Elmagd K, Fung J, Bueno J, et al. Logistics and technique for procurement of intestinal, pancreatic, and hepatic grafts from the same donor. *Ann Surg* 2000;232(5):680–687.

Fishman JA. Infection in solid-organ transplant recipients. *N Engl J Med* 2007; 357(25):2601–2614.

Hong JC, Yersiz H, Farmer DG, et al. Longterm outcomes for whole and segmental liver grafts in adult and pediatric liver transplant recipients: a 10-year comparative analysis of 2,988 cases. *J Am Coll Surg* 2009;208(5):682–689; discussion 689–691.

Mangus RS, Fridell JA, Vianna RM, et al. Immunosuppression induction with rabbit anti-thymocyte globulin with or without rituximab in 1,000 liver transplant patients with long-term follow-up. *Liver Transpl* 2012;18:786–795.

Tector AJ, Mangus RS, Chestovich P, et al. Use of extended criteria livers decreases wait time for liver transplantation without adversely impacting posttransplant survival. *Ann Surg* 2006;244(3):439–450.

Pancreas Transplantation

Fridell JA, Johnson MS, Goggins WC, et al. Vascular catastrophes following pancreas transplantation: an evolution in strategy at a single center. *Clin Transplant* 2011; DOI: 10.1111/j.1399-0012.2011.01560.x.

Fridell JA, Mangus RS, Hollinger EF, et al. The case for pancreas after kidney transplantation. *Clin Transplant* 2009;23(4):447–453.

Fridell JA, Mangus RS, Mull AB, et al. Early reexploration for suspected thrombosis after pancreas transplantation. *Clin Transplant* 2011;91:902–907.

Fridell JA, Powelson JA, Sanders CE, et al. Preparation of the pancreas allograft for transplantation. *Clin Transplant* 2011;25(2):E103–E112.

Fridell JA, Rogers J, Stratta RJ. The pancreas allograft donor: current status, controversies, and challenges for the future. *Clin Transplant* 2010;24(4):433–449.

Gruessner AC, Sutherland DE, Gruessner RW. Pancreas transplantation in the United States: a review. *Curr Opin Organ Transplant* 2010;15(1):93–101.

Humar A, Kandaswamy R, Granger D, et al. Decreased surgical risks of pancreas transplantation in the modern era. *Ann Surg* 2000;231(2):269–275.

HPB Imaging (Including IR, Ultrasound, MRI, CT, Nuclear Medicine)

Temel Tirkes and Kumaresan Sandrasegaran

Radiology offers many imaging modalities for evaluation of diseases in the abdomen; some include ultrasound, computerized tomography (CT), magnetic resonance imaging (MRI), positron emission tomography (PET) scan, and nuclear medicine. The choice of appropriate imaging modality should be made on an individual case basis depending on the lesion under question, availability of imaging facilities, and cost issues. Choosing the most appropriate imaging modality for evaluating the lesion under question depends on the information required from imaging for clinical management decisions. For example, while ultrasound might be an appropriate examination for a patient with no prior medical history and increased alkaline phosphatase and bilirubin levels, ultrasound is not an adequate screening test for hepatocellular carcinoma in a patient with cirrhosis and increased alpha-fetoprotein. Similarly, while multidetector CT (MDCT) serves as the first-line imaging modality for evaluation of liver, MRI offers an attractive radiation-free option with superior soft tissue contrast differentiation. The clinical applications and benefit of MRI are rapidly expanding due to new sequences and contrast agents. However, in most centers, MRI is still reserved as secondary imaging modality, with such indications as characterization of incidental liver lesions detected on CT or for patients with iodinated contrast allergy.

LIVER

Ultrasound

Sonography is a safe, noninvasive, quick, and inexpensive means of evaluating the liver. It can be performed at the bedside, needing little patient cooperation. The liver is ideally examined following a 6-hour fast so that gallbladder is not contracted. The normal tissue texture of the liver is homogeneous with fine echoes that appear as moderately short dots or lines. Abnormal parenchymal echogenicity is judged by comparing it to the right renal cortex. Increased echogenicity of the liver usually indicates hepatosteatosis. Ultrasound has good sensitivity for detection of focal liver lesions; however, specificity is not very high.

Duplex and color flow Doppler imaging improve the diagnostic capabilities of ultrasound by enabling the evaluation of complex circulatory dynamics of liver. Thrombosis, reverse flow, aneurysms, and fistulas are demonstrated with duplex and color flow Doppler. But color Doppler studies are usually unable to evaluate the vascularity of the liver neoplasms due to low intensity of the signals.

In liver transplant recipients, survival of the allograft depends on patency of the hepatic artery. Changes in the normal hepatic artery waveform may suggest stenosis or thrombosis in these patients. Liver transplant patients require very close follow-up for vessel patency during the immediate postoperative period.

Intraoperative Ultrasound

Acoustic attenuation by subcutaneous fat somewhat degrades the images of the transabdominal ultrasound. During intraoperative ultrasound, a high-frequency probe is directly placed on the liver surface, providing high-resolution images. The most common application of intraoperative ultrasound is during surgery in patients undergoing segmental resection for hepatic metastases. Intraoperative ultrasound can detect even the minute liver lesions and modify the surgical management of patients. Intraoperative ultrasound has been more widely utilized across the spectrum of HPB surgery (see Chapter 12).

Computed Tomography

Advances in MDCT enabled very fast scan times and improved resolution due to isotropic image acquisition. The goal of contrast enhancement is to improve lesion visibility by increasing the relative attenuation difference between the lesion and normal hepatic parenchyma. A routine contrast-enhanced CT of the liver is performed during the portal phase and is usually sufficient for detection and follow-up of most hypovascular metastatic liver lesions. Multiphasic CT is performed in the arterial, portal venous, and delayed phases. During arterial phase, hypervascular lesions including hepatocellular carcinoma and metastases from renal, breast, carcinoid, and pancreatic islet cell tumors enhance earlier than the normal liver parenchyma. These lesions may become isodense to liver parenchyma during portal venous or delayed phase. Some hypervascular lesions show lower density during portal or delayed phase called "washout" phenomenon. Detection of a hypervascular lesion that shows washout is commonly seen in cirrhotic patients with hepatocellular carcinoma. Delayed scanning has been employed to improve detection of intrahepatic cholangiocarcinoma and hepatocellular carcinoma.

Noncontrast CT scan of the liver is inferior to contrast-enhanced studies for lesion detection and is not routinely performed except in certain specific situations. Patients with liver disorders that diffusely alter hepatic attenuation, such as hepatosteatosis, hemochromatosis, and amiodarone toxicity should be evaluated with noncontrast CT. Noncontrast liver CT may be indicated for evaluation of calcified lesions calcification (such as metastases from mucinous colon carcinoma), or hemorrhage (in lesions like hepatocellular adenomas).

Magnetic Resonance Imaging

The recent development of rapid acquisition techniques with excellent image quality and tissue-specific contrast agents has made MRI the most accurate imaging modality for the evaluation of liver disease (Fig. 31.1). Traditionally T1- and T2-weighted sequences were performed with suppression of the body fat; however, many novel pulse sequences are being developed to decrease scan time and increase signal-to-noise ratio. MRI is often superior to CT or ultrasound in lesion characterization but usually reserved as a second-line modality secondary to cost.

Magnetic resonance contrast agents are crucial in liver lesion detection and characterization. There are many MR contrast agents with different properties. Examples of extracellular contrast agents include the gadolinium chelates, gadopentetate dimeglumine (Gd-DTPA) and gadoterate meglumine (Gd-DOTA). These agents function similar to iodinated CT contrast agents by rapidly diffusing from the intravascular space to the extracellular space. Hepatobiliary specific agents such as gadoxatate (Gd-EOB-DTPA) and gadobenate dimeglumine (Gd-BOPTA) increase the signal intensity of the normal liver and hepatocyte-containing lesions such as focal nodular

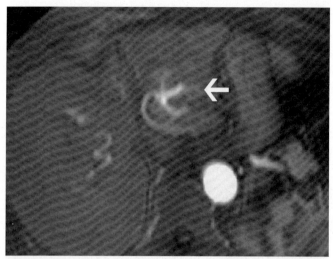

A

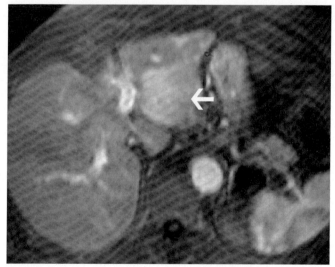

B

FIGURE 31.1 Hepatocellular carcinoma visualized by multiphasic contrast-enhanced MRI of the liver. **A.** Arterial phase of the study shows a mass within the left lobe of the liver enhancing earlier than the rest of the liver parenchyma (*arrow*). Note the prominent intra-tumoral arterial network. **B.** Portal venous phase of the examination shows that the mass is relatively hypervascular (*arrow*) compared to the surrounding liver parenchyma.

(*Continued*)

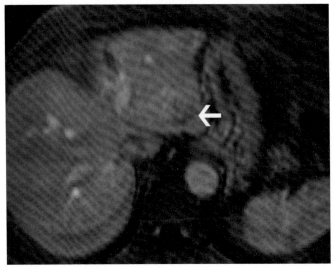

C

FIGURE 31.1 (Continued) C. Delayed phase of the study shows that enhancement characteristic of the mass has excreted the contrast earlier than the liver parenchyma and now shows relatively less enhancement (*arrow*). Early contrast uptake and early contrast clearance is called "washout phenomenon" and is a characteristic of hypervascular malignancies.

hyperplasia. This increased signal intensity improves the contrast difference between the liver parenchyma and nonhepatocellular lesions (such as metastases) during the delayed phase images.

Positron Emission Tomography Scan

The liver demonstrates diffusely increased fludeoxyglucose (FDG) activity physiologically and is used as a qualitative comparison point for other foci of uptake in the body (e.g., pancreatic and gallbladder lesions). Activity that is equal to or greater than that in the liver raises concern for pathologic processes. Overall, most metastatic tumors are FDG avid and readily detectable using PET-CT. FDG-PET imaging of hepatocellular carcinoma is somewhat limited due to the activity of glucose-6-phosphatase, which is found in varying degrees in this tumor. Hepatocellular carcinoma is more FDG avid than the liver in approximately 55% of cases; it is equal to or less avid in 30% and 15% of cases, respectively. Generally, PET detects only 50% to 70% of hepatocellular carcinomas, but is useful in detection of distant metastases (extrahepatic disease) as well as in evaluation of recurrence. In FDG avid hepatocellular carcinoma, PET-CT imaging is helpful for staging, especially in the assessment of distant metastatic disease.

GALLBLADDER

Ultrasound

Real-time transabdominal sonography is the most widely used diagnostic examination for the gallbladder since it is quick and easy to perform. The gallbladder is visible on sonograms in virtually all fasting patients despite

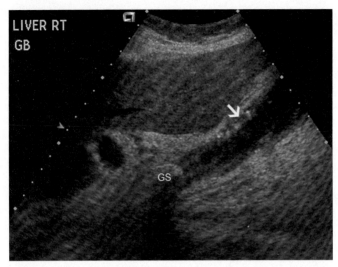

FIGURE 31.2 Abnormal gallbladder by ultrasound. Gray-scale image of the gallbladder and liver is shown. There is a round gallstone (*GS*) located within the neck of the gallbladder; note the posterior shadowing seen as black. There is abnormal and irregular gallbladder wall thickening (*arrow*). Comet tail artifacts visualized in the gallbladder wall indicates adenomyomatosis of the gallbladder. This is a diagnosis specifically made by the ultrasound.

body habitus or clinical condition. The success rate of obtaining a diagnostic study is very high; therefore, ultrasound should be considered as the first line of study for primary gallbladder pathology (Fig. 31.2). The examination can be performed at the bedside and, since no ionizing radiation is used, is safe in pregnant and pediatric patients.

Computed Tomography

The gallbladder in fasting patients is nearly always identified on CT scans of the upper abdomen. Although calcified gallstones are frequently visible, CT is not used as a primary examination for detecting gallstones because of its lower sensitivity for gallstones and higher cost compared with ultrasound. The main indication for CT in gallbladder disease is for the diagnosis and staging of gallbladder carcinoma and evaluation of the complications of cholecystitis such as perforation and pericholecystic abscess.

Cholescintigraphy

Cholescintigraphy is used primarily for the diagnosis of acute cholecystitis. This study is performed by injecting Technetium-99m iminodiacetic acid (^{99m} Tc-IDA) compounds intravenously, and the tracer is taken up by the liver and rapidly excreted into bile without undergoing conjugation, allowing visualization of the gallbladder and bile ducts. Serial images are obtained up to 1 hour. Delayed imaging up to 4 hours and possibly 24 hours may be necessary in some instances. Nonfilling of the gallbladder on cholescintigraphy indicates functional obstruction of the cystic duct and is highly sensitive and specific for the diagnosis of acute cholecystitis in the appropriate clinical setting (Fig. 31.3). Other uses for scintigraphic evaluation of the biliary tract include assessment of gallbladder ejection fraction, patency or bile leak after cholecystectomy, or biliary enteric anastomoses.

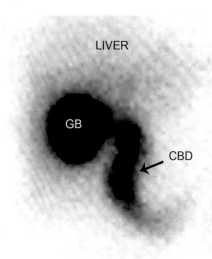

FIGURE 31.3 Normal cholescintigram. Frontal view taken 60 minutes after injection of radioisotope shows normal filling of the gallbladder (*GB*). There is excretion of radioisotope into the common bile duct (*CBD*) as well. These findings exclude possibility of acute cholecystitis with very high specificity. Normal uptake within the liver is seen as well.

Long-term function of Roux-en-Y biliary–enteric anastomosis may be evaluated by scintigraphy with delayed imaging.

BILIARY AND PANCREATIC DUCTAL SYSTEM

Ultrasound and CT, because of wide availability and ease of performance as well as high diagnostic accuracy, are the first-line imaging techniques for evaluation of the biliary tree. Magnetic resonance cholangiopancreatography (MRCP) is assuming a larger role as a rapid, accurate, and noninvasive method of evaluating the bile ducts. Currently, MRCP is replacing diagnostic endoscopic retrograde cholangiopancreatography (ERCP) in many instances. Biliary scintigraphy has a limited role in biliary imaging, used mainly for confirming acute cholecystitis and identifying bile leaks.

Ultrasound

Evaluation of the bile ducts in search of stones, masses, or obstructions is one of the main applications for ultrasound. Real-time ultrasound readily depicts dilated biliary ducts, which, in most instances, is indicative of biliary obstruction. The extrahepatic bile duct can be seen in most patients regardless of body habitus or clinical condition. The most distal common bile duct (CBD) is more difficult and frequently impossible to image by transabdominal ultrasound because of overlying gas in the duodenum and colonic hepatic flexure.

Computed Tomography

Although ultrasound continues to be used as the initial screening test for biliary disease, CT is as effective as is sonography in determining the caliber of intra- and extrahepatic ducts. In addition, because of more complete delineation of the total length of the CBD, CT may be more useful than sonography for precisely defining the site and cause of biliary obstruction. Also, if ultrasound results are equivocal, CT may be used to refine the data or confirm anatomy. In addition, CT can often differentiate benign from malignant causes of obstruction and can provide guidance for biopsy and staging of malignancies. CT cholangiography, using oral or intravenous cholecystography agents, has been widely used in Europe and has been used on a limited basis in some centers in the United States to evaluate ductal pathology.

Magnetic Resonance Cholangiopancreatography

MRCP is the most effective, safe, noninvasive MR imaging technique for evaluation of the pancreaticobiliary ductal system. The usefulness and accuracy of MRCP have been established in the evaluation of suspected pancreaticobiliary pain, choledocholithiasis, malignant obstruction, congenital anomalies, and postsurgical alterations of the biliary tract and pancreas. Contrast administration is not necessary in the evaluation of patients with suspected choledocholithiasis.

MRCP is mainly based on acquisition of heavily T2-weighted images, with variants of fast spin echo (FSE) sequences; however, examination should also include routine MRI images for a complete evaluation. The diagnostic accuracy of MRCP is comparable to that of ERCP in the evaluation of choledocholithiasis, malignant obstruction, and anatomic variants of the pancreaticobiliary tract (Fig. 31.4). Visualization of the pancreatic duct is often substantially improved with the use of the hormone secretin,

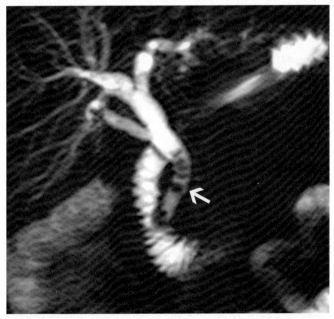

FIGURE 31.4 Choledocholithiasis visualized by MRCP. Coronal MRCP image shows multiple filling defects (*arrow*) within the distal common bile duct causing intra- and extrahepatic ductal dilatation.

which stimulates the pancreas to secrete a significant amount of fluid while transiently increasing sphincter of Oddi tone. Utilization of secretin is recommended in cases where detailed evaluation of the pancreatic duct is desired. Although the role of MRCP in the evaluation of biliary diseases is expanding, the major disadvantage of MRCP is that it is purely diagnostic and does not provide an access for therapeutic intervention. MRCP is the modality of choice for follow-up after some pancreatic operations such as pancreatoduodenectomy, where ERCP is challenging.

Percutaneous Transhepatic Cholangiography and ERCP

Percutaneous transhepatic cholangiography (PTC) and ERCP are invasive methods and usually reserved for patients requiring interventions such as biliary drainage, stone extraction, stent placement, stricture dilatation, and biopsy. Both techniques allow direct opacification of the biliary tree but require invasive access and have limited diagnostic use. The choice of procedure for direct cholangiography depends on a number of factors: the clinical situation, the potential for therapeutic intervention, and the availability of a skilled endoscopist or interventional radiologist. Both procedures allow transformation of a diagnostic study to a variety of therapeutic maneuvers. The overall complication rate for PTC is 3.5%, which less than the 10% complication rate seen with ERCP.

PANCREAS

The pancreas is one of the most challenging organs to image in the abdomen. The small size of the organ and its deep location requires high-resolution imaging. Comprehensive imaging of the pancreas should show pancreatic and biliary ductal anatomy, help detect and characterize parenchymal disease, delineate extrapancreatic extension of a mass or inflammatory process, and evaluate the vascular anatomy.

Ultrasound

Sonography is a practical and inexpensive option for evaluation of the pancreas, but it is operator dependent and usually limited in patients with large body habitus. Ultrasound examination of the pancreas is best performed on the fasting patient to reduce the amount of gas and food in overlying bowel. Without patient preparation, the overlying gastric air commonly obscures this organ, particularly the tail of the pancreas. Intraoperative sonography is very useful.

Computed Tomography

MDCT is the first-line imaging technique for the pancreas. It is unaffected by bowel gas or large body habitus and is widely available, fast, and relatively easily performed. Multiphasic studies are the primary modality used for evaluation and posttreatment follow-up of the pancreatic adenocarcinoma and hypervascular pancreatic tumors including islet cell tumors. However, CT can be confounded by a morphologic overlap and is insensitive in differentiating cystic neoplasms. In such cases, MRI of the pancreas is recommended for further evaluation.

MRI with MRCP

MRI with MRCP examination is commonly performed together for a complete evaluation of the pancreas. MRI has an advantage over CT by better depicting the internal morphology of pancreatic cysts due to the superior soft tissue contrast. This improved resolution facilitates recognition of septa, nodules, and depiction of the duct. Disadvantages of MRI include

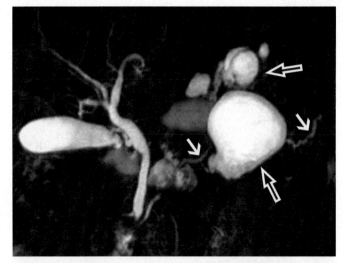

FIGURE 31.5 Pancreatic cystic neoplasms imaged by MRCP. This coronal maximum intensity projection image shows multiple round cystic lesions arising from the pancreas (*open arrows*) most likely representing an IPMN. The main pancreatic duct appears normal (*short arrows*). MRI with MRCP provides superior image depiction compared to other cross-sectional modalities such as CT.

lower spatial resolution, insensitivity to detect calcifications, and motion-related artifacts. The contraindications to the use of MR contrast agents are severe allergy, pregnancy, and end-stage renal dysfunction.

Cystic lesions in the pancreas constitute a diverse category including inflammatory lesions as well as neoplasms ranging from benign lesions to low-grade indolent neoplasia to frankly malignant tumors. One of the most common diagnostic challenges in characterization of cystic pancreatic neoplasms is distinguishing isolated side branch intraductal papillary mucinous neoplasm (IPMN) from other cystic lesions such as mucinous cystic neoplasms or pseudocyst (Fig. 31.5). Ductal dilation may provide evidence of chronic pancreatitis, but it may also indicate that an IPMN is of the main duct or mixed type. These types of IPMN are more likely to be malignant than is the more common side-branch type; therefore, a cytologic evaluation may be necessary in these patients. Improvement in the visualization of the duct has been reported with the use of the hormone secretin, which stimulates the pancreas to secrete a significant amount of fluid, while transiently increasing the tone of the sphincter of Oddi. MRCP is also valuable providing noninvasive evaluation of the chronic pancreatitis by showing the ductal ectasia, atrophy, or strictures with upstream dilatation (Fig. 31.6).

PET Scan

CT and MRI are used primarily to image pancreatic ductal adenocarcinoma, but they may be limited in the setting of enlargement of the pancreatic head without discrete mass or mass-forming pancreatitis. Metabolic imaging may be applied to improve preoperative diagnostic accuracy and potentially limit adverse outcomes from inappropriate surgical interventions. Studies have demonstrated the relatively high sensitivity and specificity

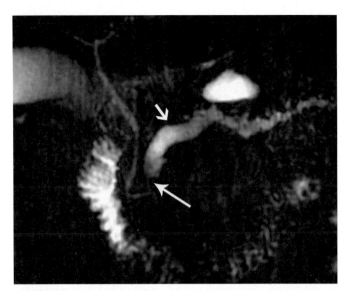

FIGURE 31.6 Pancreatic duct stricture visualized by MRCP. Coronal MRCP image demonstrates marked dilatation of the main pancreatic the duct within the body and tail (*short arrow*). This dilatation is clearly secondary to a stricture within the head of the pancreas (*long arrow*).

of PET in distinguishing benign and malignant lesions in the pancreas in comparison to CT. The primary challenge faced by PET–CT in the imaging of pancreatic cancer pertains to altered glucose metabolism created by glucose intolerance and diabetes seen in these patients. This clinical situation may create false-negative findings in patients who are hyperglycemic or have inadequately controlled blood glucose levels. False negatives may also result when the tumor is less than 1 cm, such as in small ampullary carcinomas. False positives are mainly the result of inflammation secondary to pancreatitis.

Suggested Readings

Gore RM, Levine MS. *Textbook of gastrointestinal radiology,* 3rd ed. Philadelphia, PA: Saunders/Elsevier, 2008.
Semelka RC. *Abdominal-pelvic MRI,* 2nd ed. Hoboken, NJ: Wiley-Liss, 2006:1427, xi
Siegelman ES. *Body MRI,* 1st ed. Philadelphia, PA: Saunders, 2005:527, ix
Webb WR, Brant WE, Helms CA. *Fundamentals of body CT,* 2nd ed. Philadelphia, PA: Saunders, 1998:363, xii.

Endoscopy in HPB Surgery Including ERCP and EUS

Wesley D. Leung and Gregory A. Coté

INTRODUCTION

Gastrointestinal endoscopy offers a multitude of diagnostic and therapeutic options for patients with pancreatic disease. Pancreatobiliary endoscopy derives from endoscopic retrograde cholangiopancreatography (ERCP) and endoscopic ultrasound (EUS), although gastroduodenal stenting is increasingly utilized for patients with unresectable pancreatic cancer and gastric outlet obstruction as well. This chapter reviews the indications, benefits, and limitations of ERCP, EUS, and gastroduodenal stenting, with a particular focus on pancreatic cancer and chronic pancreatitis (CP).

ENDOSCOPIC RETROGRADE CHOLANGIOPANCREATOGRAPHY

ERCP is an endoscopic technique that emerged in the 1970s where a side-viewing upper endoscope (a.k.a., duodenoscope) is advanced per oral to the level of the major and minor papilla, allowing instruments to access the bile and pancreatic ducts under endoscopic and fluoroscopic guidance. Traditionally, these ducts are opacified after the injection of iodinated contrast and visualized fluoroscopically. In certain circumstances such as complex choledocholithiasis or indeterminate strictures, a single-operator, fiberoptic cholangiopancreatoscope or mother–daughter scope can be advanced into the pancreatobiliary ducts for direct visualization. In its nascence, ERCP was a diagnostic tool in an era where cross-sectional imaging of the pancreas and bile ducts was extremely limited. Now, ERCP is primarily reserved for therapy, including stone extraction, stricture dilation, or biliary drainage. ERCP has substantial morbidity that mirrors some low- to moderate-risk surgical procedures, including acute pancreatitis (5% to 15%), hemorrhage (1%), cholangitis (1%), perforation (0.5%), and rarely death (0.1%).

ENDOSCOPIC ULTRASOUND

EUS combines a flexible endoscope with an ultrasound transducer (newer models are electronic, although older versions are mechanical) that permits full-thickness visualization of the gastrointestinal wall and surrounding structures, including the pancreas and extrahepatic biliary tree. Radial echoendoscopes provide a circumferential view at right angles to the scope shaft, whereas linear echoendoscopes yield a 270-degree oblique view that is in the same plane as the scope shaft, permitting the passage of instruments under ultrasound guidance. EUS-guided fine needle aspiration (EUS–FNA) can be performed through a linear echoendoscope with limited risks of bleeding, perforation, and infection, the latter occurring rarely in the setting of cyst aspiration. Most complications from EUS and ERCP are managed medically and are self-limiting, but serious complications such as severe necrotizing pancreatitis, hemorrhage (refractory to endoscopic and/or percutaneous treatment), and perforation may require surgical intervention.

PREPROCEDURE EVALUATION

EUS and ERCP are performed most commonly on an outpatient basis. The procedures can be performed with moderate sedation in some cases, although facilities are increasingly utilizing monitored anesthesia care or general anesthesia as the preferred approach. For elective cases, patients should fast for 2 hours (clear liquids) and 8 hours (solid food) before the procedure. Ideally, anticoagulants (e.g., warfarin) and antiplatelet agents (e.g., clopidogrel) should be held for 5 to 7 days, particularly in the setting of EUS–FNA or ERCP with sphincterotomy. As a general rule, an international normalized ratio (INR) less than 1.5 and platelet count greater than 50,000 are preferred, particularly if therapeutic maneuvers are anticipated (i.e., endoscopic sphincterotomy or EUS–FNA). Aspirin ≤325 mg by mouth daily probably does not impact the risk of postprocedure hemorrhage.

For ERCP, patients are preferably sedated in the prone position to optimize fluoroscopic visualization and to keep the duodenoscope in a stable "hockey-stick" configuration at the level of the papilla (Fig. 32.1). Patients undergoing EUS are typically sedated in the left lateral position, similar to a standard esophagogastroduodenoscopy (a.k.a., upper endoscopy). Following either procedure, patients who are at a moderate to high risk for

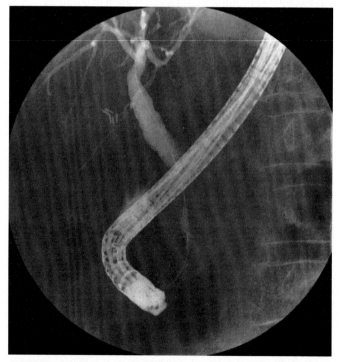

FIGURE 32.1 Endoscopic retrograde cholangiopancreatography. A retrograde cholangiogram is performed with the duodenoscope in a "hockey-stick" configuration in the second portion of the duodenum. This patient is a 53-year-old woman with idiopathic CP and jaundice. She has segmental narrowing in the intrapancreatic segment of the bile duct consistent with a CP–induced bile duct stricture.

complications should be kept fasting or advanced to clear liquids only and resume normal diet the next morning in the absence of concerning signs/symptoms. Patients who are at low risk of complications can gradually advance their diet over 4 to 6 hours.

ERCP IN THE SETTING OF PERIAMPULLARY MALIGNANCY

With improvements in cross-sectional imaging and EUS, the role of ERCP for the diagnosis of periampullary malignancy (distal cholangiocarcinoma and pancreatic ductal adenocarcinoma [PDAC], in particular) is increasingly limited. ERCP remains the procedure of choice for biliary drainage, if indicated, and is a medium for obtaining tissue samples.

Periampullary malignancies may present with a bile duct stricture that can be challenging to distinguish from a benign bile duct stricture, such as from CP. Malignant biliary strictures often have a length greater than 10 mm, a ragged contour, fixed filling defect, and/or shouldering above the stricture (abrupt transition in appearance from normal to stricture) (Fig. 32.2). The malignant potential of proximal common hepatic duct or bifurcation strictures is generally higher than that of distal bile duct strictures, often due to cholangiocarcinoma or portal lymphadenopathy causing extrinsic compression.

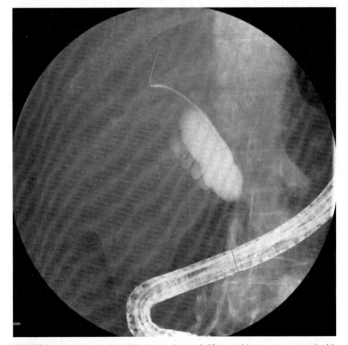

FIGURE 32.2 Malignant distal bile duct stricture. A 63-year-old woman presented with painless jaundice and was found to have a pancreatic head mass on EUS performed immediately prior to ERCP. EUS–FNA confirmed the presence of PDAC. Retrograde cholangiogram reveals a discrete common bile duct stricture with abrupt "shouldering" of the upstream, dilated common hepatic duct. This cholangiogram is highly suggestive of a malignant bile duct stricture, as in this case.

Tissue Sampling

ERCP-based tissue sampling is usually performed with a cytologic brush or forceps biopsies. The sensitivity of cytologic brushings from bile duct strictures is approximately 30% to 40% and specificity approaching 100%. Brush cytology in primary biliary tumors has a higher sensitivity than in extrinsic tumors (pancreatic or metastatic) (80% vs. 35%). Fewer studies have addressed the yield of cytologic brushings of pancreatic ducts. The accuracy is estimated to be 72%, and using a technique of collecting pancreatic juice above a stricture, a sensitivity and specificity of 93% and 100%, respectively, can be obtained. However, risks of pancreatitis and hemorrhage in the upstream pancreatic duct should be considered. In patients with PSC, diagnosing malignancy can be difficult, and cholangiography increases the specificity and positive predictive value for cholangiocarcinoma when combined with tumor markers (carbohydrate antigen 19-9) and cross-sectional imaging. There is no clinically significant difference in diagnostic yield between cytologic brushes produced by different manufacturers.

The sensitivity of forceps biopsy ranges from 43% to 88% with specificity similar to brush cytology (approaching 100%). Flexible forceps permit easier biliary cannulation than do stiffer ones. The combination of cytologic brushing and forceps biopsy increased sensitivity by 15% in one report but a smaller benefit in another study. Another study found that combination of cytologic brushing, forceps biopsy, and endoscopic fine needle aspiration was more sensitive (73% to 77%) than was each approach alone. Aspiration of bile for cytologic analysis is rarely used because of low sensitivity of 6% to 32%.

In some cases, methods such as digital image analysis (DIA) and fluorescence in situ hybridization (FISH) can improve the sensitivity of cytology alone. DIA quantifies the amount of cellular DNA by measuring the intensity of nuclei stained with a dye that binds to nuclear DNA. FISH uses a fluorescently labeled probe to detect chromosomal abnormalities in cells. FISH increases sensitivity of cytology to a greater degree than does DIA. However, there is the potential for false positives with either technique, particularly in cases of primary sclerosing cholangitis (PSC). Therefore, a positive FISH alone in the absence of a positive cytology specimen needs to be considered with the rest of the clinical picture.

Miniature endoscopes can be used to visualize the bile (cholangioscopy) and pancreatic (pancreatoscopy) ducts. Traditional mother–daughter systems required two operators to maneuver the duodenoscope and the cholangioscope independently. A single-operator, fiberoptic cholangioscope (Spyglass, Boston Scientific Corp.) is available; while this facilitates direct visualization of the bile and pancreatic ducts, its impact on confirming the presence or absence of malignancy remains unclear.

TREATMENT OF JAUNDICE

The location of malignant biliary obstruction influences the efficacy of endoscopic biliary drainage (distal better than perihilar). The endoscopic management of proximal bile duct strictures (bismuth II–IV) and bile duct obstruction are not discussed in this review. ERCP is typically preferred to percutaneous transhepatic cholangiography (PTC) for biliary drainage because an external drain is avoided. The short-term (<90 day) success of ERCP in achieving biliary drainage in the setting of distal bile duct obstruction is 80% to 90%. Complications may occur in up to 10% of patients, including cholangitis, perforation, bleeding, and post-ERCP pancreatitis. Plastic biliary stents are relatively inexpensive and easily removable compared to self-expandable metallic stents (SEMS). However, SEMS have a larger diameter (8 to 10 mm as opposed to 7 to 10 Fr for plastic) and are thus less likely to occlude prematurely (median patency rates of 6 to 9 months for SEMS as compared to 3 months for plastic stents).

In patients with locally advanced or metastatic PDAC, the goals of biliary drainage are palliation of symptoms and to permit systemic chemotherapy with a normal or near-normal serum bilirubin. The treatment of jaundice will undoubtedly relieve pruritus (if present) and may improve other symptoms such as anorexia and indigestion. For cases of unresectable disease, an endoscopic approach is safer than is surgical bypass but with reduced durability. Long-term patency of SEMS is superior to that of plastic stents due to their larger diameter; SEMS should be placed in patients having a life expectancy of greater than 3 months. The majority of patients in the United States with potentially resectable periampullary malignancy undergo preoperative biliary drainage despite a lack of evidence that it reduces postoperative complications. This practice may be explained in part by a delay in surgical consultation and concern for higher risk of perioperative complications in the setting of jaundice. Older studies suggest jaundice may be a predictor of postoperative infection and renal and nutritional complications. Experimental studies demonstrate improved nutritional status and immune function and reduced endotoxinemia after biliary decompression. Prospective studies evaluating the role of preoperative biliary drainage have excluded patients with deep jaundice (serum total bilirubin ≥10 to 15 mg/dL), where the benefits of drainage are expected to be the highest. Furthermore, the duration between preoperative biliary drainage and surgery is often less than 4 weeks despite evidence suggesting normalization of hepatocyte function after 6 weeks of decompression.

Treatment of Gastric Outlet Obstruction

Duodenal obstruction from pancreatic cancer typically is not present at diagnosis but may develop in 15% to 20% of patients. To avoid this complication, many surgeons create a prophylactic palliative gastrojejunostomy with a biliary bypass in those who are deemed to be unresectable at exploration. Endoscopic placement of a self-expandable, gastroduodenal metallic stent has lower morbidity compared to surgical gastrojejunostomy and comparable short-term efficacy but lower long-term (>3 to 6 months) efficacy due to tumor ingrowth within the interstices of the stent. In a study comparing patients who underwent surgical gastrojejunostomy with endoscopic stenting, patients who underwent endoscopic palliation had similar median survival (94 vs. 92 days) but shorter hospitalization (4 vs. 14 days), which led to overall lower cost ($9,921 vs. $28,173).

ERCP IN THE SETTING OF CHRONIC PANCREATITIS

ERCP has evolved from a diagnostic to a therapeutic tool for patients with CP as a result of advances in magnetic resonance cholangiopancreatography (MRCP), computed tomography (CT), and EUS. Pancreatic ductal changes on ERCP can be classified by the Cambridge classification as equivocal (type I), mild to moderate (type II), and severe (type III). The classification has been shown to correlate with the severity of exocrine insufficiency. However, some patients with early CP have a normal pancreatogram. Achieving a definitive diagnosis in this population is challenging and requires the incorporation of other imaging and pancreatic function testing.

Pain from CP is probably multifactorial, although one suggested mechanism is pancreatic ductal hypertension due to pancreatic duct obstruction from a stricture or stone. Therapeutic ERCP can alleviate pain and recurrent pancreatitis flares with serial dilation of pancreatic duct strictures or stone extraction. Similar to the treatment of benign bile duct strictures, pancreatic duct strictures are managed with serial dilation and placement of one or more plastic stents until the stricture is obliterated. This usually requires three or more ERCPs occurring every 2 to 4 months for up to 1 year. Pancreatic stones are more easily removed if they are small, few in number, closer to the head of the pancreas, and not impacted. For either stricture or stone management, a pancreatic sphincterotomy is usually required. Stones upstream to the tail from a pancreatic duct stricture require stricture dilation before extraction. Other options for stone removal include direct pancreatoscopy, electrohydraulic lithotripsy, and extracorporeal shock wave lithotripsy (ESWL). Notably, ESWL alone may be as effective as ESWL combined with ERCP for therapy of pancreatic duct stones. Although studies have shown endoscopic therapy may improve pain, in CP, the short- and long-term efficacy of endoscopic treatment are inferior to surgical interventions aimed at relieving obstruction and achieving pain relief.

ERCP IN THE SETTING OF ACUTE PANCREATITIS

The role of ERCP in the early management of patients with acute pancreatitis is limited. In patients with gallstone pancreatitis, urgent ERCP (to be performed within 72 hours of presentation) is indicated only in the setting of concomitant acute cholangitis or severe acute pancreatitis with biliary obstruction. The benefits of early ERCP remain controversial. One meta-analysis concluded early ERCP reduced complications but not mortality in severe biliary pancreatitis and had no benefit in mild pancreatitis. Two other meta-analyses found no benefit in morbidity or mortality from early ERCP in biliary pancreatitis.

For all patients with suspected gallstone pancreatitis, those having a high risk for common bile duct (CBD) stones should undergo CBD imaging prior to discharge. High suspicion would include the presence of stones or ductal dilation on cross-sectional imaging or persistent elevation in cholestatic labs (alkaline phosphatase, direct bilirubin). Patients at intermediate risk should undergo less invasive imaging of their extrahepatic biliary tree in lieu of diagnostic ERCP, including EUS or MRCP. For stones less than 4 mm, EUS is more sensitive, specific, and cost-effective than is MRCP. If EUS or MRCP confirms the presence of choledocholithiasis, ERCP should be performed soon thereafter.

The role of ERCP with sphincter of Oddi manometry in patients with idiopathic, recurrent acute pancreatitis requires clarification. A recent prospective randomized clinical trial suggested no incremental benefit of pancreatic sphincterotomy over biliary sphincterotomy alone in this population. The benefit of empiric biliary sphincterotomy is debatable and also requires further investigation. Individually, or in combination, MRCP and EUS have largely replaced ERCP in diagnosing less common causes of recurrent acute pancreatitis, including pancreas divisum, intraductal papillary mucinous neoplasm, and ampullary lesions, among others.

ENDOSCOPY IN THE SETTING OF PANCREATIC FLUID COLLECTIONS

Pancreatic duct disruption and fluid collections may occur in the setting of acute or CP. In properly selected cases, endoscopy can obviate the need for percutaneous drains and surgery by promoting internal drainage. A pseudocyst is an organized fluid collection, consisting of pancreatic juice enclosed by a nonepithelialized tissue. Many pseudocysts can be managed without intervention (even if over 6 cm) unless they enlarge or become symptomatic. Traditional surgical drainage of pseudocyst carries a 10% morbidity rate and 1% mortality; therefore, radiologic and endoscopic drainage compete with surgery as first-line treatment. Endoscopic drainage can involve either transpapillary or transmural (transgastric, transduodenal) placement of stents. A transpapillary approach is used for smaller pseudocysts communicating with the main pancreatic duct, whereas larger pseudocysts or those not clearly communicating with the pancreatic duct are drained transmurally. Pseudocyst drainage is usually performed after allowing the cyst wall to mature for at least 4 to 6 weeks after the onset of acute pancreatitis.

Transpapillary Drainage

Ongoing pancreatic duct disruption may heal in 78% to 92% of cases with stent placement across the disruption. Success rates plummet to 23% to 44% with transpapillary stents that do not bridge the leak (Fig. 32.3). Technical success may be lower for tail disruptions and definitely in the setting of complete pancreatic duct disruption.

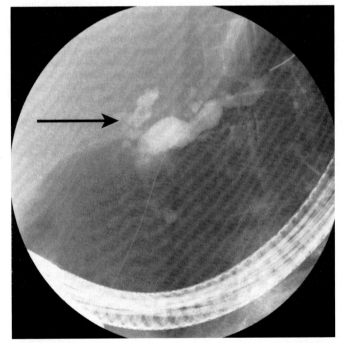

FIGURE 32.3 Severe CP with low-grade fistula. A 45-year-old woman with severe alcohol-induced CP presented with abdominal pain and pancreatic ascites. ERCP confirmed the presence of a low-grade leak from the pancreatic head (*arrow*) with severe CP changes in the main pancreatic duct and its side branches. The leak resolved following pancreatic sphincterotomy and placement of a 7-Fr plastic pancreatic duct stent.

Transmural Drainage

The goal of transmural drainage is to create an internal communication between the pseudocyst and the gastric or duodenal lumen. Traditionally, endoscopic cystogastrostomy involved piercing an endoscopically visible bulge using a needle knife catheter and electrocautery. The risk of bleeding is reduced from 15.7% to 4.6% if a Seldinger technique (advancing a guide-wire through a 19-gauge needle) is used. After obtaining access to the cyst cavity, the opening is balloon dilated, and several pigtail stents are placed. Cyst localization by EUS facilitates drainage, particularly in the setting of a pseudocyst that is not causing an endoscopically visible bulge; EUS has a higher technical success and lower morbidity versus a non-EUS–guided approach. In addition, EUS can determine if the distance between cyst and GI tract is ideal, identify intervening blood vessels, and quantify the volume of necrotic debris within the cyst.

Necrotic debris within a pseudocyst often necessitates débridement: Endoscopically, this entails entering the cavity with an endoscope and removing necrotic debris using a variety of instruments. A retrospective study suggested that, for patients with walled-off pancreatic necrosis (WOPN), endoscopic necrosectomy was superior to endoscopic cystogastrostomy alone for resolution of necrosis, decreased need for adjunctive surgical or per-cutaneous drainage, and recurrence. A step-up approach was recently com-pared to open necrosectomy as first-line treatment for patients with proven or suspected infected WOPN. Patients were randomized to primary open necrosectomy and continuous postoperative lavage or to a step-up approach (percutaneous/endoscopic drainage and if no clinical improvement repeat drainage followed by video-assisted retroperitoneal debridement (VARD) followed by open necrosectomy). Another recent trial compared endoscopic necrosectomy to VARD and open surgery in the treatment of infected WOPN. Pancreatic necrosis should ideally be addressed in the context of a multidis-ciplinary team including pancreatic surgeons and endoscopists.

ERCP FOR THE MANAGEMENT OF POSTOPERATIVE COMPLICATIONS

The most common postoperative biliary strictures occur following liver transplant and, less commonly, cholecystectomy. In general, the manage-ment of benign bile duct strictures involves serial dilation using graduated increasing size of balloons, followed by the placement of multiple plastic stents in parallel to keep the stricture patent. For strictures involving the com-mon hepatic duct, short-term success rates are generally greater than 90% and have reasonable durability, with recurrence rates of approximately 10%.

Bile duct strictures occurring after liver transplant have an incidence of 4% to 16% and can be classified as anastomotic or nonanastomotic. Most anas-tomotic strictures occur within 12 months of liver transplant. Those occurring within 6 months of surgery respond well to endoscopic balloon dilation and short-term (3 to 12 months) plastic stenting. Patients presenting greater than 6 months postoperatively require multiple endoscopic procedures to serially dilate and upsize the number/maximum diameter of stents. Superior resolu-tion rates are observed with higher total number of stents placed. In patients with Roux-en-Y choledochojejunostomy, PTC is usually preferred to ERC since patients require multiple procedures for serial dilation and endoscopic access to the biliary anastomosis is challenging with Roux-en-Y anatomy.

ENDOSCOPIC ULTRASOUND

EUS for Tissue Sampling

EUS plays an important role in tissue diagnosis to confirm the presence of pancreatic cancer and rule out metastatic lesions to the pancreas

(11% in one study) or surrounding structures and to diagnose nonmalignant processes such as autoimmune or CP. In general, EUS–FNA is the most accurate diagnostic modality with sensitivity 80% to 95% and specificity of 100% compared to CT or transabdominal ultrasound–guided FNA (sensitivity 62% to 81%). In the setting of CP, sensitivity of EUS decreases to 73%. EUS–FNA is also more accurate than is CT or magnetic resonance imaging at detecting pancreatic masses ≤1.5 cm. The needle tract for EUS–FNA of pancreatic head lesions lies within the surgical resection margin and thus has a lower risk of tumor seeding. This is not the case with lesions of pancreatic body and tail, but to date, no data definitively show EUS–FNA negatively impacts the likelihood of complete surgical resection or postoperative recurrence. A decision to perform an EUS–FNA of a pancreatic mass should be made in conjunction with a hepato-pancreatic-biliary (HPB) surgeon: If the patient is a surgical candidate and the pretest probability of cancer is greater than 90%, direct referral to surgery is also reasonable.

EUS for Staging

The accuracy of EUS for locoregional staging of pancreatic malignancy is operator dependent. A prospective clinical trial demonstrated EUS had no incremental value over contrast-enhanced CT scan in determining the resectability of a pancreatic mass. A recent review of studies comparing EUS and CT for preoperative staging of pancreatic cancer determined that it is unclear which modality is superior for both tumor and nodal staging, though this is less likely to impact on surgical management. A recent meta-analysis evaluating the accuracy of individual EUS criteria for vascular invasion had 73% sensitivity and 90% specificity.

EUS for Pancreatobiliary Drainage

The technical success of deep biliary cannulation by skilled endoscopists during ERCP is greater than 90%. The development of EUS-guided antegrade cholangiopancreatography refers to two different approaches to pancreatic drainage: EUS rendezvous or direct EUS intervention. These techniques have recently emerged as salvage methods for failed biliary cannulation, although their utilization is only available in selected centers. During rendezvous, EUS is used to access the bile duct transgastrically using a 19-gauge or 22-gauge FNA needle. A guidewire is then advanced through the needle and into the duodenum, followed by exchange of the echoendoscope for a duodenoscope to complete the ERCP procedure. Successful drainage occurred in 56% of patients in a recent cohort. Direct intervention via EUS involves creating an enterobiliary or enteropancreatic fistula. Here, EUS is again used to direct an FNA needle into the bile or pancreatic duct and advancing a guidewire across the obstructing lesion. Instead of switching to a duodenoscope and completing the procedure via ERCP, passage or balloon dilation of the EUS needle track is performed followed by deploying a stent directly. In one report, this technique had a 71% success rate but a 16% complication rate, including self-limited pneumoperitoneum and mild to severe pancreatitis. These techniques remain experimental and should not be performed in routine practice. However, advances in EUS-based devices are expected to expand the role of EUS-based therapy in the future.

EUS for Palliation of Pain

The celiac plexus is one of several purported locations mediating pain from the pancreas. Celiac plexus neurolysis (CPN) utilizes ethanol injection to ablate the celiac plexus in cases of refractory abdominal pain due to pancreatic cancer, whereas a celiac plexus block (CPB) involves the injection of a local anesthetic with or without steroid to achieve a temporary

(3 to 6 month) block in patients with CP. CPN or CPB can be achieved via surgical and transcutaneous approaches with small but potentially significant morbidity. EUS-guided CPN/CPB is technically feasible given the plexus location adjacent to the celiac artery takeoff from the descending aorta. While the celiac artery origin is easily identified during EUS, celiac ganglia are only visualized in a minority of cases (Fig. 32.4). For patients undergoing celiac block, a recent trial suggested the addition of triamcinolone did not increase the proportion of patients who reported significant pain relief or reduce self-reported pain scores compared to injection of a local anesthetic alone.

A recent meta-analysis suggests that EUS–CPN is safe and effective for patients with pancreatic cancer and CP. In pancreatic cancer, nearly 80% of patients experience pain relief after EUS–CPN; pain reduction lasts approximately 20 weeks. Early consideration (i.e., during the initial diagnostic procedure in select patients) for EUS–CPN should be made in patients with unresectable PDAC with abdominal pain requiring opioids, as it is associated with less pain and opioid requirements. In CP, the response rate and durability are lower with EUS–CPB, with 55% of individuals having a significant response rate initially but only 10% reporting a sustained response after 24 weeks.

ERCP IN THE SETTING OF POSTOPERATIVE ANATOMY

ERCP for patients with postoperative anatomy (i.e., status post pancreatoduodenectomy, Roux-en-Y gastrojejunostomy, antrectomy with Billroth I/II reconstruction) is challenging. The optimal therapeutic approach (endoscopic, percutaneous, surgical, or some combination) remains unclear but probably relates to a combination of the indication for ERCP (biliary

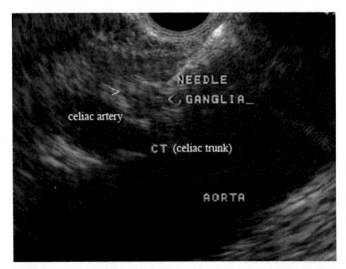

FIGURE 32.4 EUS-guided CPB. An EUS–FNA needle can be inserted into a celiac ganglion, typically located anterior to the celiac artery takeoff from the aorta. Factors associated with a better response to CPB include direct injection of celiac ganglia (when visualized) and absence of tumor invasion of the celiac plexus. (Reproduced from Coté GA, Sherman S. Endoscopic palliation of pancreatic cancer. *Cancer J* 2012;18(6):584–590.)

or pancreatic and the overall urgency for the procedure), specific anatomy (length of Roux limb), and patient preference. For patients who have undergone Roux-en-Y gastric bypass for weight loss, endoscopy obviates the need for percutaneous catheters but has a lower technical success rate. If an endoscopic approach is recommended, patients with bariatric-length Roux limbs who require pancreatic duct therapies (e.g., sphincter of Oddi dysfunction, pancreatic duct stones, or strictures) should undergo surgical placement of a large-bore ($\geq$30 Fr) gastrostomy tube into the gastric remnant to facilitate ERCP access. On the other hand, based on limited data, patients requiring short-term bile duct therapy (e.g., CBD stones) may be approached endoscopically (i.e., double balloon enteroscopy) if the anticipated success rate is greater than 80%.

For patients with a native papilla and short ($\leq$30 cm) Roux limb, a transoral approach using a duodenoscope can be attempted but is often unsuccessful. Alternatively, a colonoscope or small bowel enteroscope may be used to perform ERCP, but the number of ERCP accessories is limited by the longer length of these scopes. For patients with a native papilla and long Roux limb, surgical gastrostomy–assisted ERCP has higher success rates than has deep enteroscopy (balloon-assisted, spiral enteroscopy) but with higher morbidity (primarily related to complications from the surgical gastrostomy tube). For patients without a native papilla (i.e., bilioenteric/pancreatoenteric anastomosis) and a short Roux limb, a forward-viewing colonoscope or enteroscope can be used successfully in most cases.

CONCLUSION

Pancreatobiliary endoscopy represents an important component of the diagnostic and therapeutic management of patients with pancreatobiliary disease. Ideally, the majority of patients will be served by a multidisciplinary approach early in their disease course, combining the expert opinions of abdominal radiology, medical oncology, and gastroenterology with hepatobiliary–pancreatic surgery. A collegial working relationship between pancreatobiliary endoscopists and their surgical colleagues is critical since patients often require interventions from both disciplines. To that end, surgeons should recognize the potential benefits and limitations of pancreatobiliary endoscopy.

Suggested Readings

Anderson MA, Ben-Menachem T, Gan SI, et al. ASGE standards of practice committee: management of antithrombotic agents for endoscopic procedures. *Gastrointest Endosc* 2009;70(6):1060.

Andriulli A, Loperfido S, Napolitano G, et al. Incidence rates of post-ERCP complications: a systematic survey of prospective studies. *Am J Gastroenterol* 2007;102(8):1781.

Bakker OJ, van Santvoort HC, van Brunschot S, et al; Dutch Pancreatitis Study Group. Endoscopic transgastric vs surgical necrosectomy for infected necrotizing pancreatitis: a randomized trial. *JAMA* 2012;307(10):1053–1061.

Cahen DL, Gouma DJ, Nio Y, et al. Endoscopic versus surgical drainage of the pancreatic duct in chronic pancreatitis. *N Engl J Med* 2007;356:676–684.

Costamagna G, Tringali A, Mutignani M, et al. Endotherapy of postoperative biliary strictures with multiple stents: results after more than 10 years of follow-up. *Gastrointest Endosc* 2010;72(3):551–557.

Coté GA, Imperiale TF, Schmidt SE, et al. Similar efficacies of biliary, with or without pancreatic, sphincterotomy in treatment of idiopathic recurrent acute pancreatitis. *Gastroenterology* 2012;143(6):1502–1509.

DeWitt J, Devereaux B, Chriswell M, et al. Comparison of endoscopic ultrasonography and multidetector computed tomography for detecting and staging pancreatic cancer. *Ann Intern Med* 2004;141(10):753–763.

Hosono S, Ohtani H, Arimoto Y, et al. Endoscopic stenting versus surgical gastroenterostomy for palliation of malignant gastroduodenal obstruction: a meta-analysis. *J Gastroenterol* 2007;42(4):283–290.

Moss AC, Morris E, Mac Mathuna P. Palliative biliary stents for obstructing pancreatic carcinoma. *Cochrane Database Syst Rev* 2006;(2):CD004200. Review.

Moss AC, Morris E, Leyden J, et al. Malignant distal biliary obstruction: a systematic review and meta-analysis of endoscopic and surgical bypass results. *Cancer Treat Rev* 2007;33:213–221.

Petrov MS, van Santvoort HC, Besselink MG, et al. Early endoscopic retrograde cholangiopancreatography versus conservative management in acute biliary pancreatitis without cholangitis: a metaanalysis of randomized trials. *Ann Surg* 2008;247:250–257.

Puli SR, Reddy JB, Bechtold ML, et al. EUS-guided celiac plexus neurolysis for pain due to chronic pancreatitis or pancreatic cancer pain: a metaanalysis and systematic review. *Dig Dis Sci* 2009;54:2330–2337.

van der Gaag NA, Rauws EA, van Eijck CH, et al. Preoperative biliary drainage for cancer of the head of the pancreas. *N Engl J Med* 2010;362:129–137.

van Santvoort HC, Besselink MG, Bakker OJ, et al; Dutch Pancreatitis Study Group. A step-up approach or open necrosectomy for necrotizing pancreatitis. *N Engl J Med* 2010;362(16):1491–1502.

Varadarajulu S, Christein JD, Tamhane A, et al. Prospective randomized trial comparing EUS and EGD for transmural drainage of pancreatic pseudocysts. *Gastrointest Endosc* 2008;68:1102–1111.

Wang Q, Gurusamy KS, Lin H, et al. Preoperative biliary drainage for obstructive jaundice. *Cochrane Database Syst Rev* 2008:CD005444.

Yim HB, Jacobson BC, Saltzman JR, et al. Clinical outcome of the use of enteral stents for palliation of patients with malignant upper GI obstruction. *Gastrointest Endosc* 2001;53:329.

33

HPB Trauma

Chad G. Ball

Injuries to the liver, extrahepatic biliary tree, and pancreas are often deadly and always challenging. This area is also commonly referred to as the "surgical soul." They will engage all of your senses, test your skills, and demand great teamwork from you and your colleagues.

HEPATIC INJURIES

Although textbooks are often filled with a complex hierarchy of operative interventions and maneuvers for treating hepatic trauma, the vast majority of liver injuries are treated nonoperatively. This process involves diagnosis with cross-sectional imaging (CT), serial clinical observation, and laboratory (hemoglobin, white blood cell count [WBC], and liver function tests/enzymes) monitoring. This algorithm allows the clinician to successfully treat and predict both the initial injury and potential complications such as delayed/ongoing hemorrhage and interval formation of a biloma. Clearly, any patient who presents with hypotension and/or peritonitis (i.e., concurrent injuries) requires emergent operative therapy.

Management

Preoperative Considerations

The dominant challenge with hepatic trauma is management of the hemodynamically unstable patient with ongoing hemorrhage from a high-grade liver injury. These patients often present in physiologic extremis and therefore require damage control resuscitation techniques. Early recognition of their critical condition, as well as immediate hemorrhage control, is essential to survival.

Patients with major injury caused by blunt trauma or right upper quadrant penetrating mechanisms must undergo an immediate F.A.S.T. (i.e., Focused Assessment with Sonography for Trauma) examination in the trauma bay to confirm the presence of large-volume intraperitoneal fluid. This exam is repeatable and can be used to reevaluate patients in urban centers who present immediately following their injuries. Massive transfusion protocols as part of a damage control resuscitation must be initiated early during the patient assessment process. If the patients rapidly stabilize their hemodynamics, they should undergo an emergency CT scan of the torso (blunt and gunshot). If they remain clinically unstable, however, patients must be transferred to the operating theater without delay. Hemorrhage control is the dominant driver in these patients. Collateral issues such as optimal intravenous access, imaging of other areas (brain, spine, bones), and fracture fixation are important but, nevertheless, secondary priorities. In summary:

1. In hemodynamically stable patients without CT evidence of a hepatic arterial blush or other reasons to proceed to the operating theater, admission and close observation are warranted.

2. In hemodynamically stable patients with a hepatic arterial extravasation/blush, immediate transfer to the interventional angiography suite (or hybrid O.R.) is mandated for hepatic angiography and/or portography with selective embolization. Autologous clot or absorbable embolization medium is optimal.

3. In patients with persistent hemodynamic instability, immediate transfer to the operating theater for laparotomy is essential. Delays will lead to loss of life.

Operative Care and Technical Tips

The patient should be rapidly prepared and draped with available access from the neck to the knees. Vascular instruments and balloons must be open and ready within the theater. A midline laparotomy from xiphoid process to pubic bone should be performed with three passes of a sharp scalpel. The peritoneal cavity should be packed in its entirety with laparotomy sponges for patients with blunt liver injuries. The falciform ligament should be left intact to provide a medial wall against which to improve medial packing pressure. The right upper quadrant (and midline vascular structures) should be evaluated prior to any intraperitoneal packing for penetrating injuries. If hemorrhage continues, an early Pringle maneuver (clamping of the porta hepatis with a vascular clamp) is mandated. This is both diagnostic and potentially therapeutic. If bleeding continues despite application of a Pringle clamp, a retrohepatic inferior vena cava (IVC) or hepatic venous injury is likely. Critically injured patients in physiologic extremis do not tolerate extended Pringle maneuvers to the same extent as patients with hepatic tumors undergoing elective hepatic resection. Forty minutes represents the upper limit of viability. If the liver hemorrhage responds to packing (which describes the vast majority of cases 85% to 99% depending on the series) but continues to hemorrhage when unpacking is completed, the patient should be repacked and transferred to the ICU with an open abdomen once damage control of concurrent injuries is complete. Cover the liver with a plastic layer of sterile x-ray cassette material to avoid capsular trauma upon eventual unpacking. Topical hemostatic agents are also helpful. If control of the liver hemorrhage is dependent on maintenance of a Pringle maneuver despite packing (i.e., the retrohepatic IVC hematoma has ruptured), call for senior assistance, mobilize the right lobe, and suture the IVC or hepatic veins with 4-0 Prolene on SH needles or 5-0 Prolene on RB1 needles (assuming that a replaced left hepatic artery is not the source of inflow occlusion failure). These patients may also require total vascular exclusion (TVE) of the liver (complete occlusion of the infrahepatic IVC, suprahepatic IVC, porta hepatis (Pringle maneuver), as well as an aortic cross-clamp within the abdomen). If TVE is pursued without concurrent clamping of the aorta, the patient will arrest due to a lack of coronary perfusion. I prefer to obtain suprahepatic IVC control within the abdomen in patients with a normal length of IVC inferior to the diaphragm. An alternate option includes access of the IVC within the pericardium itself (i.e., as it enters the heart). This 2-cm length of IVC is easily accessible by opening the pericardial sac after dividing the diaphragm. Alternatively, the suprahepatic IVC can also be accessed from the thorax if a thoracotomy has already been performed. Veno–veno bypass is also a theoretical option but rarely used due to a lack of transplant training for most trauma/general surgeons.

In the case of central hepatic gunshot wounds or deep central lacerations where access and exposure are difficult, ongoing hemorrhage should be stopped with balloon occlusion. Either a Blakemore esophageal balloon or variant (red rubber catheter with overlying Penrose drain and two silk occlusion ties) is exceptional at stopping ongoing bleeding at the bottom of deep central hepatic injury tracts (including retrohepatic IVC injuries). These should be deflated approximately 72 hours after the initial placement. If hemorrhage continues, they should be left in situ for 2 to 3 additional days. Although unusual, penetrating injuries to the hepatic artery may require ligation (assuming the portal vein is intact). Portal vein injuries should ideally be repaired with 5-0 or 6-0 Prolene once control is obtained. Clamps above and below the injury are essential for visualization. Alternate damage control options for portal vein injury include TIVS (temporary intravascular shunt) with a small chest tube conduit and ligation (assuming the hepatic artery is intact). Return to the operating suite in patients with packed abdomens should occur in 48 to 72 hours (assuming hypothermia, coagulopathy, and acidosis are corrected). If an atrial–caval shunt is contemplated, two experienced surgical teams (one for the chest and one for the abdomen) are essential. The decision to pursue this shunt must be made early in the exploration process as they rarely result in patient salvage.

Postoperative Management and Complications

Complications following hepatic trauma include both early (bleeding and abdominal compartment syndrome) and late (infected hematoma, bile leak, liver failure, and associated ileus) diagnoses. Delayed laparoscopic washout with copious irrigation and insertion of a closed suction drainage catheter is particularly helpful in patients who have large collections of infected hematoma and/or bilomas. This is decidedly more common in high-grade hepatic injuries (8% to 10% risk of biloma in grade III to V injuries). If a bile leak persists, then placement of an intrabiliary stent via endoscopic retrograde cholangiopancreatography (ERCP) is helpful in lowering biliary pressure and encouraging closure of the leak. As a result, successful "nonoperative" therapy requires access to percutaneous drainage, laparoscopy, ERCP, and/or angiography in selected cases. It should also be noted that gunshot wounds with right upper quadrant trajectories (i.e., thoracoabdominal) can be treated nonoperatively in the context of normal hemodynamics and the absence of peritonitis. Concurrent injuries to the duodenum and transverse colon must be ruled out however (i.e., triple-contrast CT). Furthermore, one must also monitor for the development of a bronchobiliary fistula. Most bronchobiliary fistula can be successfully treated with a biliary stent and appropriate drainage. Hepatic failure typically occurs in response to shock liver and/or inflow occlusion (Pringle) required at the time of the operative procedure. Standard supportive care for hepatic failure is indicated.

Outcomes and Follow-up

Planned surveillance cross-sectional imaging (e.g., CT) is not required for major liver injuries (as opposed to splenic injuries). Repeat imaging should be based on any deterioration in laboratory tests or patient symptoms. The appropriate delay in time to return to physical/combat sports is debatable following major hepatic injury. Despite a known 4- to 8-week hypertrophy response following elective hepatic resection, the time to regeneration and complete organ healing is unclear in the context of hepatic injuries.

Conclusion

If diagnosis and therapy are rapid, patients who present in physiologic extremis as a result of major hepatic hemorrhage have a good chance of survival in the context of a prolonged hospital stay. Complications must be managed appropriately and without delay.

EXTRAHEPATIC BILIARY TRACT INJURIES

Extrahepatic biliary tree (common bile duct and gallbladder) injuries are incredibly uncommon. They are also relatively simple to treat relative to the context of nonelective (i.e., laparoscopic cholecystectomy) injuries. Diagnosis typically occurs within the operating theater at the time of urgent exploration for concurrent injuries. Trauma to the biliary tree is suspected upon identification of bile within the peritoneal cavity. If the diagnosis is delayed, a biloma will form in the setting of a typically sterile field. As a result, patient symptoms will consist of nausea, mild right upper quadrant discomfort, and often an ileus. The WBC and bilirubin levels may also be elevated. These patients require identification of the biloma with either ultrasound or CT, in addition to subsequent percutaneous drainage and cholangiography. In scenarios of very small partial-thickness common bile duct injuries, placement of an intrabiliary stent via ERCP may be sufficient. With any significant injury, however, immediate control of sepsis and subsequent, appropriately timed exploration by an HPB surgeon is warranted.

Management

Preoperative Considerations
In the setting of a hemodynamically stable patient with a delayed diagnosis of an extrahepatic biliary tract injury, complete cholangiography is essential prior to exploration. An experienced colleague and/or team approach is also crucial.

Operative Care and Technical Tips
Any injury to the gallbladder is an absolute indication for cholecystectomy. Although primary repair is occasionally described in very large series, it is almost never indicated. A full-thickness common bile duct injury is generally an indication for a standard Roux-en-Y hepaticojejunostomy to minimize the long-term risk of anastomotic strictures. In the setting of small, partial-thickness sharp (i.e., noncautery and nongunshot) injuries, primary repair with T-tube drainage/control may also be a viable option.

Postoperative Management, Complications, and Follow-up
Although most high-volume hepatobiliary surgeons do not utilize closed suction drainage for their hepaticojejunostomies, injury in the context of patients with additional trauma and physiologic stressors may provide an indication for drainage in some scenarios. The dominant long-term potential complication remains stricture of the biliary anastomosis. Stricture is particularly plausible in the context of hepaticojejunostomies required for very youthful patients with a long life expectancy. It also mandates a detailed discussion with the patient prior to discharge (i.e., risks and symptoms associated with stricture—cholangitis, jaundice). These patients are often amenable to dilations of their anastomoses with either an endoscopic or a percutaneous approach.

Conclusion

Injury to the extrahepatic biliary tree is unusual. Cholecystectomy is indicated for any trauma to the gallbladder. Full-thickness common bile duct injuries require a Roux-en-Y hepaticojejunostomy, whereas minor partial-thickness injuries can occasionally be treated with primary repair and decompression.

PANCREAS INJURIES

As with hepatic trauma, injuries to the pancreas can be challenging to even the most experienced trauma/general surgeon. Pancreatic injuries are divided into injuries of the left (body/tail) and right (head) organ. Clearly, injuries to the right pancreas place adjunctive structures (i.e., portal vein, IVC, aorta, duodenum, bile duct) at risk as well.

Management

Preoperative Considerations
Absolute indications for operative exploration of a suspected injury to the pancreas include (1) hypotension, (2) diffuse peritonitis, and (3) obvious full-thickness organ disruption in the pancreatic neck/body/tail on cross-sectional imaging.

Operative Care and Technical Tips
All pancreatic hematomas should be opened and explored to define the integrity of the pancreatic capsule. All segments and surfaces of the pancreas can be directly inspected by utilizing standard exposure maneuvers (Kocher maneuver, division of ligament of Treitz, entry into the lesser sac, medial mobilization of the tail of pancreas and spleen). If a disruption in the pancreatic capsule is noted (grade I or II), a closed suction drain must be placed adjacent to the injury. If a pancreatic laceration/hole is noted in the setting of an intact main pancreatic duct, a viable omental plug or patch should be combined with closed suction drainage. In general, injuries with disruption of the main pancreatic duct at any location to the left of the superior mesenteric vein/portal vein (SMV/PV) should undergo a distal pancreatectomy (grade III). Endoscopic (ERCP)-based pancreatic duct stenting across a truly disrupted main pancreatic duct fails almost uniformly. Similarly, a Roux-en-Y pancreaticojejunostomy to the pancreatic segment distal to the transaction is typically fraught with complications and fistula due to the soft texture of an otherwise normal gland.

Defining the integrity of the main pancreatic duct can be challenging. Ultrasonography has become incredibly valuable for surgeons who are trained to evaluate pancreatic gland anatomy. In the absence of this skill, however, intraoperative cholecystocholangiography remains the best alternative option. Utilize a combination cocktail of both methylene blue and radioopaque contrast material (± fentanyl) when obtaining images.

Injuries to the right pancreas (head) with main duct disruption typically require a pancreatoduodenectomy. In the context of damage control resuscitation due to massive hemorrhage, the initial surgery does not typically allow for either a completed resection or reconstruction. As a result, the "trauma Whipple" is usually performed in two stages. The second procedure (completion of resection and reconstruction) should be performed within 24 hours. More specifically, if reexploration is delayed beyond 24 hours, the viscera become so edematous that reconstruction is extremely challenging due to limited mobility of the pancreatobiliary limb and difficult, sloppy anastomoses. It should also be noted that most combined pancreaticoduodenal injuries do *not* require a Whipple procedure. In these patients (i.e., with ampullary, common bile, and pancreatic duct integrity), procedures such as pyloric exclusion with gastrojejunostomy or the Cali triple tube decompression are superior options. It must be reemphasized that the "bailout" maneuver for pancreatic head trauma remains drainage (closed suction or negative suction dressing) with early reexploration in conjunction with experienced pancreatic surgeons.

Postoperative Management and Complications

Regardless of the technique, up to 25% of distal pancreatectomies will generate a pancreatic leak and subsequent fistula. This fistula rate may be higher in the setting of trauma due to the impact of concurrent injuries and physiologic stress/exhaustion. Soft texture, contaminated fields, and bruised pancreas glands make surgery of the pancreas in the injured population challenging and fraught with complications. Wrapping the pancreas stump with viable omentum may be helpful. Octreotide has not been reliably shown to reduce the time to closure of pancreatic fistulas in injured patients. In addition to these early consequences, delayed endocrine insufficiency (i.e., diabetes) is also a concern. It is clear that upon removal of 60⁺% of pancreatic tissue in young trauma patients, approximately half will go on to achieve glucose intolerance, and up to 25% will develop diabetes.

Conclusion

Injuries to the pancreatic head typically involve catastrophic concurrent injuries to the surrounding organs and vasculature. Damage control scenarios demand drainage once ongoing hemorrhage is stopped. Injury to the left pancreas most commonly requires a distal pancreatectomy. Maintaining control of a postoperative pancreatic fistula is essential at all times.

Suggested Readings

Ball CG, Dixon E, Kirkpatrick AW, et al. A decade of experience with injuries to the gallbladder. *J Trauma Manag Outcomes* 2010;4:3.

Ball CG, Wyrzykowski AD, Nicholas JM, et al. A decade's experience with balloon tamponade for the emergency control of hemorrhage. *J Trauma* 2011;70:330–333.

Chinnery GE, Krige JE, Kotze UK, et al. Surgical management and outcome of civilian gunshot injuries to the pancreas. *Br J Surg* 2012;99.

Feliciano DV. Biliary injuries as a result of blunt and penetrating trauma. *Surg Clin North Am* 1994;74:897–907.

Kozar RA, Feliciano DV, Moore EE, et al. Western Trauma Association/critical decisions in trauma: operative management of adult blunt hepatic trauma. *J Trauma* 2011;71:1–5.

Pachter HL. Prometheus bound: evolution in the management of hepatic trauma—from myth to reality. *J Trauma* 2012;72:321–329.

Pachter HL, Feliciano DV. Complex hepatic injuries. *Surg Clin North Am* 1996;76:763–782.

Subramanian A, Dente CJ, Feliciano DV. Management of pancreatic trauma in the modern era. *Surg Clin North Am* 2007;87:1515–1532.

34

Interventional Radiology Support of HPB Surgery

Robert L. King and Matthew S. Johnson

Tremendous advances in interventional radiology (IR) technique have benefitted the interventional radiologist and surgeon alike. A close relationship with IR physicians is crucially important to ideal HPB surgery practice and management of complex HPB patients. Multiple IR techniques play important roles in preoperative diagnosis, patient optimization (i.e., biliary drainage, portal vein embolization), definitive treatment (e.g., percutaneous ablation, transarterial treatment of liver tumors), and rescue of HPB patients from postoperative complications (e.g., treatment of pseudoaneurysms, drainage of intra-abdominal abscess).

The goal of this chapter is to familiarize HPB practitioners with specific IR techniques: percutaneous biliary stenting, transjugular intrahepatic portosystemic shunting (TIPS), portal vein embolization (PVE), percutaneous radiofrequency ablation (RFA), transarterial treatment of liver tumors, percutaneous drainage of intra-abdominal abscess, and transarterial treatment of pseudoaneurysms (PSAs).

PERCUTANEOUS TRANSHEPATIC CHOLANGIOGRAPHY AND BILIARY INTERVENTION IN THE MANAGEMENT OF BILIARY OBSTRUCTION

As endoscopic techniques have become more common in cases of biliary obstruction, percutaneous biliary interventions have decreased in frequency. Percutaneous biliary intervention continues to be useful when endoscopic techniques have failed or in instances where they are unlikely to succeed. Given the complexity and risks associated with the procedure, the decision to move forward with the percutaneous procedure is usually made with multidisciplinary expertise, including HPB surgeons, interventional radiologists, and endoscopists.

Biliary obstruction may be caused by benign or malignant pathology, and obstructive jaundice can be confirmed with ultrasound, computed tomography (CT), or magnetic resonance cholangiopancreatography (MRCP). Ultrasound may demonstrate the presence of intrahepatic or extrahepatic biliary ductal dilation and may demonstrate the level of obstruction. Contrast-enhanced CT of the abdomen is more likely to identify the level and nature of obstruction. While MRCP provides excellent three-dimensional imaging, this study should be used as an adjunct to contrast-enhanced CT given its limited ability to demonstrate surgical clips, hardware, and other anatomic landmarks. In cases where bile leak is suspected, radionuclide hepatobiliary scintigraphy may be performed. Indications and contraindications are shown in Table 34.1.

Biliary intervention can be performed with conscious sedation, deep sedation, or general anesthesia. Patients should be made NPO with clear liquids only 6 hours prior to the procedure. Patients should have intravenous access and be hydrated, as manipulation of the biliary tree can cause a patient to become septic and hypotensive, requiring rapid resuscitation.

	Indications and Contraindications to Percutaneous Biliary Intervention

Indications
1. Precisely define biliary anatomy
2. Drain obstructed bile ducts
3. Obtain tissue or bile for diagnosis
4. Manage benign strictures
5. Manage intrahepatic or extrahepatic stone disease
6. Manage biliary malignancies

Contraindications

Absolute
1. Uncorrectable coagulopathy
2. No available percutaneous access to the biliary system (e.g., colonic interposition or very high left liver remnant)

Relative
1. Ascites (consider paracentesis before or during procedure)
2. Intrahepatic processes that cause multilevel obstruction not amenable to percutaneous treatment (e.g., polycystic liver disease or widespread intrahepatic metastases)

Per Society of Interventional Radiology (SIR) guidelines, prophylactic antibiotics should be administered immediately prior to instrumenting the obstructed biliary tree. If culture data are available, antibiotic choice should be tailored to specific organisms. More recently, and in patients with previous biliary instrumentation, the incidence of resistant organism colonization in the bile is very high.

For a left biliary duct puncture, a subxiphoid approach is used. For a right puncture, a lateral approach is used with the cranial/caudal position as low as possible. Ideally, this will be below the 10th rib to avoid a transpleural puncture. The access needle is then passed through the hepatic parenchyma under fluoroscopic guidance. Contrast is injected through the needle as the needle is slowly retracted until a bile duct is opacified. Once a bile duct is identified, a cholangiogram is then performed using gentle short injections of contrast until adequate filling of the ducts is obtained. (It is not always possible to opacify central ducts from the initial access. Instead, a "regional" cholangiogram is performed to assess the local ducts and the access site.) If the initial access is acceptable—that is, the duct is entered as peripherally as possible and the central angles are favorable for placement of a catheter—it may be used for placement of a 6- to 8-Fr sheath. Alternatively, a second access may be obtained by choosing an acceptable peripheral duct, which has been opacified from the original injection. It may be necessary to intermittently inject contrast though the initial access to keep the ducts adequately opacified. A flexible guidewire is then advanced through the access needle into a central duct. The needle is removed and replaced with a 6- to 8-Fr sheath over the guidewire. A complete cholangiogram can then be performed through this sheath or through a 4- to 5-Fr catheter, if the sheath tip is not central enough to obtain adequate visualization of the central ducts. The obstruction is then crossed with a combination of a hydrophilic wire and 4- to 5-Fr catheter. The same wire/catheter combination is then advanced into the proximal jejunum. The hydrophilic wire is then exchanged for a nonhydrophilic stiff wire, the tract is then dilated to the appropriate size, and an internal/external biliary stent is then placed with the tip positioned as distal in the bowel as possible while maintaining the peripheral catheter side hole at the ductal site entry point. This position ensures that the ducts peripheral to the puncture site are not excluded from drainage. If the obstruction cannot be crossed, an external biliary drain is placed with its tip as central as possible. The catheter is then sutured to the skin and placed to an external gravity drainage bag. The internal/external stent can usually be capped the following day and may remain capped as long the patient is afebrile and without other signs of cholangitis.

Malignant strictures can be treated as above, or an indwelling stent may be placed in cases of palliation. The lesion is crossed using conventional techniques. Occasionally, cholangioplasty may be performed to facilitate crossing of the lesion with the stent. Self-expanding bare metal or covered stents may be utilized. Once the stent is in place, a repeat cholangiogram is performed to ensure free flow of contrast across the stent. When this has been confirmed, the parenchymal access tract is coil embolized.

Technical Tips

1. Puncture the biliary system as peripheral as possible to avoid ductal exclusion and injury of larger central vessels. (Fig. 34.1 shows large intrahepatic hematoma from laceration of hepatic artery.)
2. During pullback injection, small "puff" of contrast should be introduced. Contrast in the portal vein and hepatic artery will head to the periphery

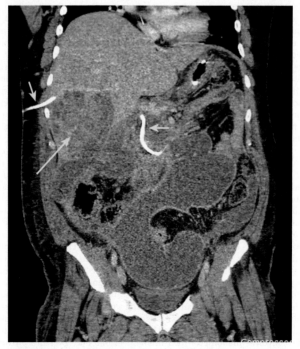

FIGURE 34.1 Coronal CT showing large intrahepatic hematoma (*long arrow*) from inadvertent hepatic artery laceration during percutaneous transhepatic cholangiography (PTC) (*short arrows*) placement.

of the liver and clear completely. The hepatic vein will clear centrally toward the heart.

3. Overinjecting a dilated infected biliary system can lead to sepsis, shock, and death.

4. If the wire does not initially advance smoothly, the entry angle of the duct may be too acute or the needle may be just outside the duct. Pulling back and repeating a more peripheral puncture will likely be helpful.

5. A short nitinol wire, increased fluoro magnification, and twirling movements of the wire may be beneficial.

6. Advancing a 6-Fr 25-cm-long sheath immediately proximal to the obstruction will allow more forward force to be placed on the coaxial catheters and guidewires.

7. The duct distal to the obstruction can be punctured, and a snare can be placed allowing through and through access.

Postprocedural Management

The patient should have his or her vital signs checked frequently immediately after the procedure. While procedure-related complications following biliary catheter placement are infrequent, bleeding from injury to the hepatic artery or portal vein is possible. This usually manifests as bleeding through or around the catheter, but would also be suggested by tachycardia with or without hypotension. Cholangiography might demonstrate communication between the catheter tract and blood vessel. Portal bleeding is usually easily treated by replacement of the indwelling catheter with a bigger catheter and/or one advanced more centrally such that its side holes no longer communicate with the portal vein. Hepatic arterial bleeding is usually treated with embolization of the injured artery. Pneumothorax and the equally uncommon bilious pleural effusion are rare complications; both are treated by catheter drainage of the pleural space.

The external or internal/external biliary catheter should undergo routine catheter care including daily site cleaning and dressing changes. Biliary catheters, whether external drains or internal/external catheters, should be flushed: Our standard procedure is to flush catheters with 10 mL of sterile saline twice a day. Bile leak around the catheter, persistent pericatheter or right upper quadrant pain, and/or difficulty flushing the catheter are all indications for cholangiography and possible catheter replacement.

Patients are observed overnight for symptomatic management and to allow for early detection of delayed procedural complications. At our institution, patients with benign bile duct strictures are normally managed with 12 months of stenting. Once the initial stent has been placed (usually 10 to 12 Fr), it is serially upsized every few months to 20 Fr as tolerated by the patient. The 12-month timeframe starts once the 20-Fr stent has been placed. The stent is exchanged every 3 months during this time. At 12 months, serum liver chemistry tests and cholangiogram are performed. If contrast flows freely through the treated stricture, a "clinical trial" is initiated. This involves placing a new catheter such that the tip is proximal to the previous stricture. The catheter is then capped for 2 weeks, at which time the patient returns for a repeat cholangiogram and serum liver chemistry evaluation. If the liver chemistry tests are stable, the cholangiogram shows resolved stricture, and the patient is doing well clinically (e.g., no fevers or signs of cholangitis), the catheter is removed. An alternative to the clinical trial to test the integrity of a treated bile duct stricture is the Whittaker test, which involves manometry measurement of bile duct pressure proximal and distal to the stricture. Patients with "definitively" treated benign bile duct strictures must have long-term annual follow-up of liver chemistry tests with their primary physician, gastroenterologist, or HPB surgeon.

Immediate Complications

1. Bleeding (subcapsular/intraparenchymal/peritoneal/pleural/biliary—hemobilia)
2. Infection (cholangitis/sepsis)
3. Bile duct perforation
4. Stent migration/malposition

Delayed Complications

1. Infection (pancreatitis/cholecystitis/cholangitis)
2. Pancreatitis
3. Bile leak in the peritoneum or pleural space
4. Stent occlusion, migration, kinking, or dislodgement
5. Biloma

The average rate of major complications is about 2%, although complication rates can vary from 4% to 25% depending on the institution and operator experience. The majority of these complications can be treated by the interventionalist. Pleural transgression is usually treated with a chest tube. A patient who is bleeding should be treated with standard resuscitative measures. In addition, coagulopathy secondary to jaundice must be corrected (administration of vitamin K and replacing plasma clotting factors). Bleeding in and around a catheter is usually due to a side hole within a blood vessel that was crossed. Advancing the catheter will stop the majority of the bleeding that is venous. If the patient continues to bleed, an arteriogram should be performed with the biliary catheter removed over a wire, maintaining access. Coil embolization distal and proximal to the bleeding arterial site is therapeutic. Infectious cholangitis should be treated with 7 to 10 days of antibiotic coverage for biliary/gastrointestinal (GI) bacteria. Additionally, a cholangiogram should be performed to ensure the catheter is functioning properly. Sepsis or septic shock requires ICU admission. Insertion-site cellulitis may suggest misplaced side holes and should be managed with cholangiography with catheter replacement, if indicated. If cellulitis is present with a well-positioned patent catheter, then antibiotics should be administered. Biliary catheter obstruction usually requires reevaluation with repeat cholangiogram and replacement. Biliary catheter dislodgement should prompt urgent evaluation as newly created tracts may close within hours. Stent occlusion can be treated with recanalization and cholangioplasty, or new stent placement.

Outcomes/Follow-up

Effective biliary drainage is established in close to 100% of bile ducts accessed in appropriately selected patients. Percutaneous drainage can successfully treat between 70% and 100% of iatrogenic bile duct injuries. Reported technical success rate for nontransplant bile duct strictures approaches 100% with transplant stenosis having a more modest success rate of 45% to 80%. The covered stent patency for biliary obstruction is 90% to 95%, 76% to 92%, and 76% to 85% at 3, 6, and 12 months, respectively.

TRANSJUGULAR INTRAHEPATIC PORTOSYSTEMIC SHUNT

A TIPS is a percutaneous technique used to treat portal hypertension and its complications. A TIPS is placed to facilitate reduction of the portal venous pressure by placing a decompressive stent between a hepatic vein and an intrahepatic portal vein (Fig. 34.2 shows TIPS). Since its inception over 20 years ago, more than 1,000 patients have been enrolled in multiple controlled trials studying efficacy and safety of the procedure. Furthermore,

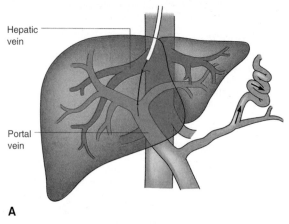

A

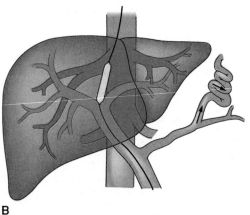

B

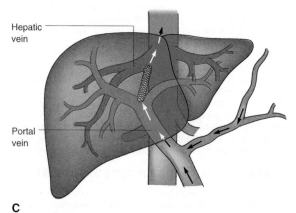

C

FIGURE 34.2 (**A-C**). Schematic of TIPS. (From Mulholland MW, Lillemoe KD, Doherty GM, et al. *Greenfield's surgery: scientific principles & practice,* 5th ed. Philadelphia, PA: Lippincott Williams & Wilkins, 2010.)

more than 1,000 papers have been published allowing for the development of guidelines to define the role of TIPS in the management of portal hypertension.

Cirrhosis is common throughout the world and may lead to ascites formation, variceal bleeding, and hepatic encephalopathy. Of these complications, variceal bleeding is the most common indication for TIPS. In fact, the mortality rate within 6 weeks of bleeding is 30%, which can most commonly be attributed to uncontrolled or early recurrent bleeding.

The model for end-stage liver disease (MELD) score was developed specifically to predict post-TIPS outcomes. This formula, which takes into account the creatinine, bilirubin, and international normalized ratio (INR), is an accurate predictor of 30-day mortality. If the MELD score is 1 to 10, the 30-day mortality is 3.7%. If the MELD is greater than 24, the 30-day mortality rises to 60%.

As the name indicates, TIPS is placed via a right internal jugular vein approach. It may be performed with moderate sedation or general anesthesia. The type of stent that is placed is operator dependent. Current evidence suggests that a PTFE-covered stent (Viatorr) may have the best long-term outcomes.

Technical success rates are greater than 95%. Hemodynamic success rates are greater than 95%. Clinical success rates are measured in terms of survival, control of bleeding, or ascites. Control of bleeding is achieved in 90%, and improved ascites control is seen in 60% to 85%.

Complications include stent malposition, hemobilia, radiation skin burn, hepatic infarction, acute TIPS thrombosis, stent stenosis (usually due to neointimal hyperplasia), liver failure, encephalopathy, heart failure, recurrent portal hypertension, and recurrent bleeding. Indications and contraindications to TIPS are shown in Table 34.2.

 Indications and Contraindications to TIPS

Indications
1. Secondary prevention of variceal bleeding
2. Refractory acutely bleeding varices
3. Refractory cirrhotic ascites
4. Portal hypertensive gastropathy
5. Gastric antral vascular ectasia
6. Refractory hepatic pleural effusion
7. Hepatorenal syndrome (type 1 or 2)
8. Budd-Chiari syndrome
9. Venoocclusive disease
10. Hepatopulmonary syndrome

Contraindications
Absolute
1. Severe or rapidly progressive liver failure
2. Severe or uncontrolled encephalopathy
3. Heart failure

Relative
1. Severe uncorrectable coagulopathy
2. Uncontrolled sepsis
3. Unrelieved biliary obstruction
4. Extensive primary or metastatic hepatic malignancy
5. Polycystic liver disease

Preoperative Evaluation

Contrast-enhanced CT is necessary to evaluate for underlying malignancy, anatomy, and patency of the hepatic and portal veins. Alternatively, a Doppler ultrasound of the liver may be performed to evaluate vessel patency. Appropriate lab work includes liver function tests and alpha-fetoprotein.

Postoperative Care

Admit for 24-hour observation, if the procedure is done electively. When TIPS is placed emergently, the patient is normally admitted to the ICU. Post-TIPS ultrasound should be ordered the following day if a bare metal stent is placed and in 1 to 2 weeks if a Viatorr (PTFE-covered) stent is used. This test is used as a baseline for future follow-up of the shunt. Changes in blood flow velocity through the stent predict potential shunt issues.

PREOPERATIVE PORTAL VEIN EMBOLIZATION

Liver resection often times is the only option that may confer long-term survival in patients with primary and secondary liver malignancies. However, patients with limited liver remnant volumes are at increased risk of postoperative liver failure and death. Preoperative PVE has emerged as a useful preoperative technique to stimulate hypertrophy of the future remnant liver (FRL) to facilitate the possibility of a major hepatectomy.

Rous and Larimore were the first to demonstrate the regenerative capacity of the liver following portal vein occlusion in the 1920s. In 1961, the first human portal vein ligation was performed during a two-stage hepatectomy. The first preoperative PVE in humans was performed in 1986. Since then, PVE has been shown to be safe and effective in inducing FRL hypertrophy in preparation for surgical resection.

Today, percutaneous transhepatic PVE is the technique of choice. PVE can be performed from an ipsilateral or contralateral approach. The choice of approach is usually based on the tumor burden within the liver, the need for segment 4 embolization, and operator preference. Many options for embolics exist, including Gelfoam, coils, Amplatzer plugs, polyvinyl alcohol particles, n-butyl cyanoacrylate and Lipiodol, or fibrin glue.

The technical success rate of PVE is 99%, and the clinical success rate is 96%. Few patients are unsuitable for hepatic resection because of inadequate hypertrophy. Regardless of approach, complications rates range from 9% to 15%. Complications include subcapsular hematoma, hemobilia, AV fistula, pseudoaneurysm, arterioportal shunt, nontarget embolization, portal vein thrombosis (of the FRL), portal hypertension, and sepsis.

Patient Selection

1. Patients with primary or metastatic liver disease, who are otherwise hepatic resection candidates, except for the following:
   a. Cirrhosis and/or advanced fibrosis and an FLR/total liver volume (TLV) < 40%
   b. Extensive chemotherapy and an FLR/TLV < 30%
   c. Normal underlying liver and an FLR/TLV < 20%
2. Patients with diabetes mellitus but without underlying liver disease may benefit from PVE, as the magnitude of postresection liver hypertrophy is usually less in these patients.
3. Patients undergoing complex hepatectomy with concomitant extrahepatic surgery, particularly pancreatectomy. In this group, studies have shown that hepatic regeneration is inversely proportional to the extent of pancreatectomy.

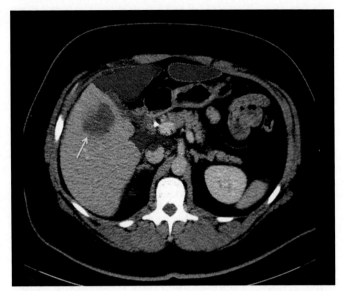

FIGURE 34.3 Preoperative volumetric analysis of a patient with right intrahepatic cholangiocarcinoma (*arrow*). Planned operation is right hepatectomy; note FLR outlined in blue.

Preoperative Workup

Volumetric 3D contrast-enhanced CT is essential for planning hepatic resection and calculating TLV and FLR. These measurements are easily calculated by dedicated abdominal radiologist (Fig. 34.3).

Postoperative Care

Admit for 24-hour observation. Patients generally do not develop postembolization syndrome as PVE leads to apoptosis as opposed to necrosis. Hydrate vigorously until the patient tolerates oral hydration. Symptomatic treatment of pain, fever, and nausea. Repeat CT is typically performed in 3 to 4 weeks to evaluate FLR hypertrophy and recalculate volumetrics.

RADIOFREQUENCY ABLATION

Image-guided percutaneous techniques for local tumor ablation offer effective treatment of select hepatic malignancies including hepatocellular carcinoma (HCC) and colorectal metastases. Although many ablation techniques exist, RFA is the primary ablative technique used currently. Traditionally, ultrasound has been the imaging modality of choice for guidance. However, hepatic lesions are not always visible by this technique. In cases where lesions are not visible on gray-scale ultrasound, contrast-enhanced ultrasound, CT, and magnetic resonance can be utilized.

The goal of RFA is to induce thermal injury to the tumor through electromagnetic energy deposition. In fact, the patient is part of a closed loop circuit that includes the RF generator, the electrode needle, and a large dispersive electrode. An alternating electric field is created within the target tumor. This agitates the tissue, which results in frictional heat around the electrode, and this generated heat is focused and concentrated around the needle electrode.

Heating of the target tissue at 50°C to 55°C for 4 to 6 minutes produces irreversible cellular damage. Temperature between 60°C and 100°C produces irreversible damage to mitochondrial and cytosolic enzymes of the cells. At more than 100°C, tissue essentially vaporizes. For adequate tumor tissue destruction, the ablative objective therapy is maintenance of 50°C to 100°C throughout the target tissue volume for 4 to 6 minutes. Slow thermal conduction through tissues, however, increases the ablation time to 10 to 20 minutes.

In order to achieve low rates of local tumor recurrence, the interventional radiologist aims to produce a 360-degree, 0.5- to 1.0-cm-thick tumor-free margin around each tumor. Hence, the diameter of the ablation must be 1 to 2 cm larger than the diameter of the target tumor.

Incidence of early major complications is 2% to 3% and includes intraperitoneal bleeding, liver abscess, intestinal perforation, pneumothorax, hemothorax, and bile duct stenosis. Late major complications include seeding of the needle tract (0.5%). The incidence of minor complications is 5% to 9% and includes pain, fever, pleural effusion, and asymptomatic self-limiting intraperitoneal bleeding. The mortality rate is 0.1% to 0.5% and commonly due to sepsis, hepatic failure, colon perforation, and portal vein thrombosis.

Indications

1. HCC: A single tumor smaller than 5 cm or as many as three nodules smaller than 3 cm each without evidence of vascular invasion or extrahepatic spread. A good performance status and Child-Pugh class A or B.
2. Secondary liver metastasis: Nonsurgical patients with metastases isolated to the liver. In limited instances, a patient with extrahepatic metastasis may be a candidate for percutaneous treatment, for example, if the extrahepatic disease is deemed curable.

Contraindications

1. Tumor located less than 1 cm to a main bile duct secondary to increased risk of stenosis of the central biliary system
2. Intrahepatic biliary dilation
3. Anterior exophytic location of the tumor, due to risk of tumor seeding
4. Untreatable coagulopathy

Relative Contradictions

1. Bilioenteric anastomosis; increased risk of hepatic abscess
2. Superficial lesions; increased rate of complications (e.g., lesions adjacent to any part of the GI tract as there is an increased risk of thermal injury)
3. Tumors located adjacent to the gallbladder; increased risk of cholecystitis
4. Pacemaker/defibrillators. Can deactivate prior to procedure

Preoperative Workup

Pretreatment imaging must define lesion(s) location relative to surrounding structures and organs. Positron emission tomography (PET) may be indicated to exclude extrahepatic metastatic disease.

Preoperative labs include alpha-fetoprotein (HCC) and carcinoembryonic antigen (colorectal cancer [CRC]), coagulation panel, and CBC.

Antiplatelet therapy should be discontinued for 5 to 10 days prior to ablation and may be restarted 48 hours postprocedure. Warfarin should be discontinued 5 days prior and may be restarted 24 hours postprocedure.

Postoperative Care

Patients are generally kept at bed rest for 2 hours and admitted for 23-hour observation.

Repeat imaging evaluation is performed 4 to 8 weeks postprocedure (Fig. 34.4). Successful tumor ablation will show nonenhancing ablation region with or without peripheral rim enhancement on CT and MR. Standard follow-up imaging and evaluation should be performed as recommended for the specific malignancy treated.

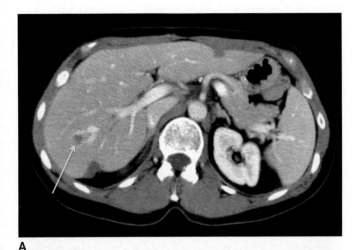

A

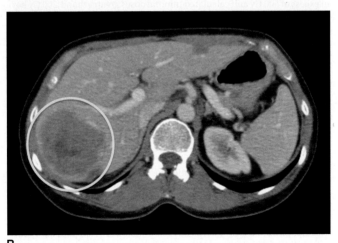

B

FIGURE 34.4 Pre- **(A)** and post- **(B)** procedural imaging of a patient undergoing percutaneous RFA to treat metastatic colorectal adenocarcinoma (*arrow*, A). Note a large, nonenhancing pattern in postablation images (*circle*, B).

TRANSARTERIAL THERAPY

Over the past 20 years, interventional radiologists have been exploring novel ways to treat cancer via the transcatheter endovascular approach. In the last 10 years, these therapies have been studied and refined such that a new branch of IR has emerged, interventional oncology. Transcatheter therapy provides clinical benefits that are distinct from the traditional medical, surgical, and radiation oncologic treatments.

Transarterial therapy includes bland embolization, chemoembolization, or radioembolization, techniques that selectively treat primary and metastatic hepatic malignancies via its nutrient arterial supply.

Bland embolization refers to the infusion of embolic particles via the nutrient artery to cause occlusion of the tumor arterioles. Chemoembolization refers to selective infusion of chemotherapeutic agents via the nutrient arterial supply, followed by injection of embolic particles to increase chemotherapy concentration by preventing chemotherapy washout. An adaptation of chemoembolization with drug-eluting beads (DEBs) has subsequently been developed. The concept includes loading the chemotherapeutic agent on a biocompatible, nonresorbable bead that is then administered via selective catheterization of the tumor's nutrient arterial supply. DEBs deliver higher and more sustained chemotherapy doses to the tumor with reduced systemic exposure.

Radioembolization refers to selective intra-arterial delivery of glass or resin microspheres loaded with the radioisotope yttrium-90. This delivery method allows for safe administration of doses that may exceed 150 Gy, whereas the likelihood of developing severe radiation-induced liver disease may exceed 50% for external beam radiation doses greater than 40 Gy. In fact, even higher doses can be attained when a "radiation segmentectomy" is performed. With this technique, high doses of radiation are delivered to one or two hepatic segments to maximize tumor irradiation and minimize exposure of normal liver parenchyma. Calculated segmental radiation doses in excess of 500 Gy and calculated tumoral doses greater than 1,200 Gy have been reported, all with very low incidence of biochemical toxicities.

Transarterial Therapy and Hepatocellular Carcinoma

The Barcelona Clinic Liver Cancer (BCLC) staging system for HCC is widely accepted in clinical practice.

Conventional transarterial chemoembolization (emulsified chemotherapeutic agent and Lipiodol followed by embolization) is the recommended first-line therapy in BCLC stage B disease without vascular invasion, cancer-related symptoms, or extrahepatic spread. Doxorubicin-loaded DEBs have similar results to conventional chemoembolization in this population, but with significantly higher administer doses of doxorubicin and significantly reduced serious liver toxicity and doxorubicin-related adverse events.

An alternative treatment option for HCC patients with BCLC stage B disease is radioembolization, which has been shown to be safe and efficacious specifically in patients with portal vein invasion.

To date, no head-to-head randomized controlled trials have compared radioembolization versus chemoembolization in HCC patients. However, a comparative effective analysis of more than 200 HCC patients treated with radioembolization and chemoembolization suggested similar survival times, with a significantly reduced toxicity profile for radioembolization.

Transarterial Therapy of Hepatic Metastatic Colorectal Cancer

Both chemoembolization and radioembolization have been used to treat patients with unresectable metastatic CRC. Radioembolization is used currently for the treatment of chemotherapy-resistant or refractory disease. Treatment of these patients should be considered in the context of the multidisciplinary group evaluation.

Transarterial Therapy of Neuroendocrine Tumors

Bland embolization, chemoembolization, or radioembolization can be used in patients with symptomatic but unresectable disease, clinically significant tumor burden, or clinically significant progressive disease.

Bland embolization and chemoembolization of neuroendocrine hepatic metastases provide significant symptomatic improvement and radiologic responses in the majority of treated patients, with encouraging progression-free survival.

Radioembolization may provide a complete response in as many as 18% of hepatic neuroendocrine tumor patients, although survival times do not differ significantly from bland embolization or chemoembolization.

Transarterial Therapy and Intrahepatic Cholangiocarcinoma

Although radioembolization and conventional chemoembolization have both been shown to be safe and effective in small series of patients with unresectable cholangiocarcinoma, no randomized control trial has been performed to date.

Preprocedure Workup

1. Tissue diagnosis or convincing clinical diagnosis
2. CT or MRI of the abdomen and pelvis
3. Exclusion of extrahepatic disease (PET-CT, bone scan, etc.)
4. Lab test: CBC, INR, creatinine, liver function tests, and tumor markers
5. Arteriography shunt study (radioembolization)

Postoperative Care

1. Twenty-three–hour observation in hospital (chemoembolization, DEBs).
2. Outpatient procedure (radioembolization)
3. Aggressive hydration.
4. Symptomatic treatment of postembolization syndrome.
5. Once the patient is tolerating oral intake and pain is controlled, the patient is discharged to home.
6. Follow-up in IR clinic in 4 to 6 weeks with imaging.

POSTOPERATIVE INTRA-ABDOMINAL FLUID DRAINAGE

Percutaneous drainage of postoperative abdominal fluid collections is one of the most commonly performed IR procedures. Furthermore, it is a well-established management option in patients who do not have another indication for immediate surgery.

Abdominal CT with or without contrast is needed to evaluate for an appropriate percutaneous window and collection size and to select the desired approach, that is, transabdominal, transgluteal, and transrectal. Patients with a limited window or small collections can be approached using CT guidance. More superficial or large collections can generally be accessed easily under ultrasound and fluoroscopic guidance. The collections are accessed with an 18-gauge trocar needle, and a stiff guidewire is placed. The drain is then placed through this access, sutured to the skin, and placed to an external drainage bag. The drain size depends on the contents of the collection to be drained. To determine content, a small volume is aspirated through the trocar needle. Generally, simple pus-filled collections require 8- to 12-Fr drains. A more complicated collection, such as a peripancreatic collection, may require 14- to 20-Fr drain.

Overall, complication rates are less than 15%, and a 30-day mortality ranges from 1% to 6% depending largely on the patient's underlying medical condition. Major complications include bleeding, septic shock, enteric fistula, peritonitis, and hemopneumothorax. Minor complications include pain, infection, pericatheter leak, catheter kinking, and dislodgement.

Indications

1. Fluid characterization
   a. Distinguish purulent fluid, bile, blood, urine, lymph, and pancreatic secretions.
   b. Determine if collection is infected or sterile.
2. Treatment of sepsis
   a. Can be curative in patients with simple abscesses
   b. Can be curative or temporizing in patients with complex abscesses
3. Relief of symptoms
   a. Alleviate pressure and pain due to size or location of collection.
   b. Obliterate recurring cysts or collections with sclerosing agents.

Contraindications

Absolute

1. Lack of safe pathway to the collection due to interposed vessels or viscera

Relative

1. Sterile collections: Prolonged catheter drainage may increase risk of secondary infection.
2. Hematoma: Increased risk of infection and poor drainage.
3. Percutaneous route requires transgression of pleura as this increases the risk of pneumothorax, empyema, and pleural effusion.
4. Tumor abscess may require lifelong catheter drainage.
5. Echinococcal cyst may elicit anaphylactic reaction if contents leak.

Preoperative Workup

CT scan to evaluate fluid collection for appropriateness. Coagulation studies. Prophylactic antibiotics (preprocedure antibiotics generally do not affect cultures)

Postoperative Care (Drain Management)

Strict record of input and output. Flush catheter twice daily with 10 mL saline to keep catheter free of complex debris. Daily dressing changes. If patient to be discharged with the drain, proper drain education should be performed.

If there is high output from the drain (>50 mL/day) beyond 4 days, the possibility of fistula to the bowel, pancreatic duct, or biliary system should be considered, and fluoroscopic-guided catheter injection may be considered.

If fluid collection persists with poor drainage, tissue plasminogen activator (tPA) or injection drain upsize may be beneficial. Typically, 6 mg of tPA is diluted in 50 mL of normal saline; up to 50 mL is injected into the drain twice daily for 3 days. The drain is clamped for 30 minutes after each injection. This technique can successfully restore drainage in up to 90%

of cases, with failure more likely in peripancreatic collections and enteric fistula.

PSEUDOANEURYSMS

False arterial aneurysms, or pseudoaneurysms (PSAs), are injuries to the arterial wall, which typically bleed into a saccular hematoma that is contained by the surrounding soft tissues. The name can be a source of confusion: PSAs are not aneurysms, but a manifestation of a vessel injury.

The prevalence of PSAs has increased over time due to increasing surgical and endovascular procedural volume. Surgery can induce PSA formation through direct trauma to an artery or through introduction of infection. Figure 34.5 shows superior mesenteric artery PSA after pancreatoduodenectomy. Arterial wall erosion from an adjacent tumor or inflammation (pancreatitis) can cause PSA.

A PSA may be asymptomatic or can cause local symptoms secondary to mass effect or adjacent tissue ischemia. The most feared complication is rupture, which can result in life-threatening hemorrhage. PSAs can communicate with and rupture into different anatomic spaces, including the pancreatic duct system, biliary tree, and gut lumen.

Clinically, a PSA can present due to its local or systemic signs and symptoms (i.e., pain) or can be detected on physical exam with signs such as a pulsatile mass, an audible bruit, or a palpable thrill. They can

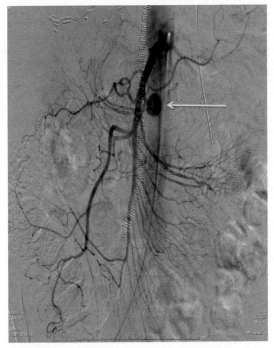

FIGURE 34.5 Angiography demonstrating large superior mesenteric artery pseudoaneurysm (*arrow*) sustained after pancreatoduodenectomy.

potentially manifest with a "sentinel bleed," such as bleeding into a drain or as a GI bleed (e.g., hematemesis, melena). The diagnosis of PSA is secured with imaging.

PSAs can be evaluated with computed tomography angiography (CTA) and magnetic resonance angiography (MRA). Both modalities can demonstrate deeper arterial structures and can be used for planning intervention. Contrast-enhanced CTA or MRA can demonstrate a contrast-opacified, saccular structure communicating with a blood vessel, with unopacified areas in the sac representing thrombus. CTA is fast and not operator dependent; however, it requires the use of iodinated contrast media, which can be nephrotoxic, as well as ionizing radiation. MRA lacks ionizing radiation but is time consuming and limited by motion and other artifacts, which makes it a suboptimal modality for PSA detection.

Another modality for imaging of PSAs is percutaneous, catheter-directed arteriography, which involves real-time, dynamic imaging of arterial flow and also allows definitive endoluminal therapeutic intervention. Catheter-directed arteriography however is invasive and also involves ionizing radiation and iodinated contrast media. Potential complications, while rare, include arterial vessel damage, including new PSA formation, dissection, rupture, thrombosis, and hematoma.

Management of PSAs has classically been surgical; however, with advances in image-guided percutaneous management, today, virtually all visceral PSAs are successfully managed with IR techniques.

The purpose of endoluminal management is PSA exclusion from the circulation. The specific endoluminal treatment depends on whether or not the blood vessel supplying the PSA is expendable or not and whether or not collateral circulation exists. If the vessel is not expendable, a covered stent can be placed across the neck of the PSA. If the vessel is expendable and is an end artery without collateral supply, the artery feeding the PSA can be coil embolized. If the vessel is expendable but has collateral circulation, the PSA must be "bracket" embolized, with coils placed in the artery central and peripheral to the PSA. Complications of endoluminal management include "nontarget" embolization, or coils migrating to unintended locations, as well as blood vessel rupture. Embolized PSAs and feeding vessels can also occasionally recanalize. Stent graft placement is relatively contraindicated with mycotic aneurysms due to risk of stent graft infection. Larger arteries have a lower risk of in-stent thrombosis than smaller arteries. A small risk of rebleeding exists after IR treatment of visceral PSA; patients should be counseled accordingly.

CONCLUSION

A diverse array of IR techniques supports HPB surgery today. Close collaboration between HPB surgeon and interventional radiologist is necessary to optimize diagnosis and treatment of complex HPB pathology.

Suggested Readings

Boyer TD, Haskal ZJ. AASLD practice guidelines: the role of transjugular intrahepatic portosystemic shunt (TIPS) in the management of portal hypertension. *Hepatology* 2010;51:306.

Cirocchi R, Trastulli S, Boselli C, et al. Radiofrequency ablation in the treatment of liver metastases from colorectal cancer. *Cochrane Database Syst Rev* 2012;6:CD006314. doi: 10/1002/14651858.CD006317.pub3

Mahnken AH, Pereira PL, de Baere T. Interventional oncologic approaches to liver metastases. *Radiology* 2013;266(2):407–430. doi 10.1148/radiol.12112544. PMID: 23362094 (Pub Med-indexed for MEDLINE)

Pitt HA, Venbrux AN, Coleman J, et al. Intrahepatic stones: the transhepatic team approach. *Ann Surg* 1994;216(5):527–535; discussion 535–537. PMID: 8185402(Pub Med-indexed for MEDLINE)

van Lienden KP, et al. Portal vein embolization before liver resection: a systematic review. *Cardiovasc Intervent Radiol* 2013;36:25–34.

Zyromski NJ, Viera C, Stecker M, et al. Improved outcomes in postoperative and pancreatitis-related visceral pseudoaneurysms. *J Gastrointest Surg* 2007;11(1):50–55.

Note: Page numbers followed by "f" indicate figures; those followed by "t" indicate tabular material.

9180533